Clinical Diagnosis in Pediatric Cardiology

MODERN PEDIATRIC CARDIOLOGY

Executive Editor

Robert H. Anderson Joseph Levy Reader in Paediatric Cardiac Morphology, Cardiothoracic Institute, Fulham Road, London SW3 6HP

Editorial Advisory Board

Anton E. Becker Amsterdam, Holland
Gordon K. Danielson Rochester, Minnesota, U.S.A.
Philip B. Deverall London, U.K.
Francis Fontan Bordeaux, France
John W. Kirklin Birmingham, Alabama, U.S.A.
Fergus J. Macartney London, U.K.
Milton H. Paul Chicago, Illinois, U.S.A.
Manuel Quero-Jimenez Madrid, Spain
Richard D. Rowe Toronto, Canada
Elliot A. Shinebourne London, U.K.
Michael J. Tynan London, U.K.

Forthcoming volumes

Atrioventricular Canal
Quero-Jimenez

Pulmonary Atresia with Ventricular Septal Defect
Macartney, Danielson, Haworth & Thiene

Paediatric Echocardiography
Hunter

The Sinus Node in Pediatrics
Yabek, Gillette & Kugler

Manual of Cardiac Catheterisation
Zuberbuhler, Neches & Park

Corrected Transposition
Losekoot & Becker

Foreword

The first major treatises on congenital heart disease in the late 1930s and early 1940s dealt largely with clinical diagnosis based on fluoroscopic and autopsy correlations. Since then the introduction and refinement of cardiac catheterization and selective angiocardiography and, more recently, of echocardiography and radionuclide studies have led to a heavy reliance on laboratory investigation in the diagnosis of heart malformations. A whole generation of physicians, though perhaps unwilling to admit the fact, has come to believe that detailed physical examination as part of the assessment of infants and children with congenital heart disease is to a large extent outmoded and has dubious reliability. For them, physical examination of the cardiovascular system seems relatively unimportant, not worthy of more than a brief period of attention and sometimes carried out for no other reason than to satisfy traditions, shortly about to be buried along with their elderly mentors.

Yet there has never been a time when physical examination better permits recognition, provides quite specific diagnosis very frequently and gives an appreciable distance in predicting the physiologic and anatomic arrangement for a large majority of young patients with heart disease. Ironically this modern bedside and technical capability has derived from the method of the pioneers — a combination of the newer accessory investigations and traditional physical methods.

To abstract key information from the huge reserve of modern clinical facts about congenital heart disease and combine that information into one concise monograph is no mean task but Dr Zuberbuhler has succeeded admirably in doing so. His position as head of one of the largest American services in pediatric cardiology, and his long experience in an environment which has contributed mightily to the subject in hand, give authenticity to the work. For those pediatricians who despair of being able to approach the specific diagnosis of congenital heart disease today amidst the bewildering technology of the 80s, this presentation has particular attraction but all who are involved in the medical supervision of children can benefit from his detailed review.

Toronto, 1981   R.D.R.

To my wife Janet, to our children and to my parents

Preface

This book was written in the hope that it will be useful to students, house officers and practicing physicians involved in the care of children with heart disease. It is not intended to be either encyclopedic or esoteric; at times complex events have been simplified, perhaps oversimplified, in the interest of brevity and clarity. The descriptions of the clinical findings are largely based on personal experience, with much assistance from colleagues and the literature. Whatever its virtues or faults, this book reflects my conviction that the clinical examination is and will remain an indispensable part of the evaluation of each child with heart disease.

I owe a considerable debt to the members of the cardiology staff at the Children's Hospital of Pittsburgh. Drs Cora Lenox, William Neches and Sang Park reviewed and criticized the manuscript and their suggestions have been invaluable. Dr James Shaver, Chief of Adult Cardiology, University of Pittsburgh, reviewed Chapter 2. These physicians, as well as other members of staff, Drs Robert Mathews, Jay Fricker and Lee Beerman, were kind enough to call the attention of the author to interesting physical findings in patients in our clinic, and many of these were included in the illustrations. Dr Sang Park was especially helpful in the selection and preparation of the illustrations. Ms Virginia Curlee, non-invasive technologist, was of great help in recording the phonocardiograms and echocardiograms and Ms Karen Hamilton helped in the preparation of the illustrations and bibliography. Ms Beverley Collins typed the several drafts of the manuscript and her help is gratefully acknowledged. I should also like to express appreciation to Ms Yen Ho, research assistant at the Brompton Cardiothoracic Institute, who prepared the diagrams.

Pittsburgh, 1981 J.R.Z.

Contents

1.	Introduction	1
2.	History	4
3.	The cardiac physical examination	6
4.	Interatrial septal defect	34
5.	Ventricular septal defect	39
6.	Patent ductus arteriosus	46
7.	Endocardial cushion defects	51
8.	Anomalous pulmonary venous connection	56
9.	Coarctation of the aorta	59
10.	Pulmonic stenosis with intact ventricular septum	64
11.	Congenital pulmonic regurgitation	71
12.	Aortic stenosis	75
13.	Aortic regurgitation	83
14.	Mitral stenosis	89
15.	Mitral regurgitation	93
16.	Tricuspid valve anomalies	99
17.	Valvar atresia	107
18.	Tetralogy of Fallot	116
19.	Transposition of the great arteries	123
20.	Arterial anomalies	134
21.	Pericardial disease	141
22.	Pulmonary hypertension	144
23.	Functional murmurs	149
24.	Conduction abnormalities	152
25.	Miscellaneous anomalies	156
26.	Differential diagnosis	165
Index		176

1

Introduction

Congenital heart disease was once regarded as a medical curiosity; rare, difficult to diagnose during life and impossible to treat. Over the past four decades a very different picture has emerged. Congenital heart disease is not rare, can be precisely diagnosed during life and, in many cases, can be effectively treated. It is, of course, less common in the population as a whole than arteriosclerotic or hypertensive cardiovascular disease, but is now more common than newly diagnosed rheumatic heart disease, at least in more highly developed countries. Congenital cardiac anomalies are estimated to occur in about 8 of every 1000 live births.

The importance of congenital heart disease is enhanced by its high rate of morbidity and mortality, most particularly in early infancy. It has been estimated that 50 percent of newborns with congenital cardiac anomalies will die in the first year of life if left untreated, and even with treatment congenital heart disease is an important cause of death in infancy. Congenital heart disease is, in fact, the single most common cause of death during the first week of life at Children's Hospital of Pittsburgh and accounts for one third of the deaths in this age group. The newborn with congenital heart disease has a more tenuous hold on life than the octogenarian with symptomatic coronary artery disease.

Diagnostic and therapeutic methods have evolved in parallel. The development of surgical techniques for the palliation or repair of cardiac anomalies stimulated the development of diagnostic techniques, and as precise diagnosis became possible during life surgeons were encouraged to extend their horizons and repair anomalies once considered uncorrectable. Although the physiologic consequences of cardiac anomalies are best defined in the cardiac catheterization laboratory, and the detailed premortem elucidation of the abnormal anatomy is by angiography and echocardiography, these techniques have not eliminated the need for a careful physical examination. Indeed, they have enhanced its value by clarifying the genesis of the abnormal physical findings associated with cardiac anomalies. Examples include the echocardiographic demonstration of the origin of the midsystolic click and late systolic murmur of Barlow's syndrome, the 'sail' sound of Ebstein's anomaly and the Austin Flint murmur of severe aortic regurgitation. Another instance is the elucidation of the determinants of width of splitting of the second heart sound by the use of micromanometer tipped catheters in the catheterization laboratory. The implications of physical findings are now more clear and the physical examination has the potential of providing more useful information than it did before the advent of these diagnostic techniques. There is, perhaps, less stimulus to do a thorough physical examination, in the expectation that cardiac catheterization will 'reveal all'. But this is unfortunate, since clinical and invasive methods compliment each other. A physician does a perfunctory physical examination on a child with congenital heart disease at his patient's peril.

Undeniably, the physical examination plays a preeminent role in the recognition of congenital heart disease, since the diagnosis is usually first suspected when a murmur is heard or when cyanosis or congestive heart failure is noted.

It is important to recognize at the outset that congenital heart disease cannot be divided into a number of discrete anomalies or combinations of anomalies, each with specific clinical findings.

Rather, there are spectra of variations of anatomy and physiologic state with corresponding spectra of clinical findings. For instance, there is no such thing as a 'typical' ventricular septal defect with a 'typical' systolic murmur. There may be a more or less 'typical' murmur of a small defect in the area of the membranous septum, or of a tiny defect in the muscular septum, or of a large defect with elevated pulmonary artery pressure, but not of a ventricular septal defect in the general sense. Similarly, there is no 'typical' clinical picture of tetralogy of Fallot. It too is a spectrum, ranging from the nearly asymptomatic young adult with no cyanosis to the desperately ill and severely cyanotic infant. There is a corresponding spectrum of auscultatory findings and both spectra ultimately depend upon the degree of severity of right ventricular outflow tract obstruction. Anatomic variation, pathophysiology, physical findings and clinical course are inextricably intertwined, and heart disease in the child can be best understood when all are considered together.

The physical findings expected with an anomaly can be profoundly altered by the presence of an associated defect. With increasing severity of isolated pulmonic stenosis, for instance, one expects the systolic murmur to become louder and longer, sometimes extending well beyond the aortic closure sound. If there is an associated ventricular septal defect (tetralogy of Fallot) the murmur instead becomes progressively softer and shorter with increasing obstruction, as more and more of the right ventricular stroke volume is shunted through the ventricular septal defect into the aorta rather than traversing the right ventricular outflow tract. In tetralogy of Fallot the murmur may actually disappear during a severe hypoxemic spell, when the right ventricular infundibulum is virtually sealed.

Not all children with congenital heart disease need undergo cardiac catheterization. Although selection of patients for invasive study may depend upon symptoms or electrocardiographic or chest roentgenographic abnormalities, the physical examination is equally important in the selection process. It is quite unusual, for example, to find cardiac symptoms in a child who does not have some indication of severe cardiac disease on physical examination. Further, an asymptomatic child with a normal chest roentgenogram and normal electrocardiogram may have congenital heart disease serious enough to require surgical repair, and in such a child abnormal physical findings form the only basis for selection for cardiac catheterization. As an example, slowly rising arterial pulses, a loud systolic ejection murmur and thrill at the high right sternal border, and an apical early systolic ejection sound indicate severe valvar aortic stenosis. Complete absence of femoral pulses and a right arm blood pressure of 180/100 constitute a severe coarctation of the aorta, even in the absence of symptoms, electrocardiographic abnormality or cardiomegaly. In combination, a soft systolic ejection murmur at the high left sternal border, fixed splitting of the second heart sound and a short mid diastolic murmur at the low left sternal border identify an interatrial septal defect which is large enough to warrant repair, even in a child who seems quite healthy. Accurate clinical diagnosis and a knowledge of the physical findings expected at the more severe end of the spectrum of an anomaly are vital to proper selection for invasive study.

Even when cardiac catheterization has been decided upon, it is quite impossible to plan to use every available hemodynamic and angiographic technique in a particular patient. Selection of the studies most likely to provide pertinent and necessary information is possible only if the physician performing the catheterization has also made a careful clinical evaluation of the patient. The study is likely to be safer and shorter if planned and executed in the light of the clinical findings. In addition, clinical findings serve as a check on data collected in the catheterization laboratory. Even in the best laboratories fallacious data are occasionally gathered, and even the most experienced cardiologist occasionally misinterprets hemodynamic data or angiograms. For example, the extent of pulmonary vascular disease may be underestimated by reliance on 'numbers' alone. The patient with a ventricular septal defect and pulmonary hypertension who has a pulmonary to systemic flow ratio of 1.5 while breathing room air and 2.5 while breathing oxygen may seem to be an acceptable, although not ideal candidate for surgical closure of the defect. If that same patient is known to have a loud single second heart sound at the high left sternal border, a short soft systolic murmur, a hemoglobin of 17g percent and a history of cyanosis with exertion, enthusiasm for surgical intervention should quickly fade. It must be realized that if the catheterization laboratory diagnosis is not compatible with the clinical picture, both the catheterization data and the physical findings should be carefully reviewed. Conclusions based on a physical examination done with care and system should not be disregarded lightly.

In a book of this sort it is difficult to illustrate adequately with the written word physical findings which depend on hearing, palpation or visible motion. An hepatic pulse tracing does not immediately translate to the 'feel' of a pulsating liver, nor does a giant 'A' wave in the jugular venous pulse tracing give quite the same impression as seeing the real thing. Nonetheless, it is as close as one can come. It is impossible to get any of the 'quality' of a murmur into a phonocardiographic illustration but the shape of a murmur can be shown and the hemodynamic events which produce the murmur, or the abnormally split second heart sound, or the gallop can be illustrated. There remains, however, a large gap between the intellectual understanding of how a particular physical finding came to be and actually appreciating that finding in a patient. The gap can be bridged only by clinical experience.

2
History

The most important function of history taking in a child with heart disease is an assessment of the impact of the cardiac anomaly on the child. The most obvious effects include physical disability, poor growth and development, actual congestive heart failure, limited exercise tolerance, and cyanosis. Less well recognized but sometimes equally important is the emotional impact, ranging from frustration at inability to participate in competitive sports to serious depression or alienation. Other important functions of the history include noting the age of the child when the cardiac anomaly was recognized, searching for a family history of congenital heart disease and assessing compliance with medical instructions.

History taking must be directed, to a degree, since certain areas must routinely be explored and may be missed if the parents are not asked specific questions. Almost all parents are eager to give as much information as possible about their child, but the physician may be tempted to turn off or redirect the conversation when it strays from a response to a direct question. Somewhere in the course of history taking, however, there should always be a time when parents are allowed, indeed encouraged, to tell what seems to them to be important about their child. Not only may valuable information about disability emerge, but one will also get a better idea of the parents' perception of the child's state, opening the door to more effective counselling and education. It is important for parents to get as clear an idea as possible of the nature of their child's anomaly and its seriousness and possible consequences. The physician can accomplish this best if he understands the parents' current knowledge, anxieties, perceptions and misconceptions about their child's problem.

Although infants with congenital heart disease may grow slowly, the poor growth may or may not be causally related to the cardiac anomaly. Indeed, unless there is a large left to right shunt with cardiomegaly or unless there is arterial unsaturation, slow growth is usually not *caused* by cardiac disease. (To put it another way, there will not be a growth spurt following repair of the defect.) Even if there is cardiomegaly and/or cyanosis, growth may not improve after successful surgery. The symmetry, or lack of it, of the growth pattern is a useful differential point, since weight, height and head circumference are not equally affected by severe congenital heart disease. Of these variables, weight is most likely to be influenced by cardiovascular stress, and if weight is below the 5th percentile while head circumference is normal the cardiac anomaly is very likely responsible for the poor growth. On the other hand, if head circumference, weight and height are all below the 5th percentile none are likely to be attributable to cardiac disease.

Parents of a child with suspected congenital heart disease should always be asked how their child breathes, how he eats, how he has gained weight and whether or not he has ever been blue, since important evidence of heart failure or of arterial oxygen desaturation may be obtained during the taking of the history. The infant in congestive heart failure feeds poorly; he typically takes a small amount of milk, rests or falls briefly asleep, and then wakes hungry and begins feeding again. With severe congestive heart failure, the infant may stop feeding entirely.

The infant with congestive heart failure may be tachypneic at rest or even after having fallen asleep. It is unwise to dismiss a parental report of rapid breathing without making an especially careful search for other evidence of heart disease, especially if the history is given by an experienced parent or by a grandmother. Unfortunately, it is not uncommon to hear from a parent that an infant now in obvious congestive heart failure had been tachypneic for some time before overt failure appeared and that the breathing pattern had been dismissed by nursery personnel or by a physician as being of no consequence.

Parents may not be aware of cyanosis in their child even if it is quite obvious to the examiner. This is especially likely if the cyanosis is constant and has developed gradually. Parents are likely to report episodic cyanosis, however, especially if it is accompanied by the respiratory distress or change in level of consciousness which occur in the hypercyanotic spells of tetralogy of Fallot (or less commonly with other varieties of cyanotic congenital heart disease). It is important to note that not all episodic cyanosis is cardiac; normal infants as well as older children may display obvious cyanosis of lips or nail beds when exposed to cold. (Parents frequently report that perfectly normal children become cyanotic after swimming.)

It is important to inquire as to the adequacy of iron intake in infants who are or who are expected to be cyanotic. If iron intake is inadequate the resulting anemia (which may be absolute or relative) may increase symptoms by reducing the oxygen carrying capacity of the blood. With tetralogy of Fallot, for instance, symptoms may be very mild with a hemoglobin level of 18 g percent, but become severe and include hypercyanotic spells if the hemoglobin drops to 10 g percent. Anemia, especially the microcytic variety which occurs with iron deficiency, may precipitate a cerebral vascular accident in a child with cyanotic congenital heart disease.

Symptoms may or may not be present in the older child with highly significant congenital heart disease. With purely obstructive lesions such as pulmonic or aortic stenosis or isolated coarctation of the aorta, symptoms tend to occur very late. In addition, children have a remarkable capacity to adapt and may not be aware of limitations when they indeed exist. The older child may also display a strong tendency to deny limitations and may compensate by attempting to maintain a high level of physical activity. On the other hand, over concerned parents frequently report easy fatigability and exercise intolerance in children with anomalies which are hemodynamically unimportant. Almost invariably the child with cardiac symptoms has other evidence of the severity of his anomaly, either on physical examination, chest roentgenogram, or electrocardiogram. (Important exceptions to this general rule include paroxysmal dysrhythmia, hypertrophic cardiomyopathy and intracardiac tumor.) If cardiac symptomatology seems inconsistent with the remainder of the clinical examination, observation of the child during exercise, either casual or during a formal exercise study, may be quite helpful. It is worth noting that chest pain in children is very rarely cardiac in origin. This fact should be made known to the worried parent.

Although episodes of syncope or of seizure activity in children are not usually of cardiac origin, the possibility of an episodic arrhythmia or of the 'long QT' syndrome should be considered in children with otherwise unexplained 'spells' and should lead to a careful cardiac physical examination and an electrocardiogram.

Although the history is less important in establishing the presence of organic heart disease in a child than it is in the adult with coronary artery disease, it is an invaluable source of information, particularly with regard to the impact of the cardiac anomaly on the child's physical state and psyche.

3

The cardiac physical examination

Three indispensable prerequisites to a good physical examination are a proper environment, a cooperative child and a conviction on the part of the physician that the examination is important. An ideal environment includes quiet and the opportunity for both the child and the physician to be comfortable. Both are easily obtained in an office setting, but may be more difficult in the hospital, where noise levels are often high and rooms crowded. Radios, television sets and conversing colleagues are common sources of ambient noise, and each should be 'turned off' before the examination begins. Most physicians find that a physical examination is most easily performed from the patient's right side, and it is better to move a bed or chair than to alter one's customary approach. A patient should always be examined from a comfortable position if at all possible.

Obtaining the cooperation, or at least the tolerance of the child may require considerable patience and skill on the part of the physician. There is usually little problem with the newborn or small infant, who is usually asleep or at least docile if well fed and dry. The older infant and young child may pose more of a challenge, and it is well to begin by asking the mother whether the child is more likely to be happy in her lap than on an examining table. It is possible to do a thorough cardiovascular examination with an infant sitting and lying in his mother's lap, and better to begin that way if the child is likely to object to the separation of an examining table. If the table is tried first and the child vigorously resists, the chances of success with a subsequent attempt in the mother's lap are appreciably lessened.

It is worthwhile getting acquainted with the child before any 'laying on of hands'. This may require little more than a smile with a six-month-old but may be more involved with an older child. Sitting down beside the mother and child and giving the child a small toy or even a tongue blade to play with is less threatening than a direct approach with a stethoscope, a strange and sometimes frightening object to a two-year-old. If the child seems to fear the stethoscope, he may be persuaded to hold and examine it by his mother and may then submit to being examined. Also, auscultation may be less threatening if a toe, leg or the abdomen is 'listened to' before the chest. (The stethoscope head should be warmed with the hand before touching the child with it.) The importance of a nonthreatening approach cannot be overestimated; a smiling and unhurried examiner is much more acceptable to a toddler than a solemn or abrupt one.

Occasionally, even with a gentle approach, young children remain uncooperative. The infant who cries vigorously during an attemped examination may respond to a bottle. Failing this, he may fall asleep if the examiner leaves the room and may remain asleep during auscultation after the examiner returns. If a window is available, a refractory toddler can sometimes be distracted by drawing his attention to a bird or cat, real or imaginary, outside the window. It is surprising how long the charade can be continued and how much information can be obtained using this simple artifice. A pre-schooler may be persuaded to cooperate simply by telling him he is 'expected' to be quiet. In the author's experience it has rarely been necessary to sedate a child to perform an adequate physical examination.

The physical examination is easily the most important non-invasive diagnostic tool for the detection and evaluation of heart disease in children. The physician who does a perfunctory physical examination, either because of lack of skill or because of his hurry to proceed to 'more objective methods' such as the chest roentgenogram, electrocardiogram or echocardiogram fails to make full use of readily available and potentially valuable information. In this chapter, the parts of the cardiac physical examination will be outlined and the physiologic basis for the various findings will be explored. When appropriate, reference will be made to other portions of the text for specific details.

THE JUGULAR VENOUS PULSE

The normal jugular venous pulse consists of 'A', 'C' and 'V' waves. The 'A' wave is caused by right atrial contraction, the pressure wave being transmitted through the venous system to the jugular veins. The 'C' wave occurs at the beginning of ventricular systole and usually appears as a hump on the descending limb of the 'A' wave. It is probably a combination of an impulse transmitted from the nearby carotid artery and a pressure wave generated by bulging of the closed tricuspid valve leaflets into the right atrium during very early ventricular systole. The 'X' descent follows the 'C' wave. It is largely due to the tricuspid valve annulus being pulled away from the right atrial cavity by the contracting right ventricle, reducing right atrial pressure in the process. As venous return continues through systole there is a slow increase in right atrial pressure, visible in the jugular veins as the 'V' wave. The 'V' wave peaks just as the tricuspid valve opens. As right atrial blood enters the right ventricle through the opened tricuspid valve, the 'Y' descent begins.

In adults it is commonly possible to see and record all of the above waves. In infants and children the venous pulse is much harder to see, both because of the shorter neck and more abundant subcutaneous tissue of the young child and because the faster heart rate common in younger individuals blurs the distinction between the waves and makes them harder to interpret. It is thus rarely possible to identify all of the 'normal' jugular venous waves in an infant. In some children and in an occasional infant an abnormal jugular venous pulse can be seen if looked for and may then give valuable insight into right heart hemodynamics.

Venous pulsations are usually more marked in the internal than in the external jugular veins, since venous valves in the external system interfere with retrograde transmission of waves from the right atrium. It is important that the neck be relaxed, since tensing of muscles may obscure venous waves. Jugular venous pulsations are strikingly dependent on the position of the patient, specifically on angulation of the trunk from the horizontal, since this angulation determines elevation of the observed vein above the right atrium. The pulsations are most obvious at the top of the 'fluid level' in the vein, or in other words at the level where the vein becomes distended by returning blood. (The vein below this point also must pulsate to a degree, but pulsations are much less obvious.) The proper angle at which the jugular venous pulse is most obvious varies from patient to patient and also from time to time in the same patient, depending upon right atrial pressure levels. Usually the veins are best seen with the patient reclining at a 15 to 30° angle, but when right atrial pressures are very high the pulsations may be seen only with the patient sitting upright. Lighting is very important, and venous pulsations are best seen when light strikes the neck tangentially, throwing the veins into relief. The veins are much less well seen in diffuse light, and if proper window lighting is not available a flashlight can be used to highlight the veins.

Visible pulsations in the neck may be of arterial or venous origin, and the distinction may occasionally be difficult, particularly if venous pulsations are unusually strong. The failure of arterial pulsations to change with position is a useful distinction and, also, venous pulsations can be damped by light pressure above the clavicle, most easily applied by stretching the skin over the area. (If pressure is too heavy, the vein will distend, since return to the heart is blocked. Even so, pulsation is eliminated.) Jugular venous waves can be timed and identified either by palpating the opposite carotid or by simultaneous auscultation of the heart. 'A' waves are, of course, presystolic and precede the carotid pulse and the first heart

8 CLINICAL DIAGNOSIS IN PEDIATRIC CARDIOLOGY

sound. 'V' waves are nearly coincident with or closely follow the carotid pulse and occur after the first heart sound.

Prominent 'A' waves result from forceful right atrial contractions and signify increased impedance to right atrial emptying. Such increased impedance is most commonly a result of the decreased right ventricular compliance which occurs with right ventricular hypertrophy (e.g. with severe 'isolated' pulmonic stenosis, primary pulmonary hypertension, or cardiomyopathy). Increased impedance to right atrial emptying also occurs with tricuspid stenosis or atresia and, in the latter entity, large jugular venous 'A' waves are presumptive evidence of a restrictive interatrial communication (Fig. 3.1). Still another cause of increased impedance to right atrial emptying is the concurrence of atrial and ventricular systole, atrial contraction then occurring while the tricuspid valve is closed. The resultant high right atrial pressure is transmitted to the jugular veins and is known as a 'cannon' wave (Fig. 3.2), one of the characteristic findings

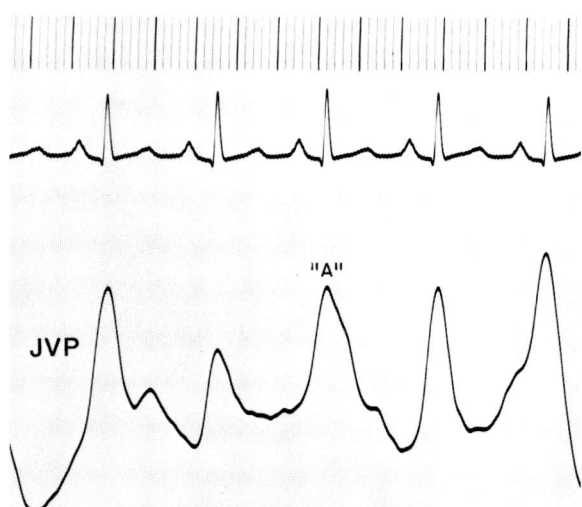

Fig. 3.1 Child with tricuspid atresia and restrictive interatrial opening. Large 'A' waves are evident in the jugular venous pulse recording (JVP).

Fig. 3.2 Child with congenital third degree atrioventricular block. Cannon waves (arrows) are seen in the jugular venous pulse (JVP) when mechanical atrial systole occurs during ventricular systole (note very short apparent PR interval).

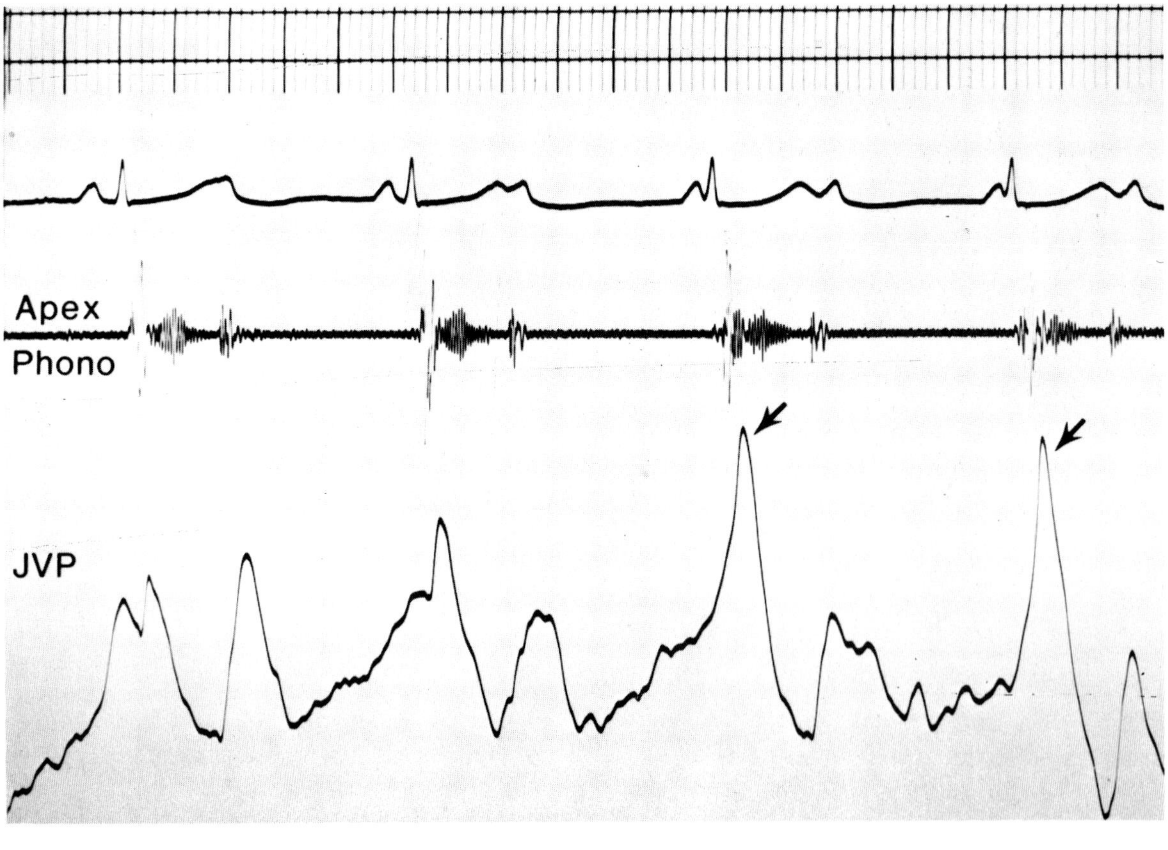

in third degree atrioventricular block. Since atria and ventricles are not electrically linked in this situation, atrial and ventricular contractions will, by chance, occasionally coincide. The intermittent nature of the large waves is characteristic, but can also occur with second degree atrioventricular block or with supraventricular premature beats, the common denominator being coincidence of atrial and ventricular systole. A long PR interval tends to make an 'A' wave more obvious, since it separates it from the subsequent carotid pulse. A short PR interval can actually be the cause of cannon waves, as they were in the early postoperative period in one of our patients who had undergone a Mustard procedure for transposition of the great arteries. Striking neck vein pulsations led to a concern that there might be partial obstruction to superior vena cava return. The presence of a junctional rhythm suggested that the pulsations might, instead, be cannon waves and the latter etiology was established when the large 'A' waves suddenly disappeared with reversion to a regular sinus rhythm.

If atrial and ventricular systole are not concurrent, a large jugular venous pulse coincident with or following the carotid pulse (or after the first heart sound if timing is by auscultation) is a 'V' wave and is generated by right ventricular systole (Fig. 3.3). Pathologic 'V' waves indicate important tricuspid regurgitation. It is important to note that significant tricuspid regurgitation can exist without producing large 'V' waves, since the right atrium enlarges with chronic regurgitation and can absorb considerable regurgitant volume without much change in pressure. The damped right ventricular impulse will not then be evident in the jugular venous pulse.

If right atrial 'A' or 'V' waves are sufficiently large the jugular pulsations may be palpated as well as seen. In the author's experience this finding has been most common in patients with either tricuspid atresia and a restrictive interatrial septal defect or with a cardiomyopathy. Palpable venous waves may also occur with severe tricuspid regurgitation and with severe 'isolated' pulmonic stenosis. Large atrial waves may be transmitted to the hepatic veins and may cause the liver to pulsate (Fig. 3.4). Hepatic pulsation must be differentiated

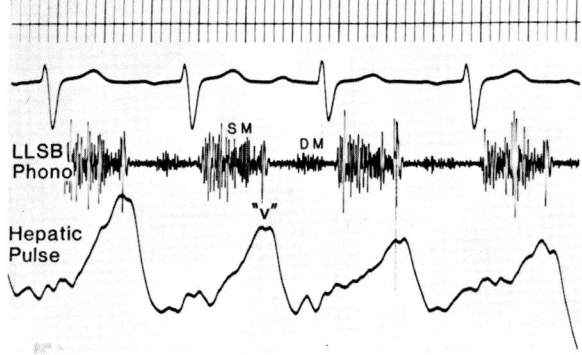

Fig. 3.4 Same child as Figure 2.3. The low left sternal border phonocardiogram shows both the systolic murmur of tricuspid regurgitation and the mid diastolic murmur of relative tricuspid stenosis. The hepatic pulse tracing shows a prominent 'V' wave.

from a transmitted cardiac impulse, and a pulsating ventral surface of the liver, felt just below the right costal margin, is more reliable evidence of large 'A' or 'V' waves than is movement of the lower edge of the liver synchronous with the cardiac impulse.

In adults, abnormal distension of the jugular veins occurs most commonly with congestive heart failure and reflects elevated right atrial pressure. The normal inspiratory fall in central venous pressure, and hence of the level of distension of jugular veins, may be lost in such a patient. If failure is severe there may be an inspiratory increase rather than a decrease in the level of distension (Kussmaul's sign). (It should be noted

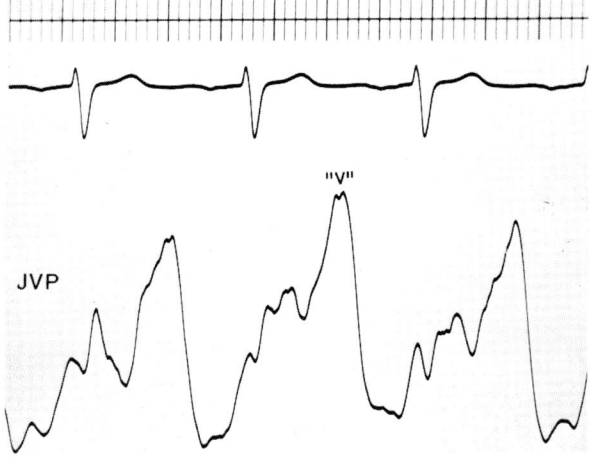

Fig. 3.3 Child with tricuspid regurgitation. A large 'V' wave is present in the jugular venous pulse recording (JVP).

that constrictive pericarditis can also produce an inspiratory increase in jugular venous distension.) In patients with borderline right ventricular function, distension may also increase when the right upper quadrant of the abdomen is compressed with the hand, quiet respiration being maintained to prevent a Valsalva maneuver. This hepato-jugular reflux occurs in patients whose 'failing' right ventricle is unable to increase its output as the abdominal compression increases systemic venous return.

In infants, congestive heart failure rarely results in obvious jugular venous pulsations or distension. If distended neck veins are present in an infant in failure, the possibility of an intracranial arteriovenous fistula should be considered. In this entity distension is related to a combination of increased right atrial pressure and to torrential venous return through the jugular venous system. In an older child, a cervical arteriovenous fistula can cause jugular venous distention, even in the absence of congestive heart failure (Fig. 3.5).

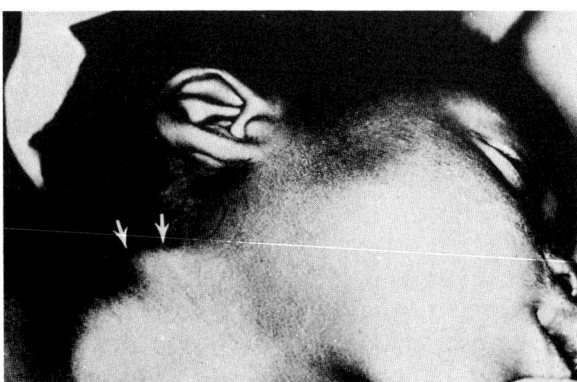

Fig. 3.5 Distended neck vein (arrows) in a child with a cervical arteriovenous fistula.

ARTERIAL PULSE

Peripheral arterial pulses should be described in terms of amplitude and symmetry. Judging the general amplitude of peripheral pulses is a subjective exercise, but attention to more distal arteries may be helpful in differentiating normal from increased pulses. Strong palmar or digital pulses, for instance, constitute good evidence that pulse pressure is increased. Pulses of increased amplitude can result from low systemic arterial resistance, as with an aortico-pulmonary artery communication (e.g. patent ductus arteriosus, aortico-pulmonary window, or persistent truncus arteriosus) or with a systemic arteriovenous fistula. Pulses are also increased when myocardial inotropy is high and most of the stroke volume is ejected in early systole (e.g. hypertrophic cardiomyopathy). Strong pulses also result from the physiologic increase in cardiac output and decrease in systemic vascular resistance which accompany fever or physical exertion. Peripheral pulses are weak when the central aortic pulse is damped by severe aortic stenosis or when there is congestive heart failure, with its low cardiac output, small stroke volume, and reflexly increased systemic vascular resistance. Striking respiratory variation in pulse amplitude suggests either pericardial tamponade or airway obstruction (Ch. 21).

To judge symmetry of arterial pulses, either the brachial, radial or axillary pulse should be felt and compared in each arm and then compared with the femoral pulses. If leg pulses are decreased or absent, a coarctation of the aorta may be assumed to be present. (Since femoral pulses may be hard to feel in the chubby infant or obese older child, it is well to check dorsalis pedis and posterior tibial pulses as well as femorals.) If a coarctation of the aorta is suspected, a femoral pulse and the brachial or axillary pulse in the right arm should be felt simultaneously. In the normal individual there is rarely enough delay in the femoral pulse to be appreciated at the bedside; with coarctation it may be obvious that the femoral pulse is not only weaker than the brachial but delayed as well (Fig. 9.2). Since the origin of the left subclavian artery may or may not be involved in a coarctation, left arm pulses may be as decreased as the femorals or may more closely resemble pulses in the right arm. Another less common cause of a stronger pulse in the right than left arm is supravalvar aortic stenosis (Ch. 12). Stenosis in a subclavian artery is a still rarer reason for a weak arm pulse. If pulses are strong in the legs but weak in the arms Takayasu's (pulseless) disease is suggested. If pulses are weak in all four extremities several possibilities should be considered. The most likely cause is low cardiac output, either because of poor myocardial function or because of obstruction to left ventricular outflow (e.g. aortic atresia or very severe aortic stenosis). A rare but curable cause of decreased pulses in both arms and both legs is a coarctation of the aorta which involves the left subclavian artery and which is associated with distal origin of the right subclavian artery. In this situation carotid and temporal pulses are strong and make the diagnosis.

BLOOD PRESSURE

Blood pressure determination is an important part of the physical examination of the child, particularly since some causes of childhood hypertension are curable and since the first evidence of adult essential hypertension may appear during childhood or adolescence.

Accurate blood pressure determination demands attention to a few details. The cuff width should be adequate, covering at least two-thirds of the upper arm. A small cuff leads to a spuriously high blood pressure estimate and should be avoided. A cuff which covers the entire upper arm from the axilla to the elbow does not distort blood pressure and is quite acceptable. The cuff should be inflated until distal arterial pulses disappear, and then deflated until Korotkoff sounds appear over the brachial artery just below the cuff, marking systolic blood pressure. With further deflation the sounds either disappear or abruptly fade, marking diastolic blood pressure. In infants, the flush technique has been advocated and does give a fairly good measure of blood pressure. In this technique, blood is expelled from the hand and forearm as the cuff on the upper arm is inflated. As cuff pressure is gradually lowered, arterial blood suddenly enters the lower arm and the skin becomes pink and 'flushed'. Even in small infants, however, blood pressure can usually be determined by auscultation or palpation and is almost certainly more accurate than blood pressure determined by the flush technique.

Ideally, blood pressure should be determined in both arms and in a leg. This is mandatory if coarctation of the aorta is suspected because of pulse asymmetry or hypertension. If a coarctation is present, blood pressure is lower in the legs than in the right arm, while pressure in the left arm is variable, depending upon whether or not the origin of the left subclavian artery is involved in the coarctation. In children, hypertension may also be due to renal arterial narrowing or renal parenchymal disease, or be of undetermined etiology (essential hypertension). Asymmetry of blood pressure is most commonly related to coarctation of the aorta, but may also accompany supravalvar aortic stenosis (Ch. 12). In this entity pressure in the right arm may be higher than in the left. (Even in normal individuals, right arm pressure may be higher than left arm; the asymmetry of supravalvar aortic stenosis is simply an exaggeration of this normal variation. To be significant, the difference in right and left arm systolic pressure should exceed 10 mmHg.) Low blood pressure is infrequently a clinical problem, unless an infant or child is obviously extremely ill and has a very low cardiac output.

Blood pressure normally varies slightly with respiration, rising with the increased intrathoracic pressure of expiration and falling as intrathoracic pressure falls with inspiration. Respiratory variation is recognized by inflating the blood pressure cuff until Korotkoff sounds disappear, then slowly deflating the cuff until sounds appear during the expiratory phase of quiet respiration and mark the upper limit of systolic blood pressure. The cuff is further deflated until Korotkoff sounds are present through the respiratory cycle, marking the lower limit of systolic blood pressure. The difference between the upper and lower limits is the measure of respiratory variation and normally does not exceed 10 mmHg. A respiratory variation in excess of 20 mmHg (paradoxical pulse) strongly suggests either pericardial tamponade or airway obstruction (Ch. 21).

PRECORDIAL MOTION

The beating heart moves within the thorax, and in some incompletely defined manner imparts movement to the thoracic wall. In the normal individual the chest wall motion is small and is well localized. The major movement (point of maximal impulse—PMI) overlies the cardiac apex, usually in the fourth or fifth intercostal space near the mid clavicular line, and is related to left ventricular contraction. Normally, there is a brief systolic outward movement which peaks at the beginning of left ventricular ejection and then subsides, followed by an inward movement, or retraction, through the remainder of systole. In the normal child there may be no obvious right ventricular impulse, or there may be a brief early systolic outward movement along the left sternal border. Precordial motion is best judged with the patient supine. The apical impulse becomes more obvious with the patient rolled to the left, since the cardiac apex moves closer to the chest wall with this maneuver, but the impulse may also be exaggerated unduly.

Precordial motion, whether normal or abnormal, is influenced by the structures lying between the heart and the skin, namely the lung and the thoracic wall. With pulmonary emphysema, for instance, more lung is interposed and precordial motion is damped; even marked ventricular hypertrophy may be inapparent in such a patient. Precordial motion of considerable amplitude, on the other hand, may be present in a normal child who has a very thin chest wall.

Abnormal precordial motion may consist of an increased amplitude of early systolic outward motion or of a prolongation of outward motion beyond early systole, or of a combination of the two. There is some tendency for volume overload to cause an increase in early systolic outward motion which is not sustained, and for pressure overload to cause a more sustained outward motion, but the correlation is not sufficiently high to be clinically very useful in the child. It is true, however, that the most strikingly abnormal precordial motion is usually observed in patients with combined pressure and volume overload of a ventricle.

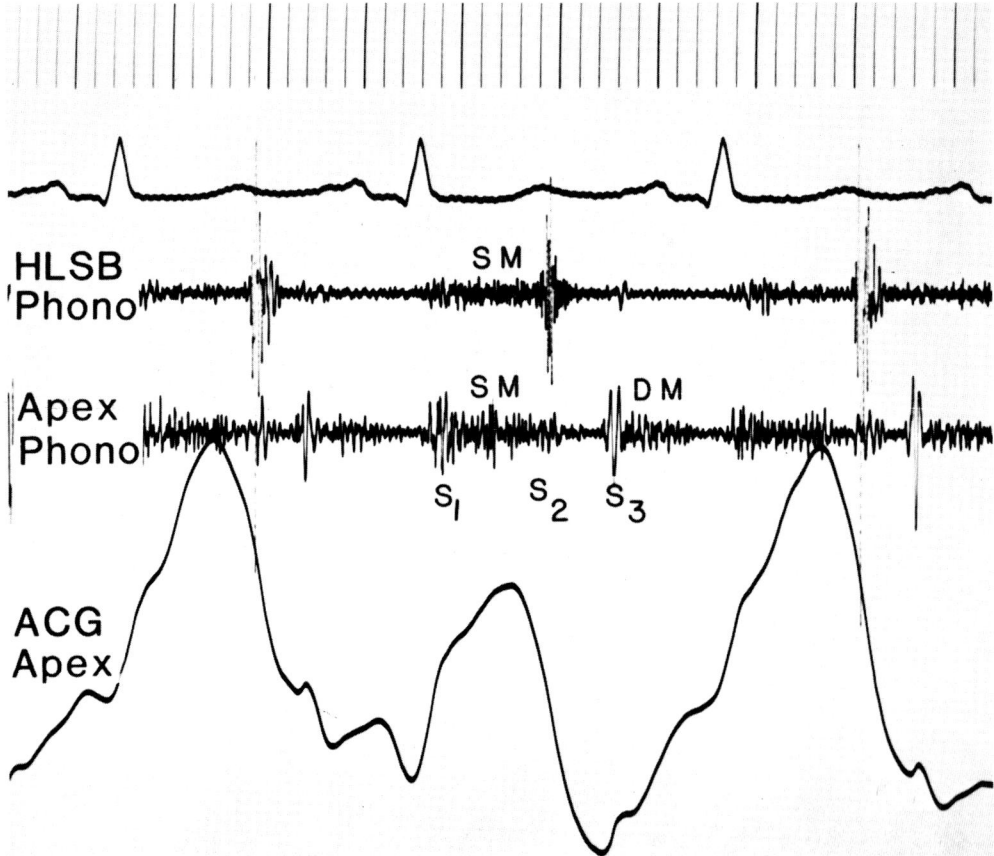

Fig. 3.6 Child with severe mitral regurgitation. Systolic and diastolic murmurs of mitral regurgitation and relative mitral stenosis, respectively, are apparent in the apex phonocardiogram. The apexcardiogram (ACG) shows a prominent and sustained systolic apical impulse.

THE ABNORMAL APICAL IMPULSE

Left ventricular hypertrophy exaggerates systolic outward motion at the apex and, in general, the greater the left ventricular hypertrophy the greater the amplitude and the longer the duration of the impulse. Left ventricular hypertrophy may be on the basis of left ventricular outflow tract obstruction, aortic or mitral regurgitation, or of a left to right shunt at ventricular or great artery level. It is usually not possible to clearly differentiate volume from pressure overload at the bedside in the child. Mitral regurgitation, in particular, may give either a pronounced but poorly sustained early systolic apical impulse or a thrust which extends through systole (Fig. 3.6). (The late systolic component has been attributed to the expanding left atrium pushing the left ventricle forward during ventricular systole.) Vigorous atrial emptying into a poorly compliant left ventricle may result in a presystolic apical pulsation ('palpable fourth heart sound') (Fig. 3.7). Such a presystolic apical impulse is most commonly appreciated in patients with obstructive cardiomyopathy, but may also be present with other causes of severe left ventricular hypertrophy.

THE ABNORMAL PARASTERNAL IMPULSE

Volume overload of the right ventricle (e.g. interatrial septal defect) typically produces a poorly sustained left parasternal lift. If there is an associated pressure overload of the right ventricle (e.g. pulmonary hypertension, pulmonary stenosis) the lift can be pronounced and sustained (Fig. 3.8). Aortic atresia also produces combined pressure and volume overload of the right ventricle, since the right ventricle provides the impetus for flow in both the systemic and pulmonary circuits. In this entity there is usually a marked left parasternal lift, which contrasts strikingly with the decreased or absent peripheral arterial pulse (Fig. 17.11). In the author's experience pure systolic overload of the right ventricle rarely produces a prominent parasternal impulse.

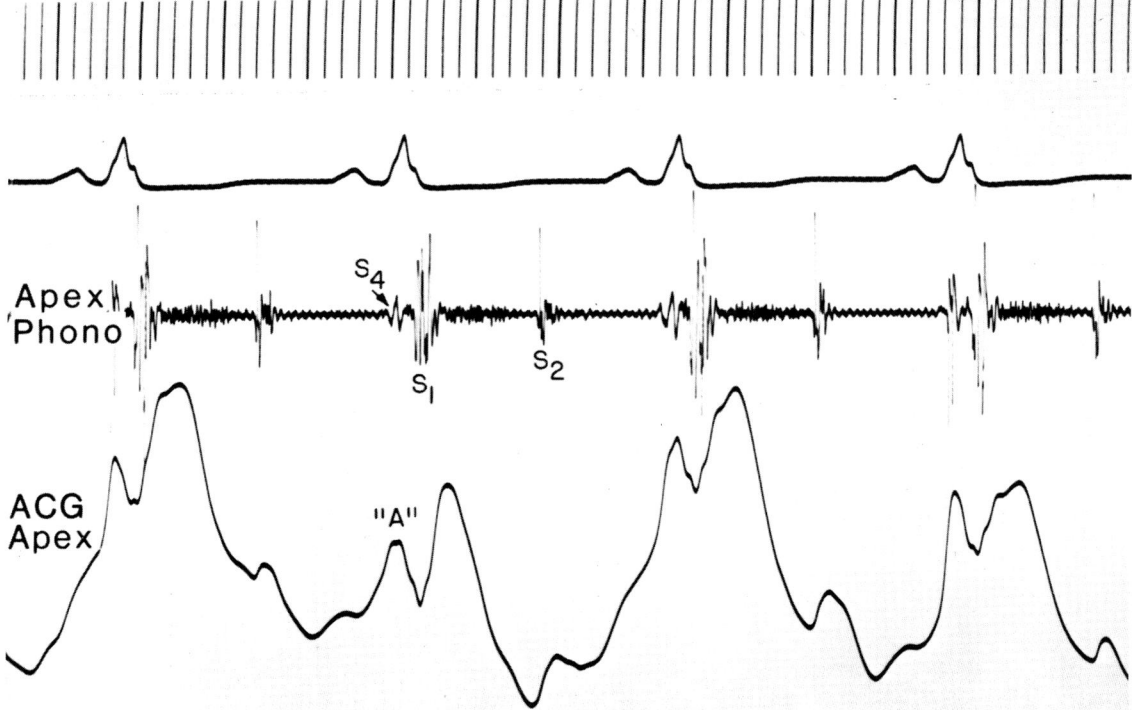

Fig. 3.7 Child with hypertrophic non obstructive cardiomyopathy. The apex phonocardiogram shows a prominent fourth heart sound (S_4) while the apexcardiogram (ACG) shows a concurrent 'A' wave.

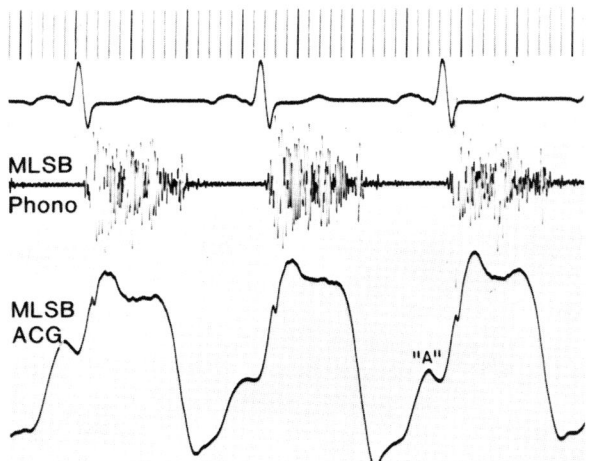

Fig. 3.8 Child with a complete endocardial cushion defect and pulmonary artery banding. There is a prominent and sustained systolic impulse as well as a presystolic pulsation ('A') in the left sternal border pulse tracing (MLSB ACG).

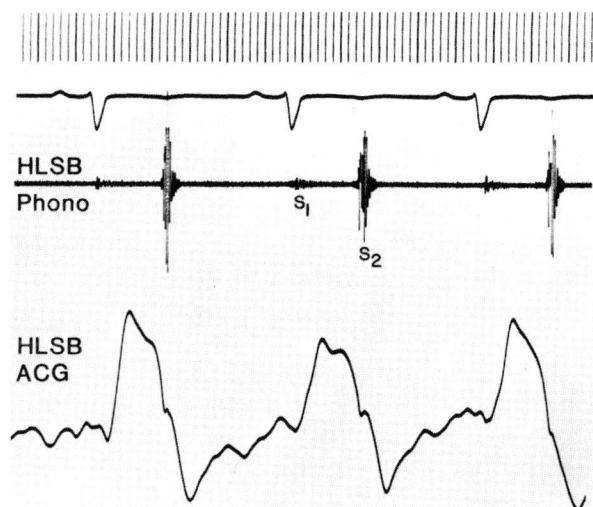

Fig. 3.9 Adolescent with a ventricular septal defect and severe pulmonary vascular disease. The phonocardiogram shows a loud single second heart sound (S_2) while the external pulse tracing over the pulmonary artery (HLSB ACG) demonstrates a prominent systolic pulsation. The dicrotic notch is concurrent with S_2.

OTHER ABNORMAL PRECORDIAL MOTION

Pulmonary artery pulsations may be palpated, or even seen, in the second intercostal space at the left sternal border in a normal but thin chested child. In older individuals, or in children with a thicker thoracic wall, such pulsations can be a valuable clue to the presence of pulmonary hypertension (Fig. 3.9). Outward systolic motion slightly lower along the left sternal border, or more lateral to it in some cases, can be produced by a right ventricular outflow tract aneurysm, itself usually a consequence of surgical repair of tetralogy of Fallot (Fig. 3.10). (The aneurysm results either from excessive resection of right ventricular muscle or from insertion of a non-contractile outflow tract patch. In either case there is a paradoxic motion of the outflow tract which is transmitted to the chest wall particularly well because of the proximity of these two structures.)

In an occasional patient with severe tricuspid regurgitation there is a systolic lateral motion of the precordium, best appreciated by viewing the patient from the foot of the bed. The motion occurs as the jet effect of the regurgitation moves the right ventricle laterally to the left during ventricular systole.

Suprasternal notch pulsations are prominent in patients with aortic regurgitation or coarctation of the aorta. In a child, a pulsatile mass just lateral to the sternocleidomastoid muscle should suggest the possibility of a cervical loop aorta.

AUSCULTATION

There are several commercially available stethoscopes which are durable and well engineered, but there are others which are not satisfactory. An acceptable instrument has at least two heads, including a bell and diaphragm. The diaphragm picks up high frequency sounds and murmurs (e.g. pulmonic ejection sound, murmur of aortic regurgitation) better than the bell. The bell, on the other hand, should be used to search for low pitched sounds or murmurs (e.g. a gallop or the murmur of mitral stenosis). It is important to remember that the transmission of low frequency sound is more efficient if the bell is applied lightly to the skin; if pressed heavily, the bell assumes the properties of a diaphragm. With the bell, a good seal to the skin is necessary and is facilitated if the bell has a rubber rim. The size of the stethoscope head is relatively unimportant, although a small diaphragm or bell makes localization of a murmur somewhat easier in an infant. Some small diaphragms, however, have relatively poor high frequency pick up and are less than adequate. If the connecting tubing of a stethoscope is too short the instrument will be awkward to use; if too long, some sound energy will be lost in transmission. Comfort is important, especially to the cardiologist who uses a stethoscope many times a day, and the choice among good stethoscopes is really one of personal preference.

The importance of a cooperative patient has already been emphasized. If the child is momentarily tranquil but it seems unlikely that this happy state of affairs will persist, it is well to use the stethoscope first, even before taking a history, since auscultation is the most difficult part of the physical examination to accomplish if the patient is crying or resistive. It is always possible to go back and listen again if diagnostic possibilities are suggested by the history or by other parts of the physical examination.

If an effort is not made to listen selectively to each part of the cardiac cycle only the most obvious sounds and murmurs will be appreciated. For instance, the loud mid left sternal border systolic murmur of a ventricular septal defect tends to obscure the faint diastolic murmur of aortic regurgitation in the same area. As another example, a very loud aortic valve closure sound may make a soft pulmonic closure sound hard to hear and it may be evident only after listening peripherally around the area where the pulmonic closure sound is usually well heard.

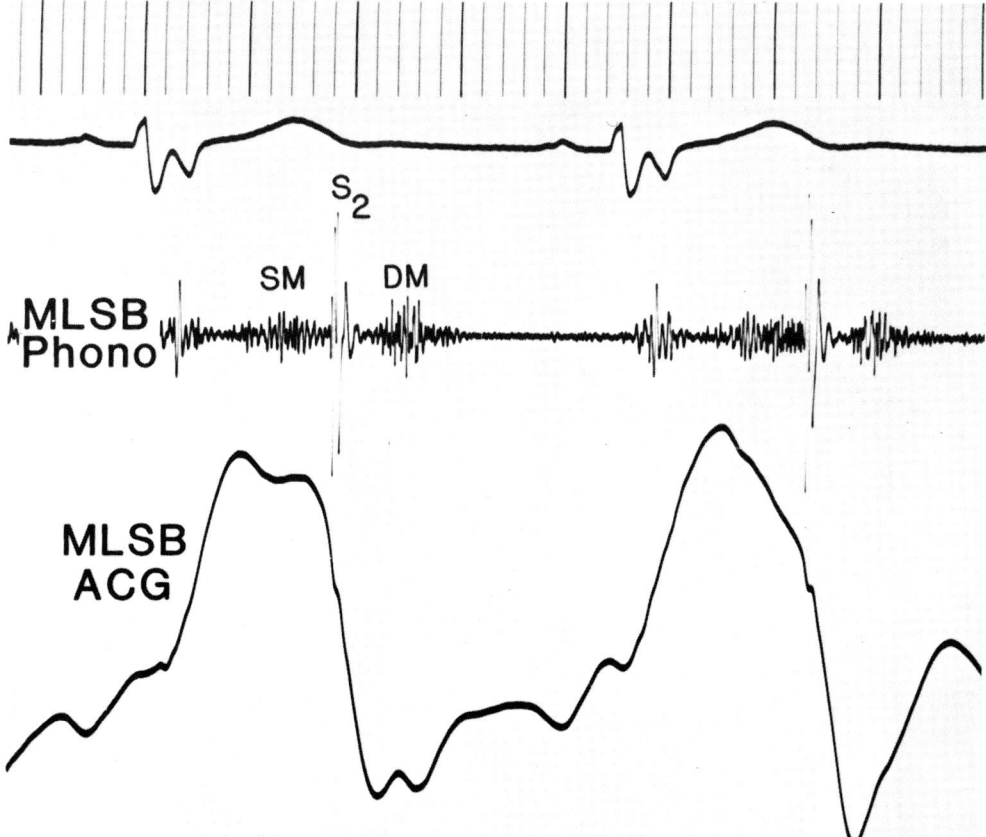

Fig. 3.10 Child with repaired tetralogy of Fallot. Systolic (SM) and diastolic (DM) murmurs of residual pulmonary stenosis and pulmonary regurgitation, respectively, are seen in the mid left sternal border phonocardiogram. The systolic pulsation of a right ventricular outflow tract aneurysm is seen in the mid left sternal border pulse tracing (MLSB ACG).

The site of maximal intensity of a murmur is important, but is not always apparent after listening to the various areas sequentially. After reaching a tentative conclusion as to the site of maximal intensity, it is well to compare the loudness of the murmur at this point with its intensity at other areas. For example, if the murmur seems loudest at the low left sternal border, compare its loudness there with the loudness at the high right sternal border and then return to the low left sternal border to listen again. Repeat the process with the other auscultatory areas, always returning to the low left sternal border for reference. Not infrequently the first impression is wrong and the murmur is found to be louder at another site. The comparison technique may also be useful in deciding whether a very faint murmur is really present or not. For example, in a patient with a large ventricular septal defect, there is often an apical mid diastolic murmur of relative mitral stenosis. Even after listening at the apex with the bell and with the patient in the partial left lateral recumbent position, it may be difficult to decide if this diastolic murmur is present or not. One should listen alternately at the apex and at the mid left sternal border, where diastole is likely to be silent. Comparison of diastole at the two areas may confirm the lack of diastolic murmur, or diastole may be obviously less clear at the apex than at the mid left sternal border, suggesting increased mitral flow.

A word about the radiation of murmurs is in order. Radiation implies preferential transmission in a certain direction. If a soft apical systolic murmur of mitral regurgitation is well heard in the left axilla, it can be said to radiate there. Similarly, the high right sternal border systolic murmur of aortic stenosis radiates to the carotids. (While a comparably loud high left sternal border murmur of pulmonic stenosis may be audible in the neck, it will be much softer there than at its site of maximal intensity.) A very loud systolic murmur originating in a ventricular septal defect may be loudest at the low left sternal border and be well heard all over the precordium and the posterior thorax, but it does not really 'radiate' since any murmur, if sufficiently loud, will be widely heard.

The attenuation of sound in travelling from its source within the heart or great vessels to the chest wall is dependent on the frequency characteristics of the sound, on the distance from the source to the chest wall, and on the characteristics of the intervening structures. High frequency sounds and murmurs attenuate more than low frequency ones, explaining the usual softness of most high-pitched sounds and murmurs and their narrow localization (e.g. pulmonic early systolic ejection sound, diastolic murmur of aortic regurgitation). A thick chest wall attenuates a murmur more than a thin one, and body habitus must be taken into account in evaluating the loudness of sounds and murmurs; a loud pulmonic closure sound is more reliable evidence of high pulmonary artery pressure in a heavy-chested adult than in an asthenic child. Closure of a posteriorly placed pulmonic valve in a patient with transposition is less well heard than that of an anterior pulmonic valve in a normal person.

Patience has been mentioned as an important factor in the performance of an adequate physical examination, patience not only in dealing with a frightened or angry child but also in checking and re-checking important physical findings. A second heart sound which seems single at first may be obviously split after 20 seconds of concentrated listening to nothing but the second heart sound. (Sometimes shutting out other sensory input by closing one's eyes helps in concentrating on auscultation.) A second heart sound which is single at the high left sternal border may be audibly split a little lower along the left sternal border or somewhat laterally from the left sternal border. In a child with a murmur of aortic stenosis an early systolic ejection sound is a nearly pathognomonic marker for a valvar locus of the obstruction. It may not be obvious at the high right sternal border or at the apex with the patient supine, yet be easily audible in the sitting position or more laterally towards the mid axillary line.

Since the findings of congenital heart disease may change rapidly, especially in the symptomatic infant, repeated examinations are often rewarding. For example, in a premature infant with both the respiratory distress syndrome and physical findings of a patent ductus arteriosus, the continuous murmur may disappear and the brisk pulses become normal, signalling closure of the patent ductus. In such a patient continued respiratory difficulties are pulmonary in origin, not cardiac.

A knowledge of the pathophysiology of congenital heart disease is necessary if one is to glean the maximal amount of usable information from the physical examination. This is especially true with auscultation, since much of auscultation consists of listening for subtleties, events that are heard only if searched for. For example, in a cyanotic newborn a continuous murmur at the high left sternal border almost always indicates a patent ductus arteriosus and very severe right ventricular outflow tract obstruction, usually pulmonary atresia. This murmur is rarely obvious, being most often very soft and high pitched and quite subtle. The importance of recognizing a ductal murmur in a cyanotic infant is obvious, since the life of such an infant may depend upon continued patency of the ductus. Another less pressing, but still important example, is the asymptomatic child with an interatrial septal defect. The most obvious physical finding is a soft high left sternal border systolic murmur, exactly like the very common innocent pulmonary 'flow' murmur heard at the same location. The presence of this murmur should always lead to a careful appraisal of the splitting of the second heart sound, including changes in the width of splitting with respiration. If splitting is 'fixed', attention should then be turned to a search for a soft medium pitched diastolic murmur or 'puff' at the low left sternal border. This murmur of relative tricuspid stenosis indicates a large left to right shunt at atrial level and the triad of a high left sternal border systolic murmur, fixed splitting of the second heart sound and the diastolic murmur is virtually pathognomonic of a left to right shunt at atrial level which is large enough to warrant surgical repair. (This initial impression will be supplemented by electrocardiogram, chest roentgenogram, echocardiogram and likely by cardiac catheterization and angiography, but is not likely to be appreciably altered by these studies.) As another example of the value of an understanding of the pathophysiology of congenital heart disease, the presence of full or bounding pulses in a newborn with congestive heart failure can be cited. Ordinarily, pulses are generally diminished with congestive heart failure unless the failure itself is a result of a large low resistance aortic run-off. Since a patent ductus is unlikely to cause failure in a full-term newborn, other causes must be searched for. In this setting, an 'aortic' early systolic ejection sound suggests a persistent truncus arteriosus; distended neck veins or a loud bruit over the head point to an intracranial arteriovenous fistula; and a to and fro left sternal border murmur indicates congenital aortic regurgitation or an aortico-left ventricular tunnel. The more one knows of the pathophysiology of congenital heart disease, the more likely it is that a given physical finding will make sense and will lead to a search for other murmurs, or pulsations, or heart sounds which will permit an accurate clinical diagnosis.

HEART SOUNDS

The events of the cardiac cycle, both in the normal and abnormal heart, produce sounds which are transmitted to the chest wall. The way in which these sounds are generated has provoked lively debate since James Hope (1846) proposed that the first heart sound was produced by 'valvar extension', 'muscular contraction' and 'muscular extension'. Over the years, convinced proponents of the 'valvar' origin of heart sounds have debated loudly and sometimes acrimoniously with equally convinced adherents of the 'muscular' theory. More recently 'acceleration-deceleration' theories have been advanced (Rushmer, 1961). Judging the merits of the several possible sources of heart sounds is beyond the scope of this book; suffice it to say that the first and second heart sounds are coincident with closure of the atrioventricular and semilunar valves, respectively. Throughout this book reference will be made to the 'pulmonic closure sound' or the 'mitral closure sound', as though the valves really generated the audible event. This does not imply complete confidence that they do; it is simply convenient.

First heart sound

Genesis and splitting

The first heart sound is normally loudest at the apex. It is usually single and is coincident with mitral valve closure as timed echocardiographically. The first heart sound may be split, the first component representing mitral valve closure and the second component tricuspid valve closure (Fig. 3.11). Audible splitting of the first heart sound is most commonly due to complete right bundle branch block, although children with this conduction abnormality not infrequently have a single first sound. The first sound is characteristically split in patients with Ebstein's anomaly of the tricuspid valve (Ch. 16). Here, the loud and delayed tricuspid component has been dubbed a 'sail' sound. (Fig. 3.12) (Fontana & Wooley, 1972). In children, a seemingly split first heart sound is often actually a first sound–ejection sound sequence (discussed further under Ejection Sounds).

Loudness

The loudness of the first sound is largely determined by the velocity of leaflet closure. Leaflets tend to close rapidly when there is increased ventricular contractility, or when closure occurs during the rapid rise of ventricular pressure, or if the leaflets are wide open at the onset of ventricular contraction.

Contractility. An increase in left ventricular contractility occurs with anxiety, exercise, hyperthyroidism or administration of sympathomimetic drugs such as isoproterinol, and the first heart sound tends to be loud in each circumstance. When left ventricular contractility is low (e.g. myocarditis, 'congestive' forms of cardiomyopathy, myxedema, or with negative inotropic drugs such as propranolol), the first heart sound is soft (Thompson et al, 1975). Alternate beat to beat variation in the first heart sound has been reported in pulsus alternans, where left ventricular contractility also varies on alternate beats (Sakamoto et al, 1966). A soft first heart sound has also been reported in patients with left bundle branch block who have a long isometric contraction time and a slow rate of rise of left ventricular pressure (Thompson et al 1975).

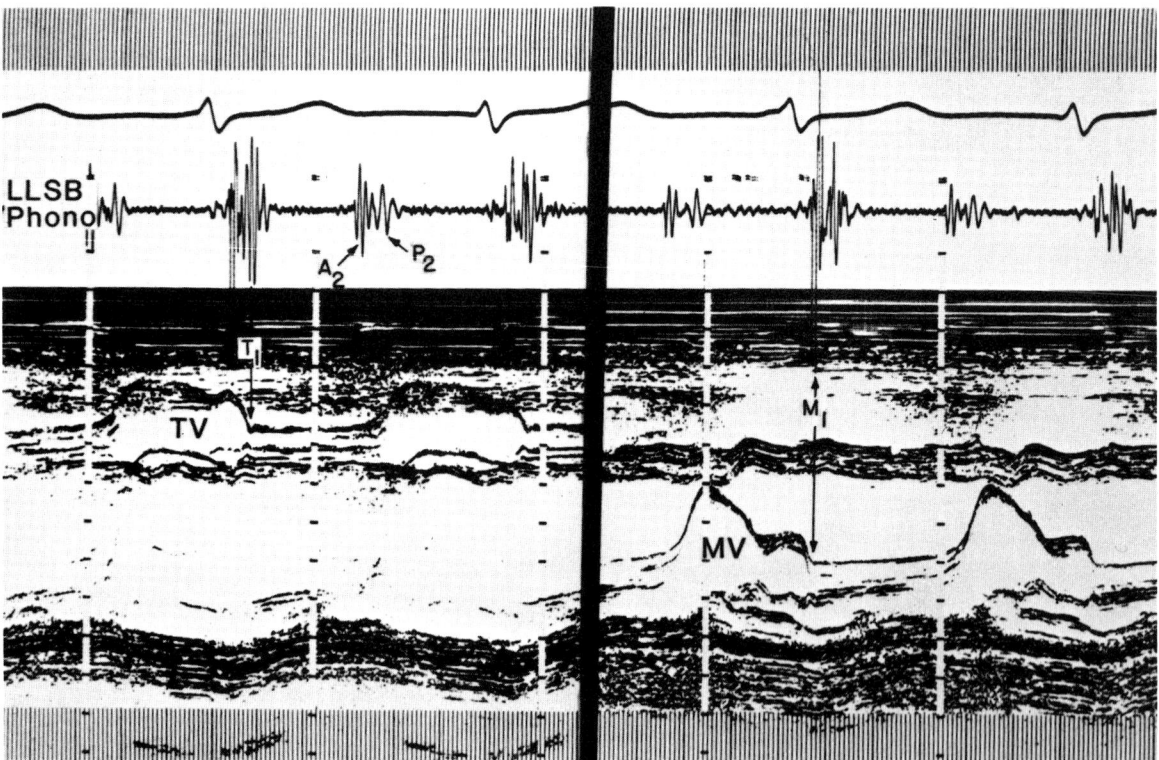

Fig. 3.11 Split first heart sound. In the left panel tricuspid valve closure is coincident with the second component (T_1) of the first heart sound. In the right panel mitral closure is coincident with the first component of the first sound (M_1).

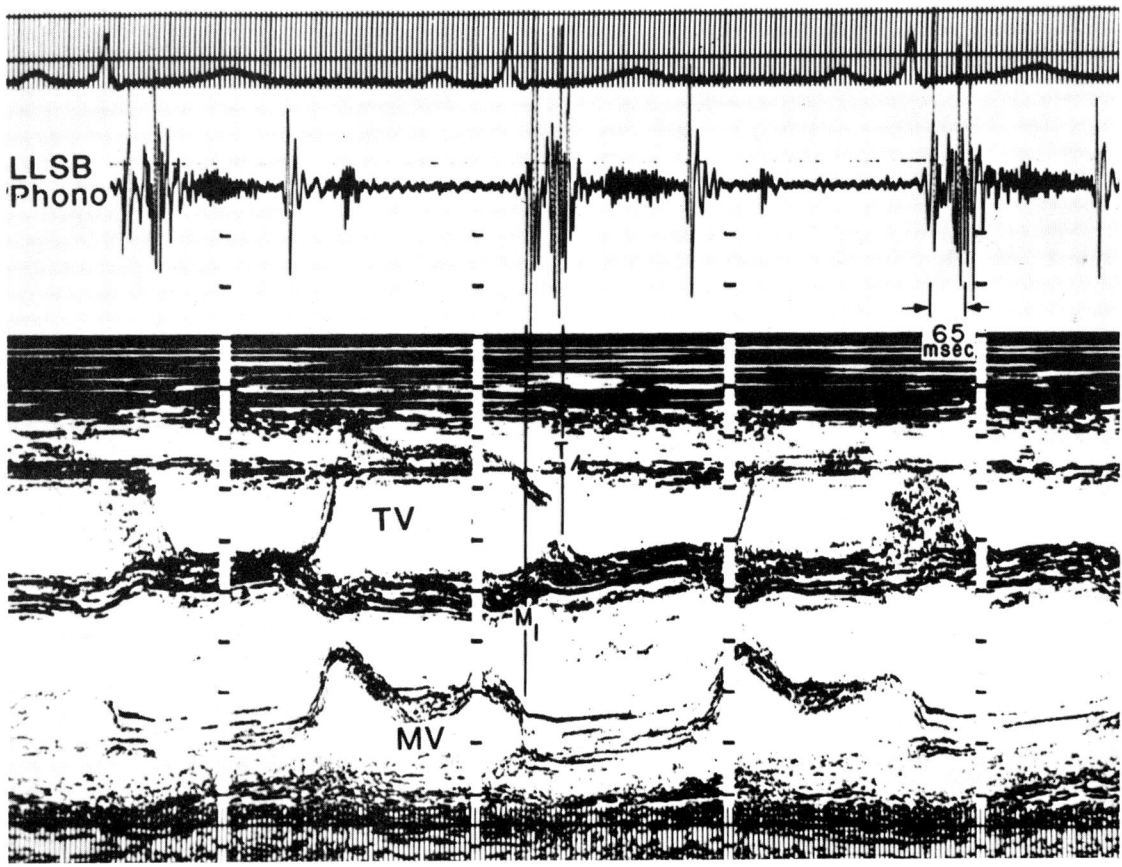

Fig. 3.12 Child with Ebstein's anomaly of the tricuspid valve. The first sound is widely split. The first component (M_1) occurs with closure of the mitral valve; the second (T_1) with late closure of the large tricuspid valve.

Leaflet position. The first heart sound tends to be unusually loud when there is a delay of mitral valve closure from the beginning of the rise in the left ventricular pressure curve to a time during its maximal rate of rise. For example, left atrial pressure is high in patients with mitral stenosis, and the cross over of left ventricular and left atrial pressure is delayed and occurs during the rapid phase of ventricular pressure rise (Criley et al, 1975). In this circumstance the first heart sound is both loud and slightly late. Another example, the well-known relationship of the loudness of the first heart sound to the PR interval, is explainable by the temporal relationship of atrial and ventricular systole. If the PR interval is long, the mitral valve tends to move toward the closed position before ventricular systole begins and the first heart sound is soft. If the PR interval is short, atrial contraction will still be propelling blood into the ventricle as ventricular systole begins. Mitral closure will then be relatively late and during the rapid rise of ventricular pressure. The first heart sound is then loud. If the PR interval varies, as it does with complete atrioventricular block, the loudness of the first sound also varies (Fig. 3.13) (Ch. 24). The first heart sound may be soft or absent in patients with severe acute aortic regurgitation (Fig. 13.6), and here the softness is due not to poor left ventricular contractility but to premature closure of the mitral valve by the regurgitation induced elevation in left ventricular end diastolic pressure (Reddy et al, 1975).

Tricuspid component. The first heart sound may be unusually loud at the low left sternal border in a patient with an interatrial septal defect, with transposition of the great arteries or with mitral

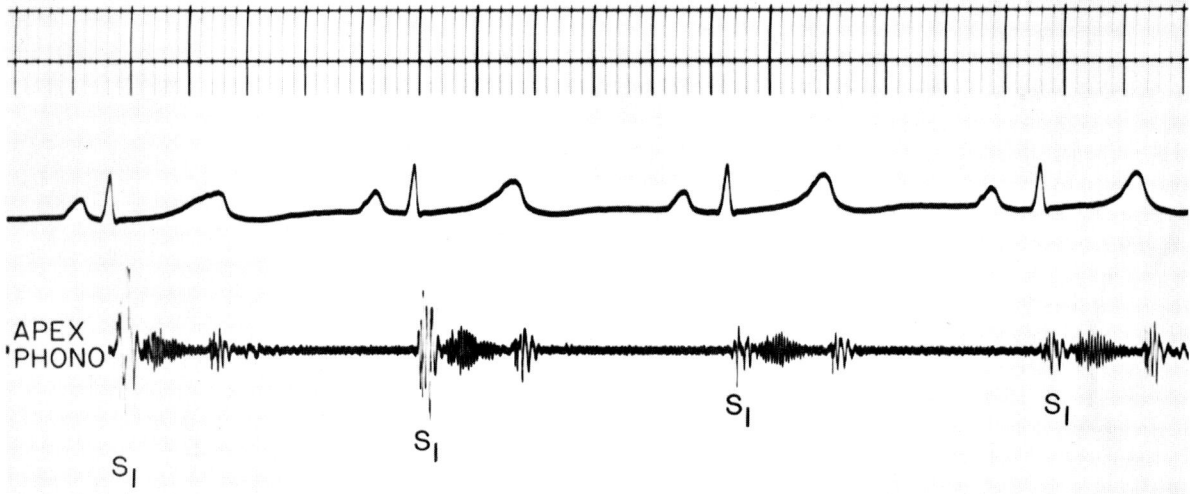

Fig. 3.13 Child with third degree atrioventricular block. As the apparent PR interval lengthens the first heart sound (S_1) attenuates.

atresia. The loudness probably results from unusually rapid closure of the tricuspid valve.

Other factors. Two other determinants of loudness of the first heart sound must be mentioned: distance from the source of the sound to the stethoscope on the chest wall and mobility of the valve itself. The first heart sound tends to be soft in a barrel-chested individual with normal hemodynamics and a normal mitral valve, and also in a patient with a heavily calcified or dysplastic valve.

Summary. In summary, the first heart sound is loud if left ventricular contractility is high, if mitral valve closure occurs relatively late and during rapid left ventricular pressure rise, or if tricuspid valve closure is unusually forceful. A soft first heart sound occurs if myocardial contractility is depressed or if mitral valve closure precedes the onset of ventricular systole.

Second heart sound

Genesis

The second heart sound is made up of aortic and pulmonic components, which are coincident with the incisurae of the aortic and pulmonary pressure tracings recorded with high fidelity catheters (Shaver et al, 1975a). Normally, both aortic and pulmonic components are separately audible in children. The auscultatory characteristics of the second heart sound are extremely useful in the evaluation of congenital heart disease, and important hemodynamic inferences can be drawn from the width of splitting, from variation of the splitting with respiration and from the intensity of each of the two components.

Splitting

The aortic component of the second sound normally precedes the pulmonic, but audible splitting depends upon separation of the two components by 20–30 milliseconds, closer splitting being heard as a single second heart sound. In normal children and in young adults the second heart sound virtually always splits with inspiration and usually becomes single with expiration. In an occasional young person the second heart sound remains audibly split during expiration if the patient is recumbent but almost always becomes single during expiration if the patient sits. The reason for this postural effect is unknown.

A small portion of the increased inspiratory separation of the aortic and pulmonic components is due to an earlier occurrence of the aortic closure sound (decreased Q-aortic closure sound interval). Most is related to a later pulmonic closure sound (increased Q-pulmonic closure sound interval). The most widely accepted explanation for this

THE CARDIAC PHYSICAL EXAMINATION   21

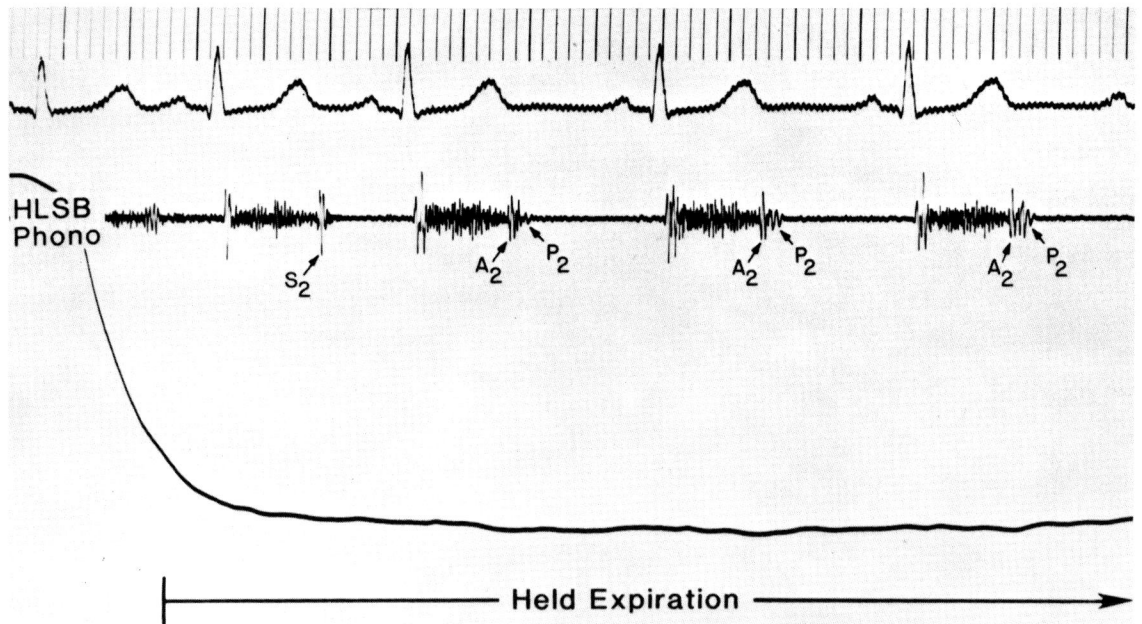

Fig. 3.14 Demonstration of physiologic splitting of the second heart sound during held expiration (see text).

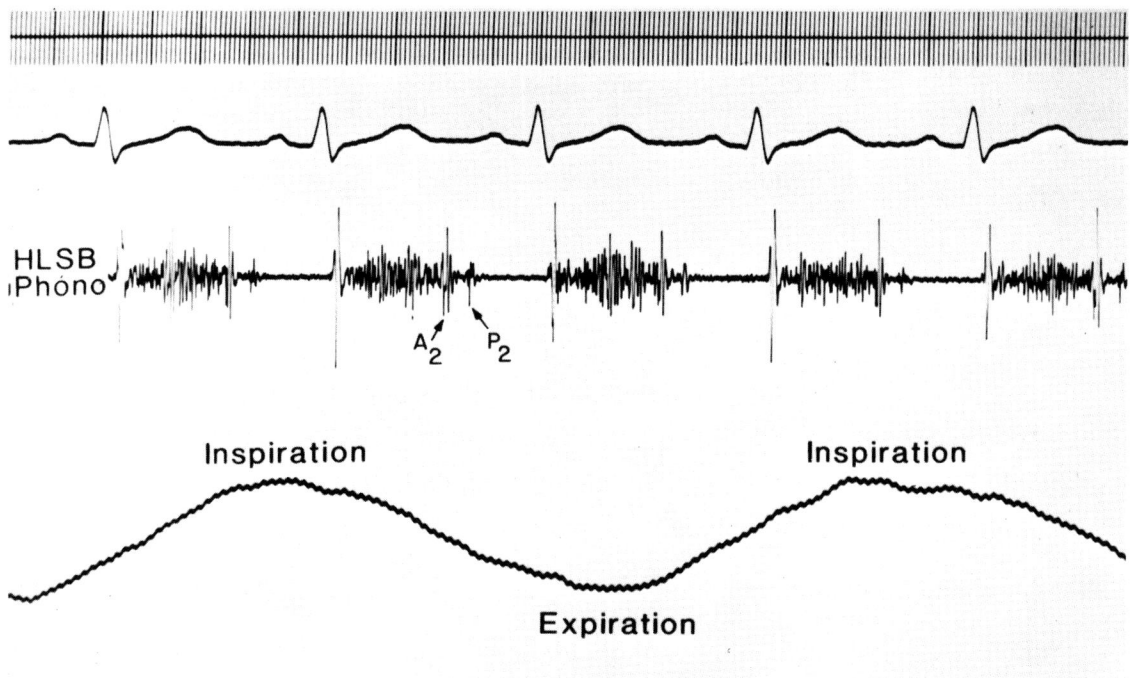

Fig. 3.15 Child with an interatrial septal defect. There is fixed splitting of the second heart sound during quiet respiration.

respiratory variation in splitting invokes an inspiratory increase in systemic venous return and right ventricular stroke volume and a consequent increase in right ventricular ejection time and delay in pulmonic closure. During expiration the opposite occurs: a decrease in systemic venous return results in a small right ventricular stroke volume and an early pulmonic closure sound, while an increase in pulmonary venous return causes a slight prolongation in left ventricular ejection time and hence a minor delay in the aortic closure sound.

A word is in order about how to listen for respiratory variation. The second heart sound may be listened to during quiet respiration and the normal pattern has been described above. In some children, respiratory noise and relatively rapid respiratory and cardiac rates make an accurate assessment of respiratory variation quite difficult, and an alternative method may be useful. The child should be asked to 'breathe in', 'breathe out', and then to 'stop breathing'. (If he is asked to 'hold his breath' he will almost invariable inspire again.)

The characteristics of the second heart sound should be noted at the end of expiration and for the next several beats during held expiration. Normally, the second heart sound is single for 1, 2 or 3 beats, then splits progressively more widely over the next few beats (Fig. 3.14).

Wide split. Several variations from the normal pattern of inspiratory split and expiratory singularity of the second heart sound occur and can be determined by either of the above auscultatory techniques. Wider than normal splitting, often with persistent splitting at end expiration, is usually attributable to electrical or mechanical delay in right ventricular systole. As examples, wide splitting is common with right bundle branch block and with pulmonic stenosis.

Fixed split. 'Fixed' splitting of the second heart sound implies a less than 20 millisecond variation in split during the respiratory cycle (Fig. 3.15). (Or as wide a split of the first beat after forced expiration as during the next several beats if the alternate method is used — see Fig. 3.16.) Fixed

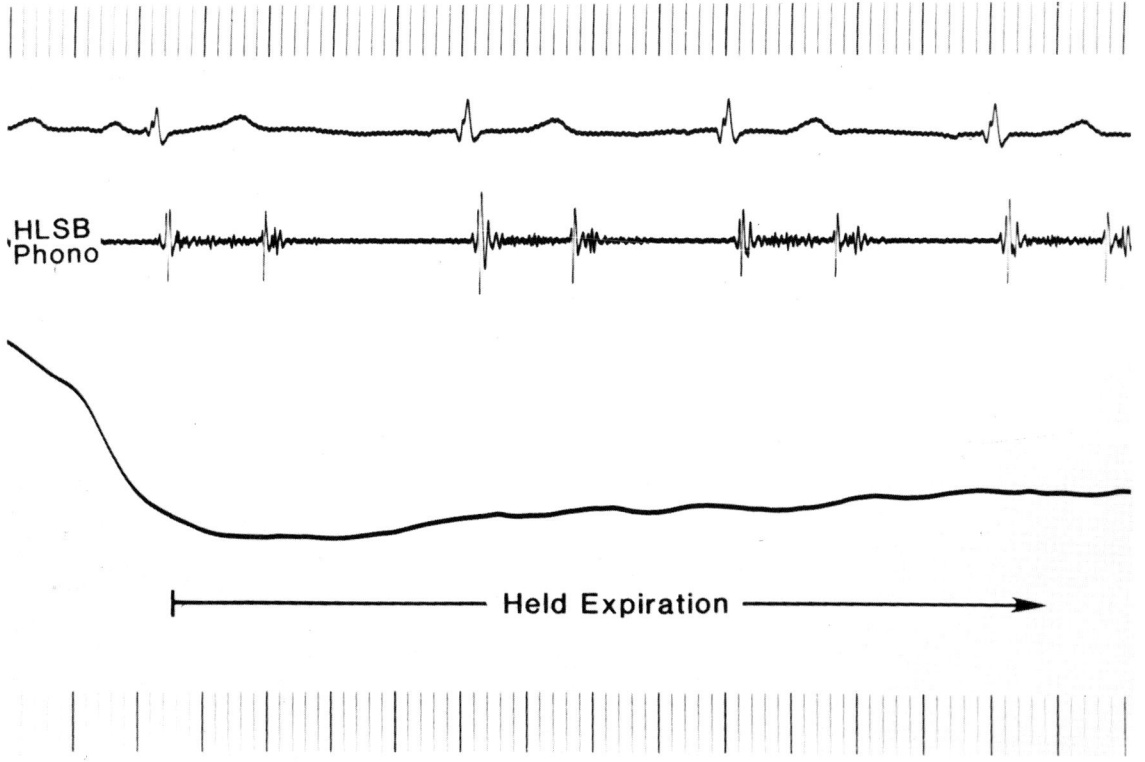

Fig. 3.16 Child with interatrial septal defect. Fixed splitting of the second heart sound during held expiration.

splitting is most common with an interatrial septal defect and is the rule if the left to right shunt is large. The fixed split has been thought to be due to reciprocal changes in systemic and pulmonary venous returns with respiration. With inspiration, an increase in systemic venous return is balanced by a decrease in pulmonary venous return and in flow to the right atrium through the atrial defect. During expiration, a decrease in systemic venous return is matched by an increase in pulmonary venous return and left to right shunting. The net result is a constant right ventricular stroke volume; there is then no change in the timing of pulmonic closure with varying phases of respiration and splitting is fixed.

Single second sound. A single second heart sound may be due either to inaudibility of the pulmonic component (e.g. pulmonic stenosis or posterior location of the pulmonary artery) or to coincidence of pulmonic and aortic closure throughout the respiratory cycle. In children, the latter is usually due to pulmonary hypertension (e.g. hypertensive ventricular septal defect), but in older adults may be normal.

Paradoxic split. The second heart sound may split with expiration and become single with inspiration. This 'paradoxical' splitting indicates a reversal in the normal sequence of aortic and pulmonic valve closure, with pulmonic now preceding aortic. With inspiration the second sound becomes single as pulmonic closure occurs later and merges with the aortic closure sound. During expiration, the pulmonic closure sound occurs relatively early and separates from aortic closure. The second heart sound is then split. (If the alternative method is used, the second heart sound is split at the end of forced expiration but progressively narrows and then becomes single over the next several beats — see Fig. 3.17.) Paradoxical splitting may be due to delay of aortic closure (e.g. left bundle branch block, aortic stenosis, left ventricular myocardial dysfunction) or, less commonly, to prematurity of

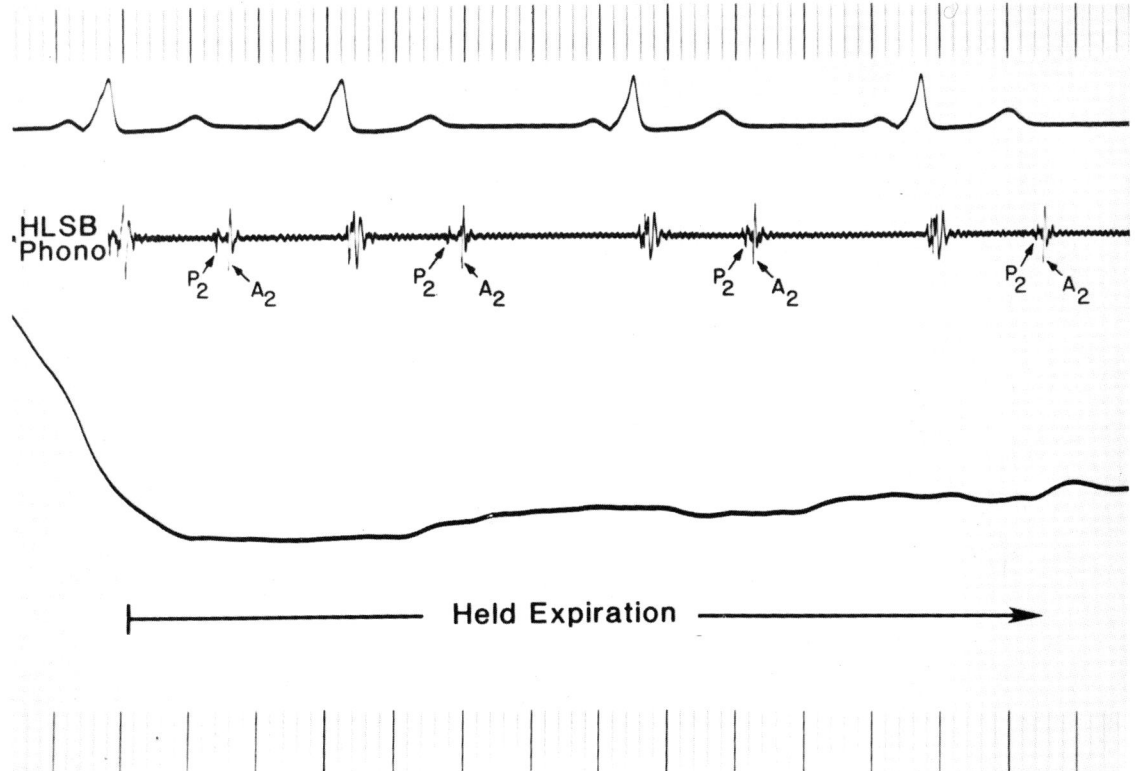

Fig. 3.17 Child with the Wolff-Parkinson-White syndrome. Width of splitting of the second heart sound gradually narrows during held expiration (paradoxic splitting).

pulmonic closure (e.g. Wolff-Parkinson-White syndrome, Zuberbuhler & Bauersfeld, 1965).

Role of impedance. There are several problems with an exclusive electromechanical explanation for variation in splitting of the second heart sound. Expiratory splitting occurs in idiopathic dilatation of the pulmonary artery and, also, may persist into the early postoperative period after atrial septal defect repair; in neither case is there electrical delay in right ventricular activation nor is there any obvious reason for prolongation of right ventricular mechanical systole. Also, in some patients with pulmonic stenosis, the width of split is out of proportion to the severity of obstruction, being quite wide with mild stenosis. Shaver (1975a) has offered an alternative explanation, emphasizing the role of impedance in the timing of aortic and pulmonic valve closure. (Impedance is the sum total of the forces which oppose forward flow and which eventually lead to cessation of flow after mechanical systole ends.) If aortic and left ventricular pressures are simultaneously recorded using equisensitive high fidelity catheters, the aortic and left ventricular pressure curves nearly track during late systole, and the aortic incisura is only slightly separated from the descending limb of the ventricular pressure curve. Simultaneous recordings of right ventricular and pulmonary artery curves in individuals with normal pulmonary artery pressure are quite different; the pulmonary artery pressure curve is delayed and the pulmonic incisura 'hangs out' beyond the right ventricular curve (Fig. 3.18). The relatively prolonged 'hang out' is thought to be related to low impedance in the pulmonary artery. The low impedance is due, in turn, to the large capacitance and low resistance of the pulmonary bed. Under these circumstances the inertia of the moving column of blood entering the pulmonary artery predominates longer and forward motion persists even after right ventricular pressure has fallen well below pulmonary artery pressure. The late pulmonic closure sound of idiopathic dilatation of the pulmonary artery, of normotensive atrial septal defect or of mild pulmonic stenosis may, in this view, be due more to the large capacitance and low resistance of the pulmonary bed than to prolongation of right ventricular mechanical systole. In fact, right ventricular systole is not prolonged in such patients with normal pulmonary vascular resistance and the width of splitting is a measure of the difference in aortic and pulmonary artery 'hang out'. Further, Curtiss (1975) has shown that the normal inspiratory delay in the pulmonic closure sound is due more to an inspiratory decrease in pulmonary impedance than to a prolongation of right ventricular systole induced by increased systemic venous return. The singularity of the second sound in many normal older adults is probably related to aging processes in the pulmonary vascular bed which increase impedance, reduce 'hang out', and therefore cause pulmonic and aortic closure to coincide (Curtiss et al, 1975).

The importance of impedance in determining the degree of separation of the dicrotic notch from the ventricular pressure curve can be shown by studies which use vasoactive drugs to manipulate impedance (Shaver et al, 1975a). The aortic 'hang out' interval increases with amyl nitrite, which lowers systemic impedance, and decreases when impedance is increased by systemic vasoconstrictors. Although aortic 'hang out' is usually so short as to have no effect on audible splitting, the dilated ascending aorta of patients with valvar aortic

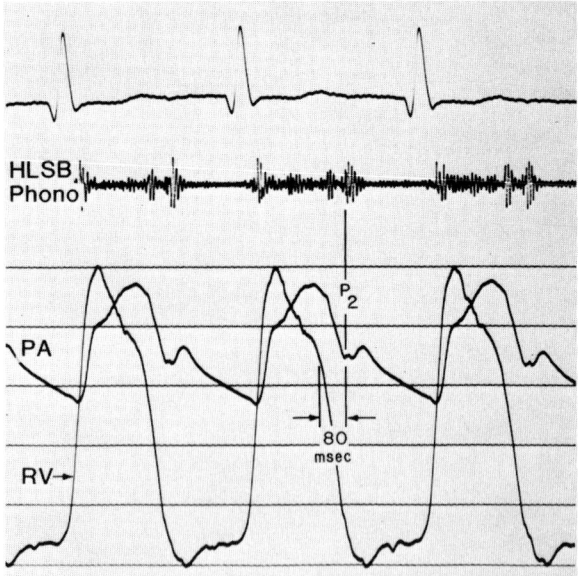

Fig. 3.18 Simultaneous right ventricular and pulmonary artery pressures in a child with a large pulmonary artery. The incisura of the pulmonary artery tracing and the pulmonic closure sound (P_2) 'hang out' beyond the right ventricular pressure by 80 msec.

stenosis may increase aortic capacitance sufficiently to cause delay in aortic closure, contributing to the single or even paradoxically split second heart sound present in some such patients.

With high pulmonary vascular resistance, pulmonary artery and right ventricular pressures nearly track in late systole, as aortic and left ventricular pressures do normally. In patients with pulmonary hypertension the width of splitting of the second heart sound is not a measure of the level of pulmonary vascular resistance, but rather of right ventricular function (Shaver et al, 1975a). The second heart sound is single in patients with pulmonary hypertension who have good right ventricular function, but when function is poor, right ventricular systole is prolonged. Pulmonic closure is then delayed and the second sound splits (Fig. 3.19). In the setting of high pulmonary vascular resistance a prominently split second heart sound is highly suggestive of severely compromised right ventricular function.

Loudness

The loudness of a semilunar valve closure sound has several determinants, including the position of the valve within the thorax, thickness of the chest wall and pressure within the respective artery. Thus, a loud second heart sound at the high left sternal border may be a loud pulmonic closure sound resulting from pulmonary hypertension, may be normal in a child with a very thin chest, or may be an aortic closure sound if the aorta is unusually positioned (e.g. 'corrected' transposition of the great arteries). The aortic closure sound is less often soft than the pulmonic closure sound, since the aorta is almost never abnormally posterior in the thorax and since, even with severe aortic stenosis, aortic pressure never falls to the low levels seen in the pulmonary artery with even moderate pulmonic stenosis.

Third heart sound

A third heart sound is a low frequency sound which occurs in early diastole, 100 to 200 milliseconds after aortic closure. It is recordable in almost all normal individuals and is commonly audible in normal children. The sound is a

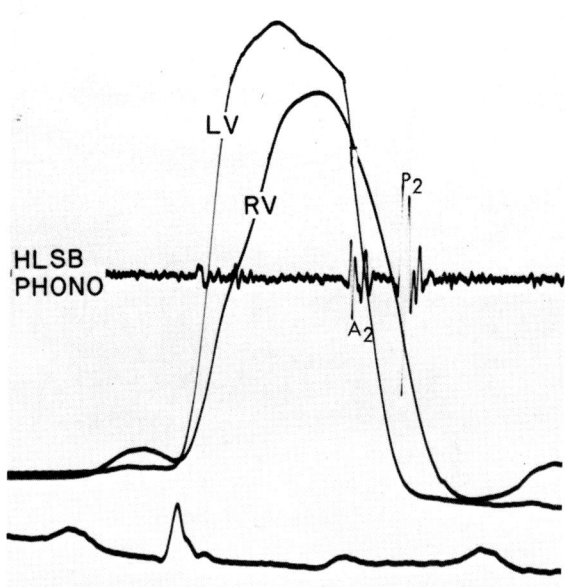

Fig. 3.19 Adolescent with pulmonary hypertension and poor right ventricular function. Peak right ventricular systolic pressure is nearly as high as left ventricular pressure. Right ventricular mechanical systole is prolonged, accounting for the delay in pulmonic valve closure (P_2) and for the wide split of the second heart sound.

consequence of ventricular vibrations induced when the rate of early diastolic filling exceeds ventricular distensibility, resulting in a sudden deceleration of the incoming stream. It is not generated by sudden diastolic tensing of an atrioventricular valve as was once thought (Shah & Jackson, 1975). In children there is no real difference between a third heart sound and a protodiastolic gallop, except that calling the event a gallop implies cardiac disease. For example, a 'third heart sound' is common in situations where rapid early diastolic filling occurs, such as exercise, anemia, fever, thyrotoxicosis, an unusually slow heart rate, or mitral regurgitation, but if there is other evidence of congestive heart failure a loud 'third heart sound' becomes, by convention, a protodiastolic 'gallop'. Gallops may originate in either ventricle. A left ventricular protodiastolic gallop is maximal at the apex and is constant through the respiratory cycle; a right ventricular gallop is prominent at the low left sternal border and may increase with inspiration (Tavel, 1978a). The differentiation of a right from a left ventricular gallop may be important. For example, a left ventricular gallop in a patient with mitral stenosis and mitral regurgitation implies predominant regurgitation, since major mitral stenosis precludes rapid early diastolic filling of the left ventricle, but a right ventricular gallop may occur with pure mitral stenosis if there is pulmonary hypertension and right ventricular dysfunction. Unusual prominence of the third heart sound is not expected when there is ventricular hypertrophy without an increase in volume or rapidity of early diastolic filling (e.g., pulmonic stenosis, aortic stenosis, coarctation of the aorta). It should be emphasized that even a loud third heart sound does not, of itself, imply heart disease in a child.

A very prominent protodiastolic sound may be present with constrictive pericardial disease (Fig. 21.3). It is known as a pericardial 'knock', tends to be earlier than the usual third heart sound (90 to 120 milliseconds after aortic closure), and results from sudden arrest of ventricular filling by the inelastic pericardium (Tavel 1978a).

Fourth heart sound

A fourth heart sound (atrial gallop) may be right or left sided and occurs when atrial systole induces a rapid pressure rise in a ventricle. An audible fourth heart sound implies lack of distensibility of a ventricle; in other words, an exaggerated pressure rise in response to the increased volume induced by atrial contraction. This lack of ventricular compliance may be related to ventricular hypertrophy (e.g. aortic stenosis, idiopathic hypertrophic subaortic stenosis, cardiomyopathy, hypertension) or to a failing and acutely dilated ventricle (e.g. myocardial disease or severe aortic or mitral regurgitation of sudden recent onset). A fourth heart sound is not heard in normal children and is uncommon with even severe valvar aortic or pulmonic stenosis. In this age group it is probably most common with the hypertrophic cardiomyopathies (Fig. 3.7).

A fourth heart sound originating in the left ventricle can best be heard with the patient in the partial left lateral recumbent position and with the bell of the stethoscope lightly applied at the apex. An audible left sided fourth heart sound is identical in timing with a presystolic impulse palpated at the apex or recorded there with an apexcardiogram (Fig 3.7). (Both fourth heart sound and presystolic impulse have a common origin and are the audible and palpable manifestations of the same event.) A right sided fourth heart sound may be accompanied by a large jugular venous 'A' wave or by a presystolic hepatic pulsation. It may increase during inspiration (Fig. 3.20) (Tavel, 1978b).

It may be quite difficult to differentiate a fourth heart sound-first heart sound sequence from a split first heart sound or from a first heart sound-early systolic ejection sound combination. A simultaneous phonocardiogram and apexcardiogram may be very helpful in identifying the presystolic timing of a fourth heart sound and of an accompanying impulse.

Summation gallop

A summation gallop occurs when atrial systole coincides with the rapid ventricular filling of early diastole. The most common cause is tachycardia, but a fusion of the third and fourth heart sounds can occur at slower rates if the PR interval is long. The intermittent 'third heart sound' heard in patients with atrioventricular block is really a summation gallop, and occurs when atrial systole, by chance, occurs in protodiastole (Fig. 24.2).

Ejection sounds

Early systolic ejection sounds may be pulmonic or aortic and originate either at a semilunar valve or in a dilated arterial root.

Pulmonic

Pulmonic ejection sounds are most common with valvar pulmonic stenosis, being the rule in all but the most severe cases. The ejection sound of valvar pulmonic stenosis has been shown to occur when the valve 'domes' into the pulmonary artery. This doming of the pulmonic valve marks the limit of excursion of the pulmonic cusps (Hultgren et al, 1969). Echocardiographically, the pulmonic ejection sound is simultaneous with the shoulder on the pulmonic valve echo which marks maximal opening (Fig.10.3). An early systolic ejection sound may also originate in a dilated pulmonary artery,

THE CARDIAC PHYSICAL EXAMINATION 27

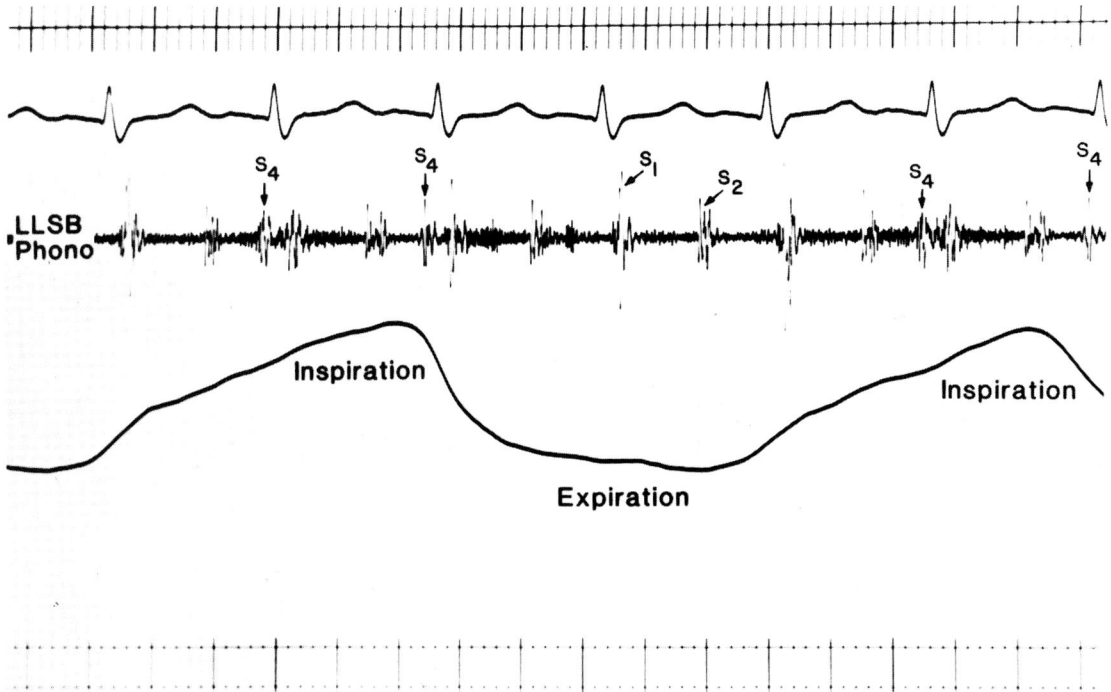

Fig. 3.20 Adolescent with hemochromatosis and cardiomyopathy secondary to thallasemia major. There is a prominent fourth heart sound (S_4) during inspiration. The respiratory variation and the low left sternal border localization of the sound suggest it is of right ventricular origin.

most commonly in the presence of pulmonary hypertension, but also occasionally in a patient with normal pulmonary pressure. Pulmonary artery ejection sounds have been attributed to a sudden checking of the pulmonary arterial wall as it reaches its elastic limits. Cineangiographically, however, there is continued expansion of the pulmonary artery well after the occurrence of the ejection sound. The exact mechanism of production of the pulmonary artery ejection sound remains in doubt.

A pulmonic ejection sound is loudest at the high left sternal border, is high pitched and clicking, and typically varies with respiration, being louder with expiration and fading or disappearing entirely with inspiration (Fig 10.4). It has been postulated that the increased systemic venous return of inspiration increases right ventricular filling and causes the pulmonic valve to float open before the rapid early systolic rise of right ventricular pressure, thus attenuating the sound of valve opening (Hultgren et al, 1969). (The hypertrophied and relatively non compliant right ventricle of moderate or severe pulmonic stenosis probably increases the tendency to presystolic opening of the pulmonic valve during inspiration.) With very severe pulmonic stenosis an ejection sound may be absent, either because of immobility of the pulmonic valve, because of presystolic opening due to transmission of a large right atrial 'A' wave to the pulmonary artery, or because the ejection sound comes sufficiently early to merge with the first heart sound. (In general, the ejection sound is earlier the more severe the valvar pulmonic stenosis.) In some patients with a pulmonic ejection sound the first heart sound is not audible at the base and the ejection sound may seem to be the first heart sound. Its high pitch and respiratory variation should identify it.

Aortic

Aortic ejection sounds may be valvar or originate in a dilated aortic root. An aortic ejection sound is usually as loud at the apex as at the high right sternal border and does not vary with respiration.

An ejection sound is present in virtually all children with valvar aortic stenosis and is a very useful diagnostic finding, since it does not occur with sub or supravalvar obstruction unless there is valvar involvement as well. As with valvar pulmonic stenosis, the ejection sound of aortic stenosis occurs as the valve domes in early systole and is the audible counterpart of an anacrotic notch on the aortic root pressure tracing (Shaver et al, 1975b). The ejection sound occurs simultaneously with maximal opening of the valve cusps on echocardiogram (Fig 3.21). Probably the most common etiology of an aortic ejection sound is a bicuspid aortic valve, and here the mechanism is the same as with valvar aortic stenosis. An aortic 'root' click coincides with the beginning of aortic pressure rise. It can be heard in some patients with a dilated ascending aorta and also in some individuals with unusually forceful left ventricular ejection (Shaver et al, 1975b).

An aortic ejection sound is not nearly as high pitched as a pulmonic one and may closely resemble a component of the first heart sound. In fact, it may be quite difficult to differentiate a first heart sound-aortic ejection sound sequence from a split first heart sound 'at the bedside'. An aortic ejection sound does tend to occur slightly later than a separate tricuspid valve closure sound but there is some overlap. The location of a 'split first sound' may help in the differential; a first heart sound which is 'split' only at the apex and not at the low left sternal border is suspect and is usually really a first sound-aortic ejection sound sequence. A high right sternal border systolic ejection murmur also argues for an aortic valve abnormality and is indirect evidence that the second component of a 'split first sound' is really an ejection sound.

Systolic clicks

Mid systolic clicks may be single or multiple and may be 'isolated' or introduce the late systolic murmur of a 'billowing' or 'floppy' mitral valve (Barlow et al, 1963) (Fig. 15.4). Both click and murmur are often intermittent and both timing and intensity may be manipulated by squatting and standing or by the Valsalva maneuver (Ch. 15).

Opening snaps

An opening snap is generated by the opening of an atrioventricular valve. It occurs as the leaflets reach the limit of their motion (Tavel, 1975) and is the atrioventricular valve equivalent of a semilunar valve early systolic ejection sound. An opening snap is most commonly due to mitral stenosis and is a very uncommon auscultatory finding in childhood, just as mitral stenosis is uncommon. The opening snap of mitral stenosis is high pitched and of short duration and is usually maximal at the low left sternal border and toward the apex (Fig. 14.1). The timing of an opening snap does not vary with respiration but is influenced by the severity of the mitral stenosis. A short aortic closure sound-opening snap interval is a sign of more severe mitral stenosis, since the greater the mitral obstruction the higher the left atrial pressure and therefore the earlier the valve opening in diastole. (This

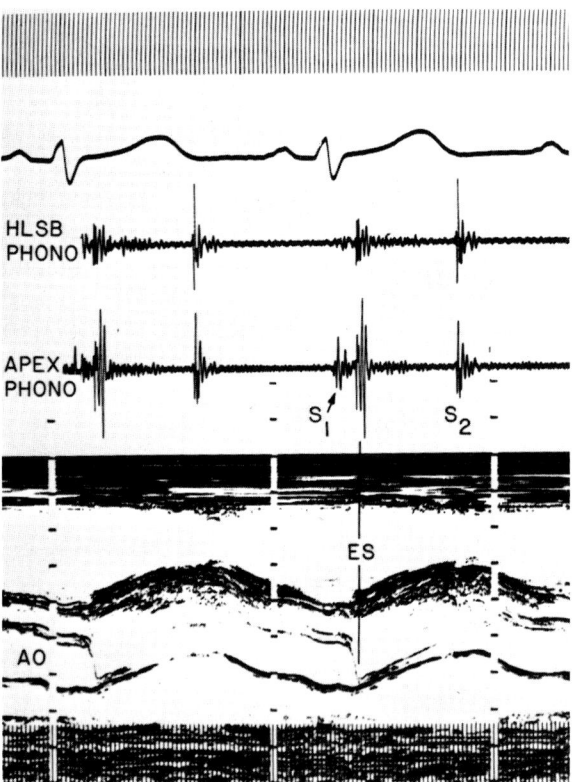

Fig. 3.21 Child with valvar aortic stenosis. The prominent ejection sound (ES) is coincident with maximal opening of the aortic cusp on the echocardiogram.

interval is also influenced by cardiac output, however, since the mitral gradient and left atrial pressure are output dependent.) An opening snap is not usually present if obstruction is mild or if the mitral leaflets are heavily scarred or calcified and therefore relatively immobile. An opening snap may be differentiated from the second component of a widely split second heart sound by its high pitch, lack of respiratory variation and maximal intensity well away from the 'pulmonic' area. Opening snaps of tricuspid origin have been reported but are very difficult to differentiate from mitral snaps (Tavel, 1975). They are exceedingly rare in childhood (Fig. 16.8).

MURMURS

Murmurs result from disturbances of laminar flow; whether turbulence (Sabbah & Stein, 1976) or some more ordered flow pattern such as the 'shedding of vortices' (Bruns, 1959) has been debated. For the sake of simplicity, in this text the term 'turbulence' will be used to describe any departure from laminar flow. Turbulence is related both to the geometry of the containing vessel or chamber and to the velocity of blood flow. Velocity, in turn, is determined by the resultant of ventricular contraction, which propels the blood, and impedance, the sum total of the forces which oppose flow. These opposing forces include resistance (viscosity plus characteristics of the peripheral vascular bed), inertia (the tendency of any mass to remain in its current state of rest or motion), and capacitance (distensibility of containing walls) (Murgo et al, 1975).

The interaction of velocity and the geometry of the structures in which flow occurs determines the presence of a gradient, and a murmur occurs only when a gradient exists. It must be emphasized that 'gradient' refers not to a peak systolic or diastolic gradient, but to an instantaneous one. For example, flow across a normal aortic or pulmonic valve results in an early systolic gradient which may produce a corresponding early systolic murmur, even though peak pressure may be equal in the ventricle and the great artery. (Both gradient and murmur can be demonstrated with high fidelity catheters positioned in the aorta and left ventricle or the pulmonary artery and right ventricle.) The early systolic gradient tends to be somewhat larger across the pulmonic than the aortic valve and a systolic murmur can regularly be recorded in the main pulmonary artery of children, even if they have no right heart abnormality. This particular murmur is very commonly audible externally at the high left sternal border and is one of the commonest 'innocent' murmurs.

In a normal individual, the early systolic gradient is related to the rate of change of velocity (acceleration) of blood in the arterial root. High velocity and acceleration result in a larger gradient and a louder murmur (Murgo et al, 1975). Increased early systolic velocity and acceleration occur with exercise, fever, thyrotoxicosis and other high output states and explain the systolic murmur heard in these conditions. A murmur which is produced in an abnormal heart is also related to a gradient, whether due to an obstructive lesion, to a restrictive septal defect or to valvar regurgitation.

Loudness

Murmurs are traditionally described in terms of loudness, timing, location, pitch, shape and quality. There are several determinants of the loudness of a murmur, including gradient, volume of flow, and distance from source to stethoscope. The relationship of gradient to velocity and geometry has already been discussed, and in general the loudness of a murmur varies with the gradient, which in turn varies with velocity of flow. For example, an increase in myocardial contractility increases the velocity of flow into the aorta or pulmonary artery in early systole and produces or accentuates a murmur, even though stroke volume may not change. As another example, with a very large ventricular septal defect there is little or no gradient between the left and right ventricle. Velocity of flow is relatively slow through such a defect and a systolic murmur is soft or absent. With a restrictive ventricular septal defect, on the other hand, a gradient exists between the left and right ventricle. Velocity of flow is high and the murmur is therefore loud.

Quite apart from velocity, volume of flow may be an important determinant of the loudness of a murmur under certain circumstances. A tiny ventricular septal defect, for instance, produces a softer murmur than a larger but still restrictive one, even though the gradient and, presumably, the velocity of flow across the defects may be similar. With the tiny ventricular septal defect, however, the volume of flow is so small that the resulting murmur is soft.

The presence or absence of a thrill should always be noted in any patient with a loud murmur. A thrill should be felt for with the portion of the palm immediately proximal to the forefinger and middle finger, as this area seems to be quite sensitive. The finger tips should be avoided, since there is a tendency to mistake heart sounds for thrills when they are used.

A murmur must always be louder at its source than at the stethoscope head, and attenuation is related both to the distance between source and sampling site and to the characteristics of the intervening structures. Thus, the murmur of pulmonic stenosis tends to be much softer in a patient with transposition of the great arteries than in one with normally related great arteries, simply because the pulmonic valve is located far posteriorly in the former and very close to the chest wall in the latter. Although sound transmits well through both air and fluid, attenuation is much greater across air-fluid interfaces. The classic auscultatory areas (to be described below) are areas where cardiac sound is relatively well heard, at least in part because there is little or no lung between heart and thoracic wall.

In an individual patient the loudness of a murmur may vary with the phase of respiration. Murmurs which arise in the right heart, such as the murmurs of pulmonic or tricuspid stenosis or of pulmonic or tricuspid regurgitation, should theoretically increase with the increased venous return of inspiration. Tricuspid murmurs commonly do show the expected variation, but pulmonic murmurs usually do not. Even an unequivocal increase in loudness of a murmur at a given point on the chest wall does not necessarily mean an increased intensity *at the source*. For example, the murmur of subvalvar pulmonic stenosis may be well heard at the low left sternal border and may increase in intensity *at that area* during inspiration. Unless it is recognized that there is a reciprocal decrease in intensity at the mid left sternal border, caused by a change in position of the heart with respect to the chest wall, the murmur may be thought to represent tricuspid regurgitation (Fig. 16.4).

Murmurs arising in the left heart might be expected to decrease during inspiration because of the slight decrease in flow and/or pressure in the left heart during this phase of respiration. Any such decrease in loudness, however, is more likely related to the attenuating effect of increased lung volume. In practice, respiratory change in intensity of murmurs arising in the left heart is rarely diagnostically useful.

The loudness of some murmurs may also change with altered positioning of the patient. The murmur of aortic regurgitation tends to be louder with the patient sitting forward with the breath held in expiration, for example, while the murmur of pulmonic regurgitation (at least the variety with normal pulmonary artery pressure) is louder in the recumbent than the sitting position. The murmur of aortic regurgitation is also regularly accentuated by squatting and attenuated by sudden standing. The murmur of a tiny muscular ventricular septal defect may also increase with squatting and decrease or disappear with sudden standing or with the strain phase of a Valsalva maneuver (Fig. 5.7), as the decreased return to the left ventricle causes a decrease in left ventricular end diastolic volume and a corresponding thickening of the septum, functionally closing the defect. The murmur of hypertrophic subaortic stenosis behaves quite differently, increasing with standing and decreasing with squatting, as the left ventricular volume increases and obstruction decreases. Although, as in the above examples, a positional change in the intensity of a murmur may be helpful in differential diagnosis, it is not often useful in labeling a murmur as functional.

The most commonly used scale of loudness of murmurs includes six grades of increasing intensity. A Grade I murmur is one that is not immediately apparent when auscultation is begun, while a Grade II murmur is quite soft but immediately audible. At the other end of the scale, a Grade VI murmur can be heard with the stethoscope held away from the chest wall and a Grade V murmur can be heard with just the edge of the tilted stethoscope head in contact with the skin. Grade III and IV murmurs are intermediate and are difficult to precisely define. Some use the presence of a thrill as the important differential point, a loud murmur without a thrill being Grade III and a loud murmur with a thrill being Grade IV. The presence of a thrill is probably not determined solely by the loudness of a murmur, however. What seems to an experienced observer to be a Grade IV murmur on the basis of its *loudness* may occasionally not have an associated thrill. Conversely, a thrill may be present with a murmur that would otherwise be labeled Grade III. It must be admitted that there is considerable inter-observer and even intra-observer variation in murmur grading, particularly with regard to Grade III and IV murmurs.

Location

In localizing a murmur, both the area of maximal intensity and direction of radiation, if any, must be noted. The classical auscultatory areas include the high right sternal border, the high, mid and low left sternal border, and the apex. The high right and high left sternal border areas are sometimes referred to as the 'aortic' and 'pulmonic' areas, respectively, but these appelations are to be avoided when dealing with congenital heart disease, since they may have no bearing on what anatomic structures underlie these areas. In tetralogy of Fallot or transposition of the great arteries, for instance, the second sound in the 'pulmonic' area is really the aortic valve closure sound. Although auscultation is most frequently productive over the classic areas, heart sounds and murmurs are occasionally well or even better heard elsewhere, including the lower right sternal border, the subclavicular areas, the neck, axillae and posterior thorax.

Pitch

Murmurs are vibrations with a considerable range in frequency, and pitch is the observer's perception of frequency. High frequency murmurs are often described as 'blowing' and are usually generated by structural anomalies associated with a large gradient and high velocity but a relatively low volume flow. Common examples include a tiny ventricular septal defect and mitral and aortic regurgitation. In each case, flow is from a high pressure area to a low pressure one; the left ventricle to the left atrium with mitral regurgitation, and the aorta to the left ventricle with aortic regurgitation. (With very severe acute mitral or aortic regurgitation there is much less gradient and the murmur is not so high pitched.) Lower frequency murmurs are commonly described as being 'harsh' or 'rough' and they most commonly arise from obstruction to right or left ventricular outflow or from a restrictive ventricular septal defect. A very low frequency murmur is often called a 'rumble', an example being the murmur of mitral stenosis.

Timing

Murmurs are either systolic, diastolic or continuous. (By convention, the latter term describes a murmur which extends through the second heart sound into diastole; it may or may not occupy the whole of the cardiac cycle.)

Systolic

Systolic murmurs can be further characterized as being early, mid, late or holosystolic (pansystolic) (Fig. 3.22). Early or mid systolic murmurs usually arise from obstruction to ventricular outflow or are innocent and unrelated to abnormal cardiac anatomy. Late systolic murmurs are most commonly due to a prolapsing mitral valve, while holosystolic murmurs usually arise from mitral or tricuspid regurgitation or from a restrictive ventricular septal defect.

Diastolic

Diastolic murmurs may also be early, mid, late or pandiastolic (Fig. 3.23). Early diastolic murmurs usually indicate semilunar valve regurgitation; mid diastolic murmurs are most commonly due to relative mitral or tricuspid stenosis; and late diastolic murmurs are usually the result of organic mitral stenosis. Pandiastolic murmurs occasionally occur with atrioventricular valve stenosis or with semilunar valve regurgitation.

32 CLINICAL DIAGNOSIS IN PEDIATRIC CARDIOLOGY

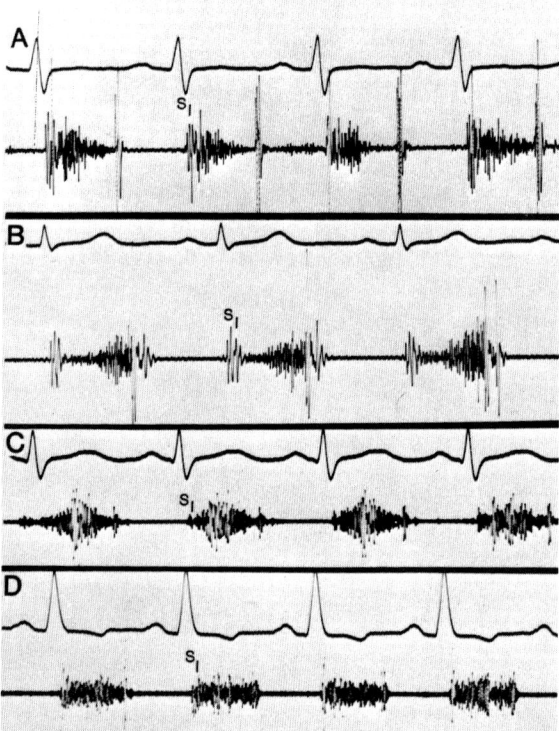

Fig. 3.22 Timing and shape of systolic murmurs.
A. Decrescendo early systolic murmur in a child with a ventricular septal defect and pulmonary hypertension.
B. Crescendo late systolic murmur in a child with a defect in an aneurysm of the membranous interventricular septum.
C. Crescendo-decrescendo murmur in an infant with pulmonic stenosis. D. Pansystolic plateau shaped murmur in a child with tricuspid atresia and a restrictive interventricular septal defect.

Continuous

Continuous murmurs most commonly occur when an artery, usually the aorta or a systemic artery, communicates with a lower pressure artery, vein, or cardiac chamber. Examples of these categories include a patent ductus arteriosus, systemic arteriovenous fistula, and a coronary-cardiac fistula, respectively.

Shape

Murmurs are also described by their shape or configuration. A commonly used classification refers to systolic murmurs as being of either 'ejection' or 'regurgitant' type. Ejection systolic murmurs do not extend entirely throughout systole and are crescendo-decrescendo. Further, the term implies origin at a semilunar valve or at another site of obstruction. The term 'regurgitant' implies backward flow across an atrioventricular valve or from the left ventricle to the lower pressure right ventricle. Regurgitant murmurs extend through systole and are usually of level intensity throughout their duration. It is probably preferable to simply describe murmurs as being plateau, crescendo, decrescendo, or crescendo-decrescendo, as they sound (Fig. 3.22), rather than to use terms such as 'ejection' or 'regurgitant' which imply origin or function. Although it is true that systolic murmurs generated by obstruction are usually crescendo-decrescendo and of 'ejection' type and that murmurs of atrioventricular valve regurgitation or of

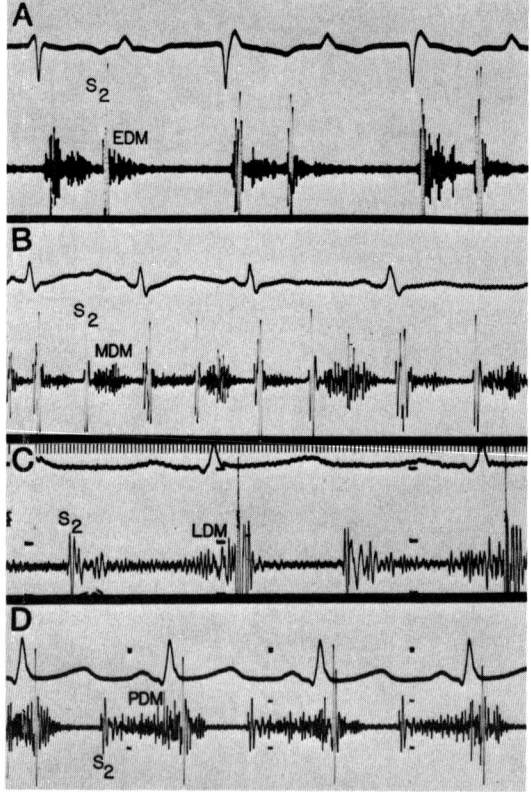

Fig. 3.23 Timing of diastolic murmurs. A. Decrescendo early diastolic murmur (EDM) in a child with pulmonary hypertension and pulmonic regurgitation. B. Crescendo-decrescendo mid diastolic murmur (MDM) in a child with 'normotensive' pulmonary regurgitation. C. Late diastolic murmur (LDM) in a child with mild mitral stenosis.
D. Pandiastolic murmur (PDM) in an infant with severe congenital mitral stenosis.

a ventricular septal defect are usually holosystolic and plateau and therefore of 'regurgitant' type, there are frequent exceptions to this general rule. Pulmonic stenosis may produce a murmur which is plateau and holosystolic (at least in terms of extending from the first heart sound to the only audible component of the second heart sound) and which, in itself, is indistinguishable from the murmur of a small ventricular septal defect. On the other hand, the murmur of a ventricular septal defect may be less than holosystolic and may be crescendo-decrescendo, mimicking the usual murmur of pulmonic stenosis.

It should be pointed out that it may be very difficult to accurately describe the exact timing and shape of a murmur if the heart rate is very rapid. One may hear murmurs described as being 'diamond-shaped and extending two-thirds of the way through systole' in a fussy infant with a cardiac rate of 170, but this much detail under such circumstances borders on glibness. One may be fortunate to be able to decide whether a murmur is systolic or diastolic, and it is important to recognize the limits of auscultation. It is in the timing of murmurs and sounds that phonocardiography has its most important clinical application.

Quality

'Quality' is another term used to describe murmurs. The 'twanging string' innocent murmur, the 'machinery' murmur of a patent ductus, the 'cooing dove' murmur of one variety of aortic regurgitation and the 'groaning' or 'honking' murmur heard in some cases with a prolapsing mitral leaflet are examples of descriptions of a murmur's quality. The quality of a murmur may be quite distinctive and be very useful in diagnosis.

REFERENCES

Barlow J B, Pocock W A, Marchand P, Denny M 1963 The significance of late systolic murmurs. American Heart Journal 66: 443

Bruns D L 1959 A general theory of the causes of murmurs in the cardiovascular system. American Journal of Medicine 27: 360

Criley J M, Chambers R D, Blaufuss A H, Freidman N J 1975 Mitral Stenosis. Mechanico-acoustical events. Physiologic principles of heart sounds and murmurs. American Heart Association Monograph No. 46. American Heart Association, New York, p 149

Curtiss E I, Shaver J A, Reddy P S, O'Toole J D 1975 Newer concepts in physiologic splitting of the second heart sound. Physiologic principles of heart sounds and murmurs. American Heart Association Monograph No. 46. American Heart Association, New York, p 68

Fontana M E, Wooley C F 1972 Sail sound in Ebstein's anomaly of the tricuspid valve. Circulation 46: 155

Hope J 1846 A treatise on the diseases of the heart and great vessels. Lea & Blanchard, Philadelphia, p 52

Hultgren H N, Reeve R, Cohn K, McLeod R 1969 The ejection click of valvular pulmonic stenosis. Circulation 40:631

Murgo J P, Altobelli S A, Dorethy J F, Logsdon J R, McGranahan G M 1975 Normal ventricular ejection dynamics in man during rest and exercise. Physiologic principles of heart sounds and murmurs. American Heart Association Monograph No. 46. American Heart Association, New York, p 92

Reddy P S, Leon D F, Krishnaswami V, O'Toole J D, Salerni R, Shaver J A 1975 Syndrome of acute aortic regurgitation. Physiologic principles of heart sounds and murmurs. American Heart Association Monograph No. 46. American Heart Association, New York, p 166

Rushmer R F 1961 Cardiovascular dynamics, 2nd edn. Saunders, Philadelphia, p 310

Sabbah H N, Stein P D 1976 Turbulent blood flow in humans: its primary role in the production of ejection murmurs. Circulation Research 38: 513

Sakamoto T, Kusukawa R, MacCanon D M, Luisada A A 1966 First heart sound amplitude in experimentally induced alternans. Diseases of the Chest 50:470

Shah P M, Jackson D 1975 Third heart sound and summation gallop. Physiologic principles of heart sounds and murmurs. American Heart Association Monograph No. 46. American Heart Association, New York p 79

Shaver J A, O'Toole J D, Curtiss E I, Thompson M E, Reddy P S, Leon D F 1975a Second heart sound: the role of altered greater and lesser circulation. Physiologic principles of heart sounds and murmurs. American Heart Association Monograph No. 46. American Heart Association, New York, p 58

Shaver J A, Griff F W, Leonard J J 1975b Ejection sounds of left-sided origin. Physiologic principles of heart sounds and murmurs. American Heart Association Monograph No. 46. American Heart Association, New York, p 27

Tavel M 1975 Opening snaps: mitral and tricuspid. Physiologic principles of heart sounds and murmurs. American Heart Association Monograph No. 46. American Heart Association, New York, p 85

Tavel M 1978a Clinical phonocardiography and external pulse recordings, 3rd edn. Year Book Medical Publishers, Chicago, p 39

Tavel M 1978b Clinical phonocardiography and external pulse recordings, 3rd edn. Year Book Medical Publishers, Chicago, p 120

Thompson M E, Shaver J A, Leon D F, Reddy P S, Leonard J J 1975 Pathodynamics of the first heart sound. Physiologic principles of heart sounds and murmurs. American Heart Association Monograph No. 46. American Heart Association, New York, p 8

Zuberbuhler J R, Bauersfeld S R 1965 Paradoxical splitting of the second heart sound in the Wolff-Parkinson-White Syndrome. American Heart Journal 70: 595

4

Interatrial septal defect

The anomaly

An interatrial communication, the foramen ovale, is a normal and necessary feature of the fetal circulation and permits passage of blood from right to left atrium. Shortly after birth left atrial pressure rises above right atrial and pushes the flap of the foramen against the interatrial septum, closing the aperture. In some individuals the foramen remains probe patent although functionally closed. An actual interatrial septal defect is less common than a probe patent foramen ovale but is one of the more common varieties of congenital heart disease.

Interatrial defects may occur in various locations in the septum. Those in the general area of the fossa ovalis are known as ostium secundum defects, while those located high in the septum near the entrance of the superior vena cava are referred to as sinus venosus defects. The latter are usually accompanied by partial anomalous pulmonary venous return but are clinically indistinguishable from the more common secundum defects. An ostium primum defect (partial endocardial cushion defect, incomplete atrioventricular canal) is another variety of interatrial septal defect, and one which may have associated mitral regurgitation. In fact, an apical pansystolic murmur of mitral regurgitation occurring in association with the physical findings of an interatrial septal defect is highly suggestive of the ostium primum variety (Ch. 7). It must be noted that the anatomic location of the atrial septal defect does not influence physical findings, since none of them originate at the defect itself.

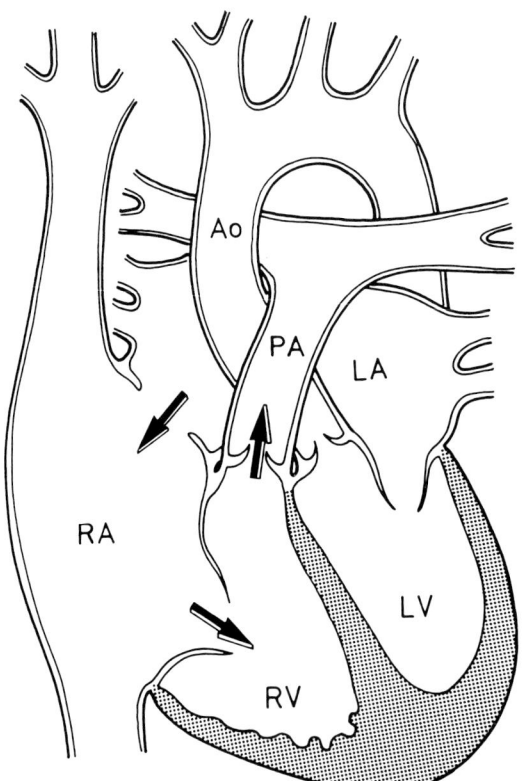

Fig. 4.1 Diagram of interatrial septal defect. There is increased flow across the tricuspid and pulmonic valves but not across the mitral or aortic valves.

Clinical course

The major direct hemodynamic consequence of an uncomplicated interatrial septal defect is an increased volume of blood flow through the right heart and pulmonary vascular bed (Fig. 4.1). Unlike large communications at ventricular or great artery level, an interatrial septal defect does not retard the rapid fall in pulmonary vascular resistance which normally occurs shortly after birth. As a consequence, right ventricular pressure is normal in almost all young individuals with this anomaly. Since the right ventricle is able to tolerate a pure volume overload for many years before showing evidence of dysfunction (Rushmer, 1958), most children and young adults with an atrial defect are without symptoms. In unoperated individuals symptoms and disability become increasingly more common beyond age 40 years (Campbell, 1970).

Physical findings

General

An atrial septal defect is usually first suspected because of abnormal physical findings, although such findings are more subtle than those associated with other common congenital cardiac anomalies — so subtle that the diagnosis is often missed in childhood. Children with an uncomplicated interatrial septal defect are not cyanotic and have normal arterial and jugular venous pulses and normal blood pressure. Although patients with this anomaly tend to be slender, there are no characteristic findings on general examination. The signs which do occur are related to an increased velocity of blood flow through the right heart and pulmonary artery and to a large right ventricular stroke volume. The latter imparts a poorly sustained outward movement to the left parasternal area and, in older children and young adults, there may be a precordial bulge. The most characteristic findings, however, are auscultatory.

Auscultation

Murmurs. The first clue to the presence of an interatrial septal defect is usually a high left sternal border systolic murmur. The murmur is generated by high velocity flow across the pulmonic valve, the interatrial defect itself being 'silent'. The murmur is crescendo-decrescendo and is soft unless there is associated pulmonic stenosis. There is nothing about this murmur to distinguish it from the functional murmur heard at the same area, or from the high left sternal border systolic murmur heard in some patients with coarctation of the aorta, or from the murmur of very mild pulmonic stenosis or of idiopathic dilatation of the pulmonary artery. The accompanying auscultatory findings, however, are distinctive. One of the most important is a short soft medium pitched diastolic murmur at the low left sternal border. This murmur is generated by rapid flow across the tricuspid valve and can be recorded in the right ventricular inflow area using a micromanometer tipped catheter (Fig. 4.2). The murmur is mid

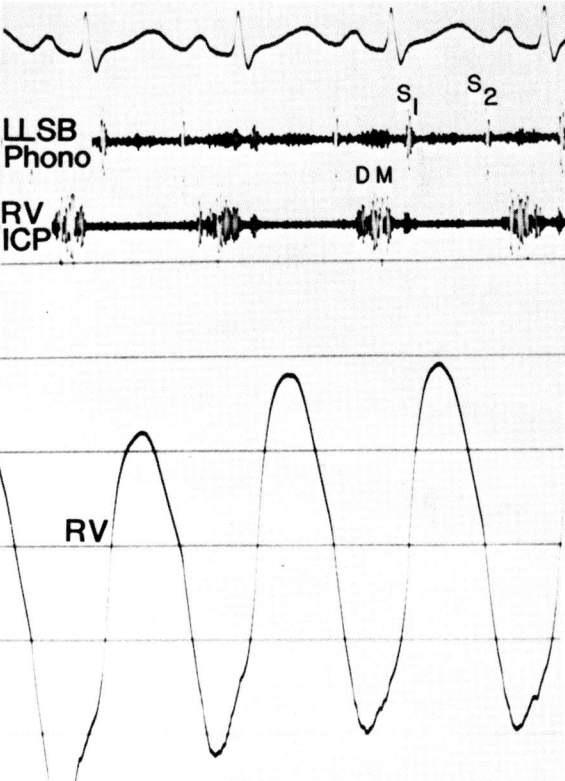

Fig. 4.2 Child with an interatrial septal defect. A prominent mid diastolic murmur (DM) is shown in a low left sternal border phonocardiogram (LLSB Phono) and on an intracardiac phonocardiogram recorded in the right ventricular inflow area (RVI ICP). Right ventricular pressure was recorded simultaneously using a micromanometer tipped catheter.

diastolic, beginning well after the second heart sound. It is often referred to as a 'rumble', but the term is a misnomer; the murmur does not resemble the apical rumble of mitral stenosis — it is not so low pitched — and is perhaps better described as a 'puff' or as being 'scratchy'. The murmur of relative tricuspid stenosis is a useful sign when present, since it indicates a pulmonary to systemic flow ratio of at least 2:1 and is therefore a useful marker for potential candidates for corrective surgery. It must be emphasized that this murmur is almost always subtle and will be missed unless specifically listened for. In patients with an atrial defect and large pulmonary blood flow, a soft systolic ejection murmur is present in the axillae and across the back. It is generated by high velocity flow in the pulmonary arteries.

A continuous murmur is occasionally generated at an atrial septal defect, but only if left atrial pressure is very high and the interatrial defect is restrictive, the combination permitting a pressure gradient between right and left atrium throughout the cardiac cycle. This murmur is heard at the mid or low right or left sternal border and has been described in patients with a small interatrial defect and either mitral atresia (Zuberbuhler et al, 1975) or severe mitral stenosis (Ross et al, 1963). It is occasionally quite loud and accompanied by a continuous thrill.

Heart sounds. Perhaps the most characteristic physical finding of an interatrial septal defect is fixed splitting of the second heart sound (Fig. 4.3). Several explanations for this phenomenon have been offered. First, right ventricular stroke volume may already be maximal and not augmentable by an inspiratory increase in systemic venous return. According to this hypothesis right ventricular ejection time does not increase during inspiration and, consequently, the timing of the pulmonic closure sound is not altered by the phase of respiration. Since the width of split does not correlate closely with the size of the left to right shunt this explanation does not seem tenable (Rees et al, 1972). Alternatively, right ventricular stroke volume might be constant throughout the respiratory cycle, increased inspiratory systemic venous return being counterbalanced by a correspondingly decreased pulmonary venous return and consequent decreased flow across the interatrial septal defect. The total return to the right atrium (and to the right ventricle) would thus be similar during inspiration and expiration and right ventricular stroke volume would remain constant, as would the timing of the pulmonic closure sound (Aygen & Braunwald, 1962). Since pulmonary venous return is known to decrease with inspiration this counterbalancing of venous returns may well play a role in fixed splitting. It does not, however, explain the fixed split which sometimes persists for a few days after surgical closure of an interatrial septal defect (Adolph & Fowler, 1970), nor does it explain persistence of fixed splitting during the temporary occlusion of an interatrial defect with

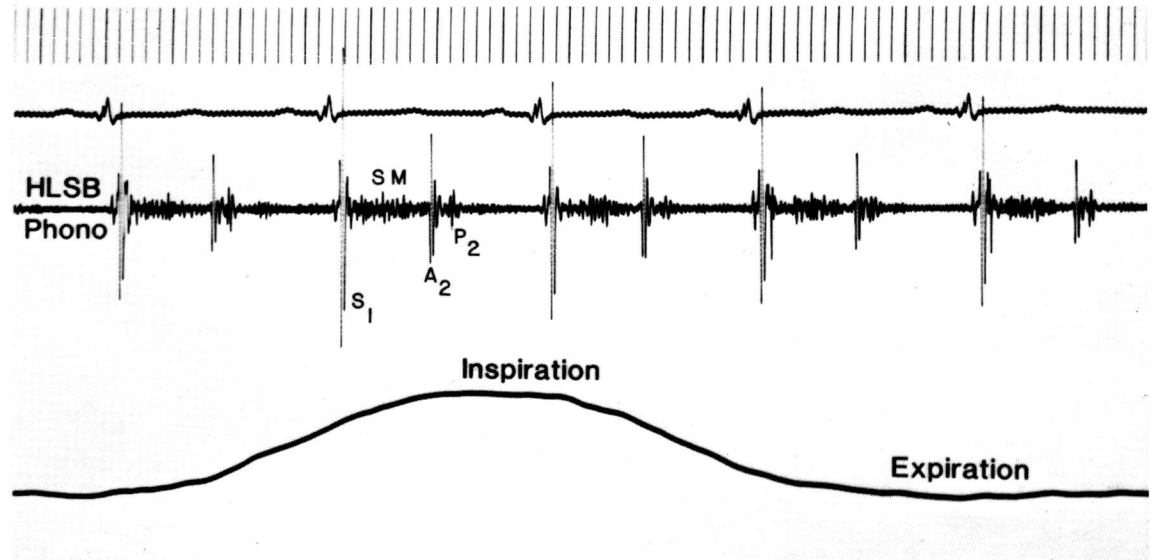

Fig. 4.3 Child with interatrial septal defect. The high left sternal border phonocardiogram shows a systolic murmur and prominent splitting of the second heart sound. The split does not vary with respiration.

a balloon catheter (Zuberbuhler, 1970). A third explanation of fixed splitting involves altered impedance. Shaver et al (1975) have shown that the down stroke of the pulmonary artery pressure curve does not track right ventricular pressure if both are recorded by high fidelity micromanometer tipped catheters. The pulmonary incisura 'hangs out' beyond the right ventricular pressure trace, especially when the pulmonary arterial tree is voluminous and pulmonary artery pressure is normal (in other words, when impedance is low). This 'hang-out' interval closely approximates the interval between aortic and pulmonary closure sounds in patients with an interatrial septal defect (Fig. 4.4). Under some circumstances, at least, wide or fixed splitting seems to be largely a function of impedance and is not due to a prolongation of right ventricular mechanical systole.

The first heart sound is often loud at the low left sternal border in patients with an atrial septal defect. This is probably due to an augmentation of the tricuspid component and may be related to prolongation of rapid tricuspid flow into late diastole, with consequent rapid leaflet closure during the more steeply rising portion of the right ventricular pressure curve.

Pulmonary hypertension

Pulmonary hypertension changes the clinical picture of an interatrial septal defect in several respects. The right ventricular impulse becomes more forceful and sustained and increased pressure in an enlarged pulmonary artery may produce a systolic impulse at the high left sternal border.

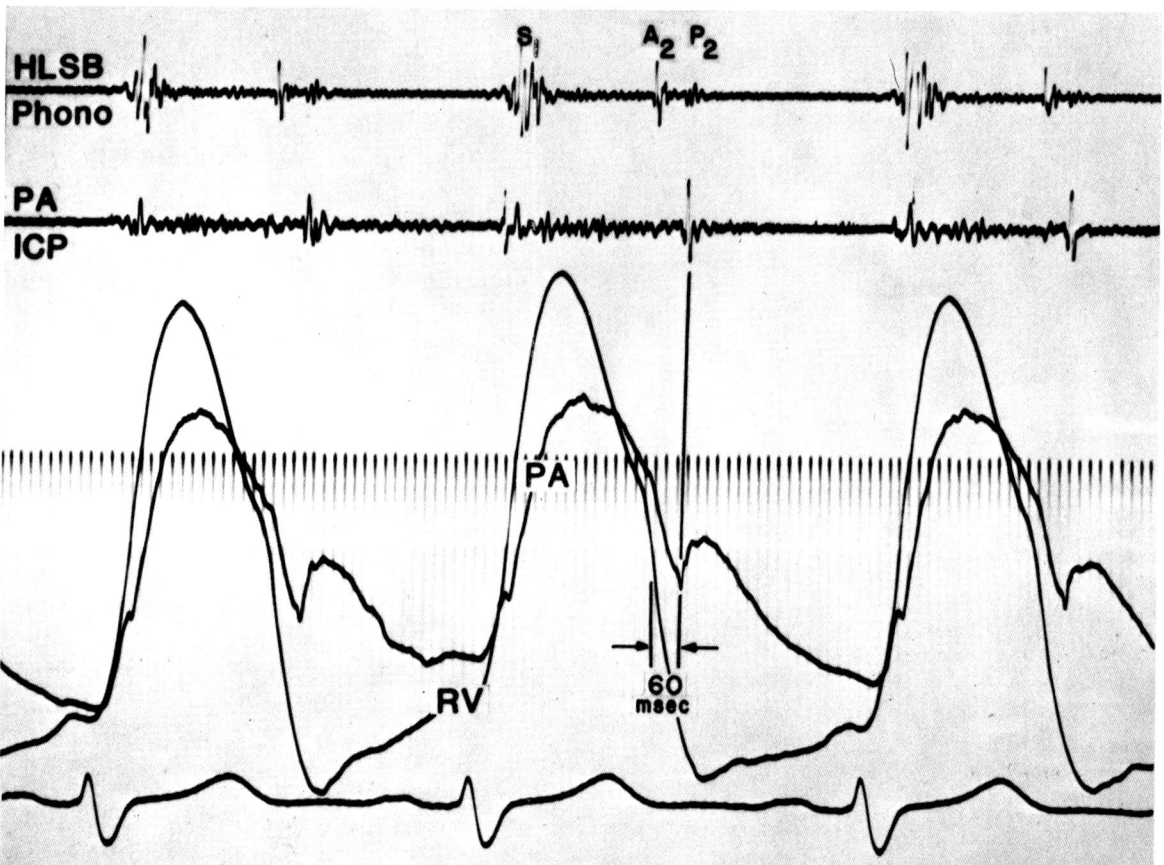

Fig. 4.4 High fidelity pressure recordings in the right ventricle and pulmonary artery of an adolescent with an interatrial septal defect. The pulmonary artery pressure is delayed and the incisura 'hangs out' beyond the descending limb of the right ventricular pressure tracing.

Right ventricular overload may also lead to tricuspid regurgitation, signaled by a high pitched systolic murmur at the low left sternal border. Pulmonary hypertension increases the loudness of the pulmonic component of the second heart sound and splitting is more likely to exist when advanced pulmonary vascular disease occurs in association with an interatrial septal defect than with a ventricular septal defect or patent ductus arteriosus.

Associated anomalies

Associated cardiovascular abnormalities may greatly influence the physical findings and the clinical course of an individual with an atrial septal defect. Any left heart abnormality which tends to impede left atrial emptying through the mitral valve will increase the magnitude of left to right shunting across the atrial septum. For example, coarctation of the aorta, aortic stenosis, or myocardial disease may raise left ventricular diastolic pressure and thereby induce massive left to right shunting at atrial level. The resulting increase in pulmonary blood flow may raise pulmonary artery pressure and thus subject the right ventricle to both a pressure and volume overload. Under these circumstances poor somatic growth and even congestive heart failure may occur in early infancy. Mitral stenosis or mitral regurgitation have similar hemodynamic consequences in patients with an atrial septal defect. (In an occasional infant symptoms occur early, even in the absence of left heart abnormalities.) In older patients the onset of left ventricular dysfunction, usually a result of coronary artery disease or hypertensive cardiovascular disease, increases the magnitude of shunting through a previously well tolerated interatrial septal defect and may result in decreased exercise tolerance or frank congestive heart failure.

Summary

An atrial septal defect is the congenital cardiac lesion which is most likely to be newly diagnosed during adult life. This delay in diagnosis is a testimonial to the subtlety of the physical findings and to the lateness of the onset of symptoms in patients with this anomaly. Although the high left sternal border systolic murmur is soft and differs in no way from a systolic murmur that may be heard in perfectly normal children, the presence of such a murmur should always lead to a careful evaluation of splitting of the second heart sound. If the second heart sound is fixedly split or persistently split during expiration, one should specifically listen for the soft mid-diastolic murmur of relative tricuspid stenosis. If the triad of a high left sternal border systolic murmur, fixed splitting of the second heart sound and a low left sternal border mid-diastolic murmur are present, there is little doubt that an interatrial septal defect exists and that there is significant left to right shunting.

REFERENCES

Adolph R J, Fowler N O 1970 The second heart sound: a screening test for heart disease. Modern Concepts of Cardiovascular Disease 39:91

Aygen M M, Braunwald E 1962 The splitting of the second heart sound in normal subjects and in patients with congenital heart disease. Circulation 25:328

Campbell M 1970 Natural history of atrial septal defect. British Heart Journal 32:820

Rees A, Farru O, Rodriquez R 1972 Phonocardiographic, radiological and haemodynamic correlation in atrial septal defect. British Heart Journal 34:781

Ross J, Braunwald E, Mason D T, Braunwald N S, Morrow A G 1963 Interatrial communication and left atrial hypertension: a cause of continuous murmur. Circulation 28:853

Rushmer R F 1958 Work of the heart. Modern Concepts of Cardiovascular Disease 27:473

Shaver J A, O'Toole J D, Curtiss E I, Thompson M E, Reddy P S, Leon D F 1975 Second heart sound: the role of altered greater and lesser circulation. Physiologic principles of heart sounds and murmurs. American Heart Association Monograph 46. The American Heart Association, New York, p 58

Zuberbuhler J R 1970 Unpublished data

Zuberbuhler J R, Lenox C C, Park S C, Neches W H 1975 Continuous murmurs in the newborn. Physiologic principles of heart sounds and murmurs. American Heart Association Monograph 46. The American Heart Association, New York; p 209

5

Ventricular septal defect

Clinical course

In our clinic, a ventricular septal defect is the most commonly diagnosed congenital cardiac anomaly. Prominent physical findings, most notably a loud systolic murmur, usually lead to recognition in early infancy, but it is important to note that the systolic murmur of a ventricular defect is not present at birth in the full term infant. The defect remains silent until pulmonary vascular resistance falls some time after birth and permits the development of the interventricular pressure gradient which is necessary for the generation of a murmur. The timing of the fall in resistance varies with the size of the defect. In the normal newborn, pulmonary vascular resistance and right ventricular and pulmonary arterial pressures fall soon after birth. A similar rapid fall occurs in the newborn with a small ventricular septal defect, and although the murmur is usually absent in the delivery room, it often appears before discharge from the newborn nursery. If the ventricular defect is large and unrestrictive, right ventricular pressure cannot fall appreciably below left ventricular pressure. The persistently high pressure in the pulmonary artery delays the fall in pulmonary vascular resistance (Rudolph, 1965). In a newborn with a large ventricular septal defect the murmur usually is not heard until the first office visit following discharge from the nursery.

Symptoms do not occur in an individual with a small defect and no therapy is necessary. Even when the defect is large there are usually no symptoms during the first month of life. Only when pulmonary vascular resistance falls, usually during the second month of life, does pulmonary blood flow increase substantially and only then may poor feeding, slow weight gain, sweating, tachypnea or frank congestive heart failure appear. The subsequent clinical course of such infants may be one of continuing congestive heart failure. In others failure may improve as the defect becomes smaller, as pulmonic stenosis develops or as pulmonary vascular resistance increases. (In each instance improvement is related to a decreased volume load of the left ventricle.)

Physical findings

General

The general physical appearance of an infant with a ventricular septal defect is normal unless a large left to right shunt has resulted in poor growth. (Weight is usually more severely affected than height.) In general, if a ventricular septal defect is small any abnormal physical findings are related entirely to the jet of blood traversing the defect during systole. With larger defects the manifestations of left and right ventricular overload, of increased flow across the mitral valve (Fig. 5.1), and of pulmonary hypertension are superimposed. There is no cyanosis and the jugular venous pulse is normal in a patient with an uncomplicated ventricular septal defect. Arterial pulses are usually normal but may be 'quick' and poorly sustained if the defect is large and the left to right shunt torrential, since ejection into the aorta is poorly sustained in the face of a large low resistance outlet from the left ventricle. In a patient with large interventricular flow the apical impulse tends to be prominent, since left ventricular stroke volume is increased. The left parasternal impulse is normal unless there is secondary pulmonary hypertension (Fig. 5.4).

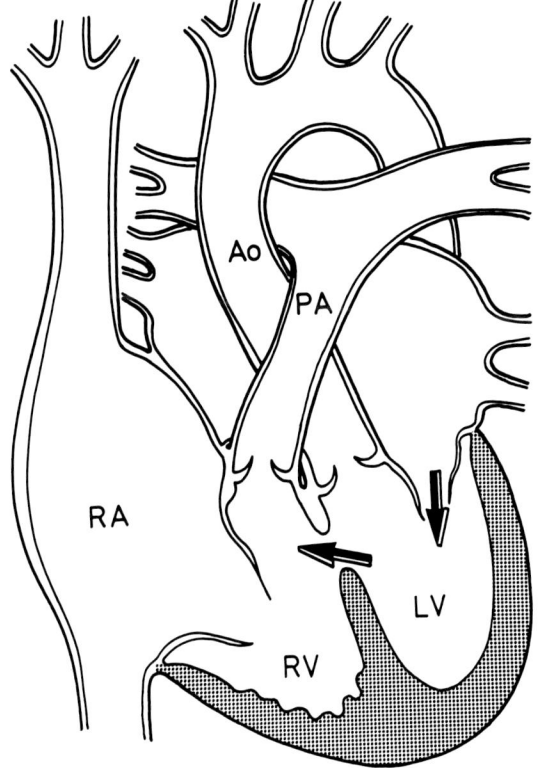

Fig. 5.1 Diagram of an interventricular septal defect. Flow is increased across the mitral valve.

Auscultation

Heart sounds. The second heart sound is usually physiologically split. The split tends to be wide if the left to right shunt is large or if the defect is supracristal (subarterial) (Steinfeld et al, 1972) and to be narrow or single if pulmonary vascular resistance is elevated (Fig. 5.4). A third heart sound is commonly heard and may be difficult to distinguish from a short mid diastolic apical rumble. A fourth heart sound is not heard in a patient with an uncomplicated ventricular septal defect.

Murmurs. A systolic murmur is the most striking physical finding in most patients with a ventricular septal defect. The characteristics of the murmur depend upon pressure and flow relationships, the intensity of the murmur varying directly both with the magnitude of the interventricular pressure gradient and with the volume of flow across the defect. These two variables are interrelated. In general a loud systolic murmur and prominent thrill are present if the defect is small enough to be restrictive, permitting a sizable interventricular pressure gradient to exist, and large enough to allow more than trivial flow. The murmur of such a defect is usually pansystolic and plateau (Fig. 5.2) but may be crescendo, decrescendo, or crescendo-decrescendo (Fig. 5.3).

The murmur of a ventricular septal defect tends to be soft and without an associated thrill at both ends of the spectrum of defect size. With a tiny defect the interventricular gradient is large but flow is very small. The resultant murmur is high pitched and soft and is holosystolic if the defect remains patent throughout systole. The murmur ends before the second sound if the defect closes during the course of ventricular contraction, as it may if it is in the muscular septum (Tavel, 1978). If the defect is very large and unrestrictive a soft systolic murmur is usually present, even though right and left ventricular peak systolic pressures are equal. In this situation, the murmur is early systolic, since the more rapid left than right ventricular pressure rise causes an early systolic gradient.

The systolic murmur generated at a ventricular septal defect is well heard in the back only if it is loud anteriorly. With large defects rapid flow

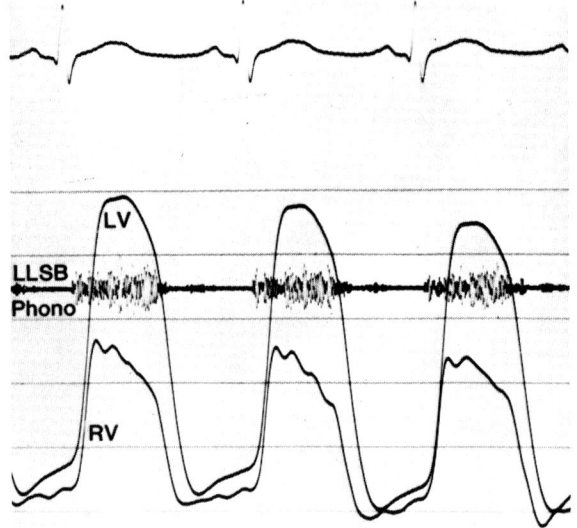

Fig. 5.2 Pansystolic plateau shaped murmur in a child with a restrictive interventricular septal defect. There is a pressure gradient across the defect throughout systole.

VENTRICULAR SEPTAL DEFECT

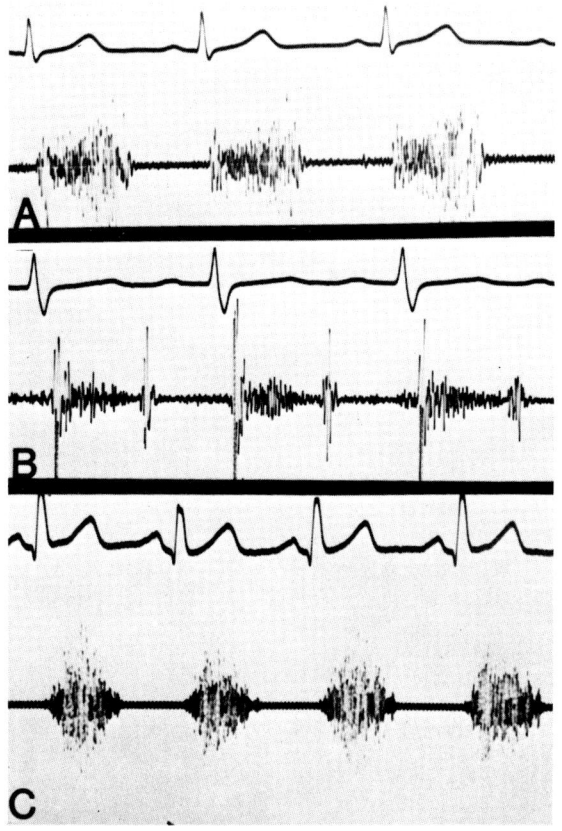

Fig. 5.3 Shape of the systolic murmur of ventricular septal defect. A. Crescendo murmur in a patient with an aneurysm of the membranous interventricular septum. B. Decrescendo murmur of a tiny defect in the muscular system. C. Crescendo-decrescendo murmur of a supracristal (subarterial) defect.

pitched, is either early systolic or pansystolic, and is maximal at the mid or low left sternal border. The murmur of a very large defect is lower pitched and physical findings indicative of pulmonary hypertension and/or large pulmonary blood flow are evident.

Ventricular septal defects may be classified anatomically as perimembranous, inlet septal, muscular septal or supracristal (subarterial) (Fig. 5.5). The anatomic location of the defect influences, to a degree, the characteristics of the associated systolic murmur. The murmurs of perimembranous, inlet septal and muscular septal defects are characteristically loudest near the fourth left intercostal space at the left sternal border, but there are exceptions. For example, the murmur of a defect in the apical portion of the muscular septum may be maximal at the apex and be indistinguishable from the murmur of mitral regurgitation. Or the murmur of a perforation in an aneurysm of the membranous septum may be loudest at the high left sternal border, since the aneurysm may direct the jet anteriorly and superiorly (Fig. 5.6). The murmur of a supracristal defect, on the other hand, is *characteristically* maximal at the high left sternal border and often

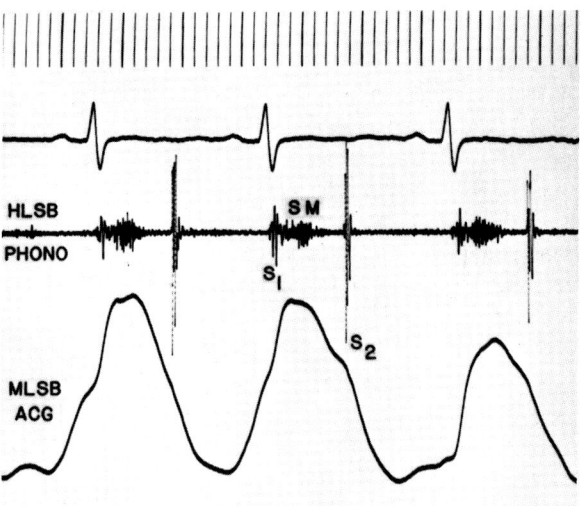

Fig. 5.4 High left sternal border phonocardiogram (HLSB Phono) and mid left sternal border apexcardiogram (MLSB ACG) in child with a ventricular septal defect and high pulmonary artery pressure. There is a soft crescendo-decrescendo systolic murmur (SM) and a prominent right ventricular lift.

through the pulmonary arteries may generate a separate soft systolic murmur which is well heard both posteriorly and at the high left sternal border.

A ventricular septal defect tends to become 'silent' in the presence of advanced pulmonary vascular disease, although a soft systolic ejection murmur may be generated in a dilated main pulmonary artery and be audible at the high left sternal border. Other signs of pulmonary hypertension, including a right ventricular lift and a loud pulmonic closure sound, are usually evident (Fig. 5.4). Although the systolic murmur of a ventricular septal defect tends to be soft at both ends of the spectrum of defect size, the very large and very small defects can easily be distinguished clinically. The murmur of a tiny defect is high

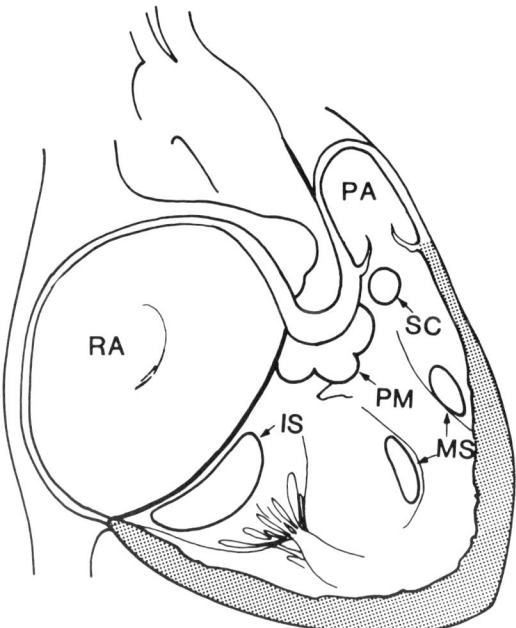

Fig. 5.5 Diagrammatic view of the interventricular septum showing the location of the several types of defect. IS — inlet septal; PM — perimembranous; SC — supracristal; MS — muscular septal.

excursion (Pickering & Keith, 1971), analogous to the early systolic sound of a doming aortic or pulmonic valve.

The usual systolic murmur of a ventricular septal defect does not vary strikingly with pharmacologic or physical manipulation, but the murmur of a very small defect in the muscular septum may change as left ventricular dimensions are altered by the Valsalva maneuver or by squatting and sudden standing (Fig 5.7). During the strain phase of the Valsalva or with sudden standing, systemic venous return to the heart decreases, left ventricular volume diminishes, and the left ventricular wall, including the septum, thickens. As the septum thickens the defect may become smaller and the murmur attenuate or even disappear.

radiates out under the left clavicle (Steinfeld et al, 1972). It is usually quite loud, sometimes Grade VI, with a prominent systolic thrill; both murmur and thrill often have a 'superficial' quality. The location and characteristics of the murmur of a supracristal defect may be very similar to those of a defect in an aneurysm of the membranous septum. The two entities may be indistinguishable clinically.

The murmur of a perimembranous, inlet septal or muscular defect which is restrictive is usually pansystolic and plateau shaped but is occasionally crescendo-decrescendo. The murmur of a supracristal defect is more commonly crescendo-decrescendo than is the murmur of a defect in other parts of the septum (Fig. 5.3C) (Steinfeld et al, 1972). The murmur of an aneurysm of the membranous septum may be crescendo (Fig. 5.3A), the late systolic accentuation presumably being related to an increase in size of a very small defect as the aneurysm expands and bulges into the right ventricle during late systole (Linhart & Razi, 1971). A septal aneurysm may produce a high pitched early systolic sound at the zenith of its

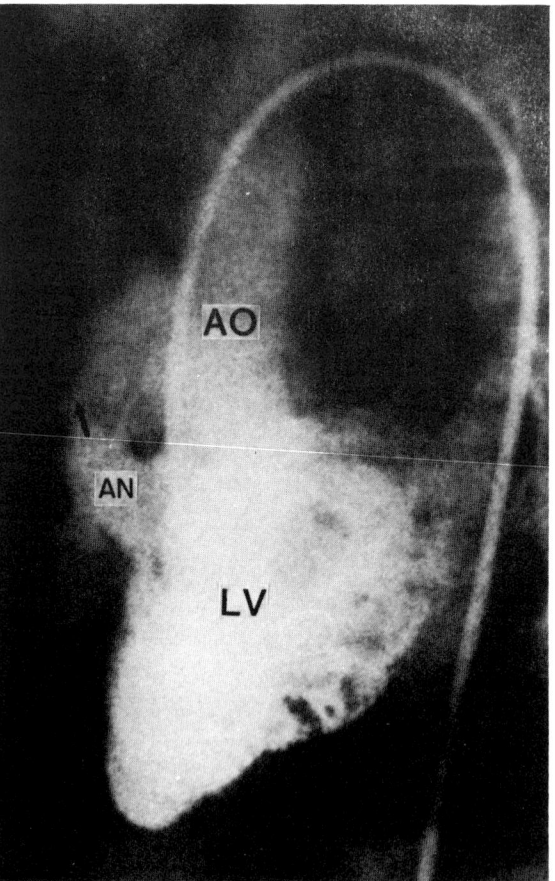

Fig. 5.6 Lateral view of the left ventricle of a child with an aneurysm of the membranous interventricular septum (AN). The jet through a small defect in the tip of the aneurysm is directed anteriorly and superiorly (arrow).

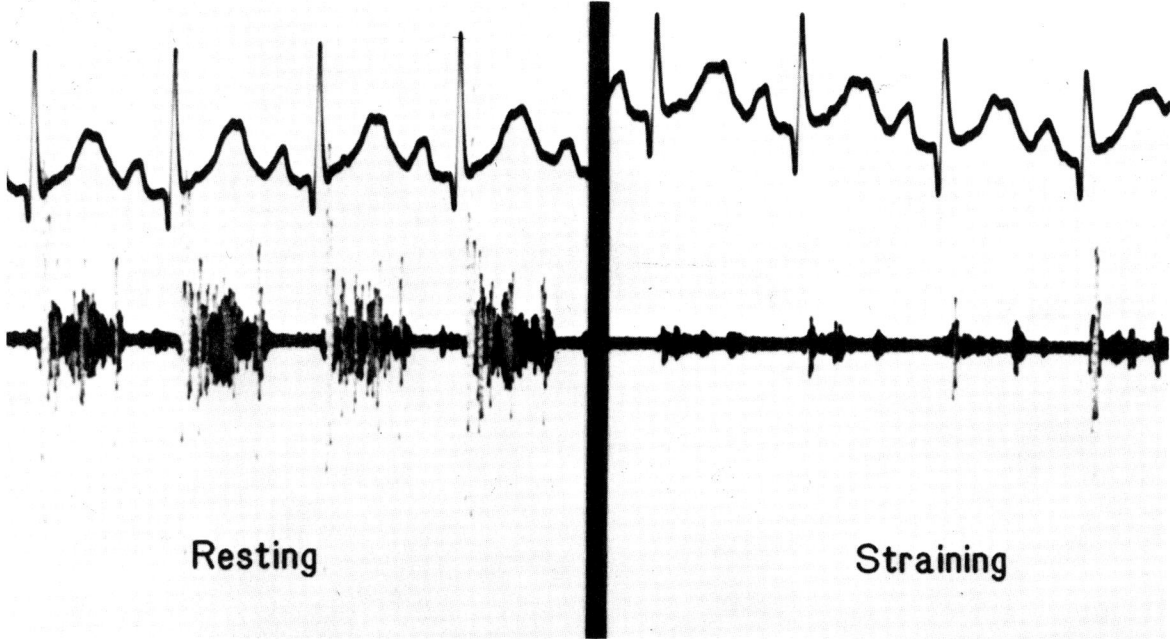

Fig. 5.7 Low left sternal border phonocardiogram in an infant with a tiny defect in the muscular septum. There is a loud systolic murmur at rest. With a Valsalva maneuver (straining induced by abdominal pressure) the murmur virtually disappears.

Conversely, left ventricular volume increases during the release phase of the Valsalva maneuver or after squatting. As the septum thins the defect may enlarge and permit greater flow, increasing the intensity and sometimes the duration of the murmur.

Any net left to right shunt across a ventricular septal defect results in an increase in flow across the mitral valve. If the return to the left atrium is sufficiently great a diastolic mitral gradient will occur and produce a murmur of relative mitral stenosis (Fig. 5.8). This apical murmur is low pitched and mid-diastolic and is most easily heard with the patient in the partial left lateral recumbent position. If it is very soft it may be appreciated only by listening alternately at the apex and at the mid left sternal border, the contrast between the 'silent' left sternal border and the apex permitting recognition of an otherwise imperceptible apical murmur. An apical diastolic murmur of relative mitral stenosis is evidence of a sizable left to right shunt and indicates that pulmonary blood flow is at least twice as large as systemic flow. The absence of an apical diastolic murmur in a patient with a ventricular defect suggests that the left to right shunt is small, either because the defect itself is small or because there is associated pulmonic stenosis or pulmonary vascular disease.

Associated anomalies

Associated anomalies may alter the expected physical findings of a ventricular septal defect. Coarctation of the aorta, for instance, may significantly increase the magnitude of the left to right shunt across a ventricular septal defect and cause congestive heart failure to appear earlier than usual, even during the first week or two of life. As another example, coexistent pulmonic stenosis attenuates the murmur of the ventricular defect by raising right ventricular pressure and reducing the interventricular gradient. If pulmonic stenosis is severe and right and left ventricular pressures are equal (tetralogy of Fallot) the ventricular defect will be 'silent'.

Differential Diagnosis

In most acyanotic patients with a ventricular septal defect the differential diagnosis is that of a mid or low left sternal border systolic murmur. If the murmur is loud and accompanied by a thrill the only anomalies likely to be confused are subvalvar pulmonic or subvalvar aortic stenosis. With these obstructive lesions the murmur is usually louder at the mid than at the lower sternal border and with subvalvar aortic stenosis the loudness of the murmur at the high right sternal border helps to differentiate it from a ventricular septal defect. The clinical differentiation of subvalvar pulmonic stenosis and a small ventricular defect may be impossible, since each entity may have either a plateau or a crescendo-decrescendo murmur, a normally split second heart sound and normal precordial activity. The chest roentgenogram and electrocardiogram may be normal, even with important subvalvar pulmonic stenosis, especially if it is due to an anomalous muscle bundle within the right ventricle.

If the left sternal border systolic murmur is soft,

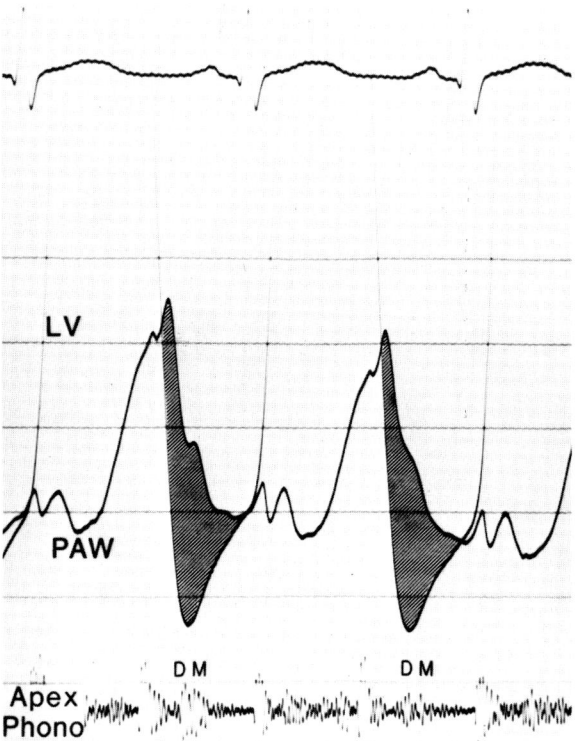

Fig. 5.8 Simultaneous left ventricular and pulmonary arterial wedge (PAW) pressures in a patient with a ventricular septal defect and large left to right shunt. The mitral gradient (hatched area) corresponds temporally with the mid diastolic murmur (DM) recorded at the apex.

the differential includes a functional murmur, tricuspid regurgitation and tetralogy of Fallot with severe infundibular pulmonic stenosis. The vibratory or 'twanging string' quality of the functional murmur serves to distinguish it from the high pitched blowing murmur of a small ventricular septal defect. Although the murmur of tricuspid regurgitation may be very like that of a tiny ventricular septal defect, incompetence of the tricuspid valve is, in infants, usually associated with pulmonary atresia or with Ebstein's anomaly of the tricuspid valve. There is then little likelihood of confusion with a small isolated ventricular defect. Tricuspid regurgitation is rare in older children but occasionally occurs in asymptomatic individuals with Ebstein's anomaly of the tricuspid valve. The widely split second heart sound, prominent third heart sound, 'sail' sound, and diastolic murmur commonly present in Ebstein's aid in the differential. In an occasional infant with tetralogy of Fallot the systolic murmur is soft, short, high pitched and maximal at the mid left sternal border. If there is no cyanosis it is easily mistaken for the murmur of a small and insignificant ventricular septal defect. The second heart sound is single, however. Splitting of the second sound should always be sought in an infant with such a murmur and its absence should raise the suspicion of a more complex anomaly. The difficulty in clinically distinguishing a tiny defect in the apical interventricular septum from mitral regurgitation or a supracristal defect from right ventricular outflow tract obstruction has already been pointed out.

Patients with either supracristal or perimembranous ventricular septal defects occasionally have associated aortic regurgitation. If the ventricular septal defect is very small, the high pitched pansystolic murmur of the ventricular defect extends to the aortic closure sound and the similarly high pitched diastolic murmur of the aortic regurgitation begins with the same sound, giving the impression of a continuous murmur at the mid left sternal border. In this situation separate systolic and diastolic murmurs can sometimes be distinguished at the low left and high right sternal border, respectively, but it may be impossible to clinically differentiate this entity from a coronary-cardiac fistula.

Summary

To summarize, most patients with a ventricular septal defect have a loud harsh pansystolic murmur and thrill at the mid or low left sternal border. Only with very small or very large defects is the murmur soft. The location of the murmur varies somewhat with the location of the defect and an apical defect may produce an apical systolic murmur which mimics mitral regurgitation. In patients with supracristal defects and in some cases of defects with a membranous septum aneurysm, the murmur is loudest at the high left sternal border and mimics the murmur of right ventricular outflow obstruction. An apical mid-diastolic murmur is generated only if there is large flow through a ventricular septal defect. A large defect without right ventricular outflow tract obstruction will have associated pulmonary hypertension, with a right ventricular lift and a loud and single or narrowly split second sound at the high left sternal border. In the late stages of pulmonary vascular disease there may be murmurs of tricuspid and/or pulmonic regurgitation.

ATRIOVENTRICULAR SEPTUM DEFECT

The anomaly

A defect in the atrioventricular portion of the membranous septum is not, strictly speaking, 'interventricular' but will be considered here. The septal portion of the tricuspid annulus, and hence the annular attachment of the septal leaflet of the tricuspid valve, crosses the membranous septum, dividing it into interventricular and atrioventricular portions. The atrioventricular part of the septum separates left ventricle and right atrium and a defect there results in flow from left ventricle to right atrium. A true atrioventricular septal defect is quite rare. It is clinically indistinguishable from the more common defect in the adjoining interventricular septum which shunts preferentially to the right atrium, either because of a cleft in the septal leaflet of the tricuspid valve or because the defect is immediately at the commissure between anterior and septal leaflets.

Physical findings

The most striking physical finding in a patient with a defect in the atrioventricular septum is a loud holosystolic plateau murmur at the lower left sternal border, indistinguishable externally from the murmur of an ordinary perimembranous defect. (Localization of the murmur to the right atrium with an intracardiac phonocatheter is strong evidence for a left ventricular–right atrial shunt, whether it be directly through the atrioventricular septum or through a defect of the interventricular septum via the tricuspid valve.) A sizable left ventricular–right atrial shunt results in increased flow across both mitral and tricuspid valves, and the murmurs of relative tricuspid stenosis and relative mitral stenosis can sometimes both be heard. The combination of a short medium pitched diastolic murmur at the low left sternal border and a systolic murmur and thrill at the same area strongly suggests a defect in the atrioventricular septum or a ventricular septal defect with tricuspid regurgitation (although organic tricuspid regurgitation may give rise to similar findings).

REFERENCES

Linhart J W, Razi B 1971 Late systolic murmur: A clue to the diagnosis of aneurysm of the membranous ventricular septum. Chest 60:283

Pickering D, Keith J D 1971 Systolic clicks with ventricular septal defects. A sign of aneurysm of ventricular septum? British Heart Journal 33:538

Rudolph A M 1965 The effects of postnatal circulatory adjustment in congenital heart disease. Pediatrics 36:763

Steinfeld L, Dimich I, Park S C, Baron M G 1972 Clinical diagnosis of isolated subpulmonic (supracristal) ventricular septal defect. American Journal of Cardiology 30:19

Tavel M E 1978 Clinical phonocardiography and external pulse recording, 3rd edn. Year Book Medical Publishers, Chicago, p 140

6

Patent ductus arteriosus

Clinical course

A patent ductus arteriosus is one of the most common congenital cardiovascular anomalies. It may exist as an isolated anomaly, be associated with other congenital cardiac defects, or be part of a syndrome (e.g. maternal rubella). The clinical course of an individual with an isolated patent ductus arteriosus is largely determined by the luminal size of the ductus. If the ductus is small the left to right shunt will be hemodynamically unimportant and congestive heart failure and pulmonary vascular disease will not ensue. If the ductus is large, congestive heart failure and pulmonary vascular disease are much more likely. The signs of congestive heart failure do not ordinarily appear during the first month of life, however, since the large aortico-pulmonary communication retards the normal post natal fall in pulmonary vascular resistance. Only when resistance eventually decreases does torrential left to right shunting precipitate failure.

Premature infants have much higher incidence of persistent patency of the ductus arteriosus than do full term infants (Danilowicz et al, 1966), presumably because of immaturity of the ductal wall. Also, unlike term infants, congestive heart failure is common during the first week or two of life, since the pulmonary arterioles are less well endowed with smooth muscle and cannot maintain a high level of resistance after inflation of the lungs at birth. Pulmonary abnormalities are also more prominent in prematures than in full term infants with a patent ductus; there is a high incidence of rales, episodes of apnea and bradycardia, respiratory insufficiency and requirement for respiratory support. The pulmonary disability may be related to increased pulmonary capillary permeability, to intrinsic lung disease, to lack of central respiratory drive, or to a combination of these factors.

If a patent ductus is very large, high pulmonary blood flow and elevated pulmonary artery pressure eventually lead to pulmonary vascular disease. The process usually requires several years, and irreversible pulmonary vascular disease related to a patent ductus has now become rare, since diagnosed cases are routinely sent for surgical interruption before vascular disease develops. Infectious endocarditis is a potential threat in any patient with a patent ductus arteriosus.

Physical findings

General

The general appearance of an individual with a patent ductus is normal unless the ductus is part of a syndrome, such as that caused by maternal rubella during the first trimester of pregnancy (Venables, 1965). (In such patients low birth weight, cataracts, deafness and mental retardation are common and permit easy recognition.)

The most important physical signs of a patent ductus arteriosus are directly related to blood flow through the ductus and are influenced by its luminal size and by the pressure gradient between the aorta and pulmonary artery. If flow is large the left ventricular stroke volume is increased and the apical impulse will be prominent. In addition, aortic run-off to the pulmonary artery reduces aortic diastolic pressure and increases pulse pressure as well as amplitude of the palpated pulse wave. Arterial pulses are normal only if the ductus is small. Cyanosis does not occur with an uncomplicated ductus and the jugular venous pulse is normal.

Auscultation

The first heart sound is unremarkable in patients with a patent ductus arteriosus. Paradoxical splitting of the second heart sound has been reported to occur (Gray, 1956) but in the author's experience splitting of the second heart sound, whether physiologic or paradoxic, has been hard to appreciate because of the continuous murmur and because of the late systolic clicks which are so common in this entity. A third heart sound may be present but a fourth heart sound is not part of the auscultatory picture.

The most common and characteristic sign of a patent ductus arteriosus is a continuous murmur. (The term 'continuous' describes a murmur which is present in systole and which extends beyond the second heart sound into diastole; it need not occupy all of the cardiac cycle.) The murmur is typically loudest in the first or second intercostal space lateral to the left sternal border and characteristically peaks in late systole and early diastole,

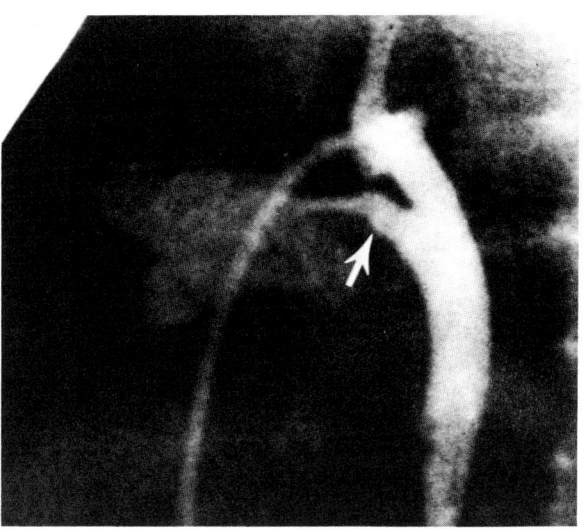

Fig. 6.2 Lateral cineangiographic frame showing an anteriorly directed jet from a patent ductus arteriosus (arrow).

when the aortic-pulmonary artery pressure gradient responsible for the murmur is maximal (Fig. 6.1). The murmur is not prominent over the posterior thorax unless it is very loud anteriorly. This is not surprising, since flow is from aorta to pulmonary artery and is thus directed toward the anterior chest wall (Fig. 6.2). As expected, intracardiac phonocardiography shows the murmur to be much louder in the pulmonary artery than the aorta (Fig. 6.3). The murmur of a very small patent

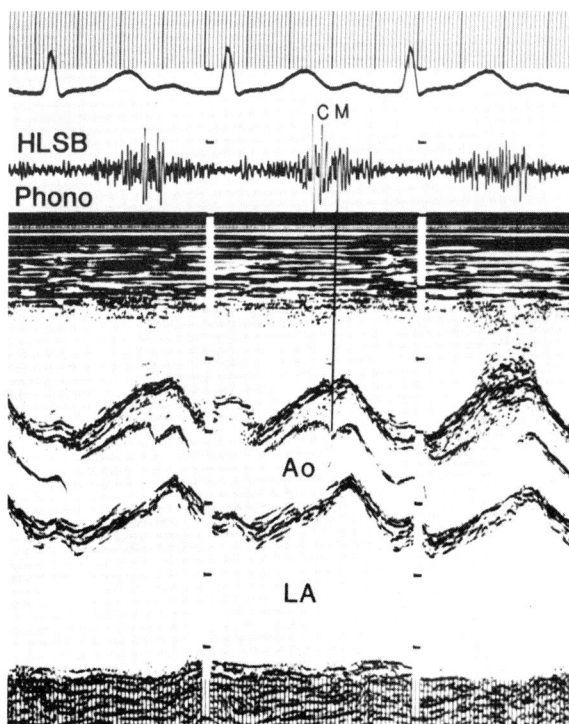

Fig. 6.1 Child with a patent ductus arterious. The high left sternal border phonocardiogram (HLSB Phono) shows peaking of the continuous murmur near closure of the aortic valve in the echocardiogram.

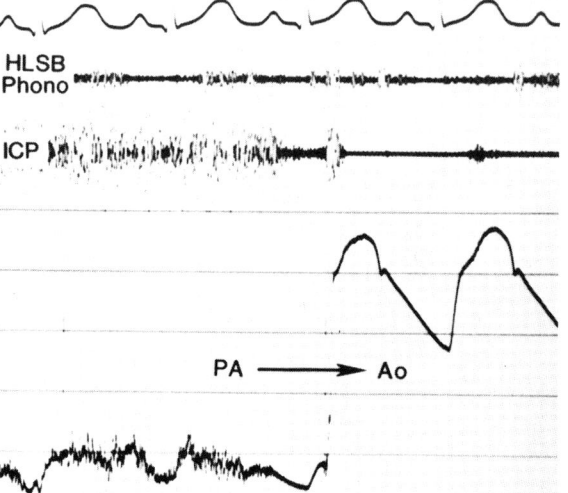

Fig. 6.3 Child with a patent ductus arteriosus. The intracardiac phonocardiogram (ICP) shows a loud continuous murmur in the pulmonary artery (PA) but not in the aorta (Ao).

ductus is soft and high pitched and may not extend completely through diastole. A larger but still restrictive ductus generates a loud continuous murmur which often is punctuated by a series of clicking sounds. If the ductus is very large and unrestrictive aortic and pulmonary artery pressures tend to equalize during diastole and the murmur ends with, just beyond, or even before the second heart sound (Fig. 6.4).

A large left to right shunt through a patent ductus arteriosus results in excessive pulmonary venous return to the left atrium. As a consequence, diastolic flow across the mitral valve may be increased sufficiently to generate a mid diastolic apical rumble of relative mitral stenosis.

In the normal newborn a ductus murmur may be transiently present during the first 24 hours of life, when pulmonary vascular resistance and pulmonary artery pressure have fallen below systemic vascular resistance and aortic pressure, respectively, and before complete functional closure of the ductus arteriosus has occurred. With persistent patency of a large ductus a continuous murmur is rarely appreciated in the newborn nursery, since pulmonary vascular resistance and pulmonary artery pressure fall more slowly in the presence of a large aortic-pulmonary communication. High pulmonary artery pressure precludes the aortico-pulmonary artery gradient necessary for a continuous murmur. The typical murmur does not appear until pulmonary vascular resistance falls, usually during the first few weeks of life.

Pulmonary hypertension

The clinical picture is quite different in the presence of elevated pulmonary vascular resistance. As pulmonary resistance approaches systemic, pulmonary artery and aortic pressures tend to track and the ductal murmur disappears. Since pulmonary flow is not increased in such patients, there is no apical rumble and the apical impulse is quiet. The elevation in pulmonary artery pressure results in an accentuated pulmonic closure sound and the second heart sound is single or narrowly split. A left parasternal lift may also be appreciated and the diastolic murmur of hypertensive pulmonic regurgitation may be heard. At this stage the clinical picture is that of pulmonary hypertension, all evidence of a patent ductus having disappeared. If pulmonary vascular resistance exceeds systemic, however, ductal flow reverses and unsaturated blood enters the descending aorta. If this right to left shunt is sufficiently large, differential cyanosis will be evident, with the lower trunk and the feet being cyanotic and the hands, lips and upper trunk remaining pink. (The left hand will also be cyanotic if the ductus 'feeds' the left subclavian artery.) Such differential *central* cyanosis is quite rare, but may be simulated by differential *peripheral* cyanosis, a much more common phenomenon which is related to poor cutaneous blood flow in the lower extremities.

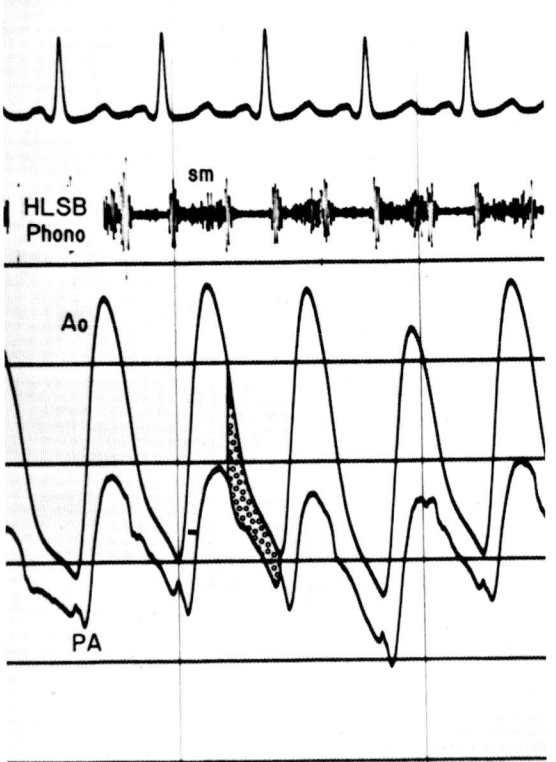

Fig. 6.4 Patient with a patent ductus arteriosus and elevated pulmonary artery pressure. Simultaneous aortic and pulmonary artery pressures show a large gradient during systole but only a small one during diastole (stippled area), and the murmur is only systolic.

Associated anomalies

Associated cardiovascular anomalies influence the clinical picture of a patent ductus arteriosus. For instance, a patent ductus may be 'silent' in the presence of a large and unrestrictive ventricular septal defect, since aortic and pulmonary artery pressures are similar. As another example, pulmonic stenosis may be difficult to recognize in the presence of a large patent ductus arteriosus, both because the pulmonic stenosis murmur is masked by the continuous murmur of the ductus and because pulmonary artery pressure is raised by inflow through the ductus, reducing the gradient between the right ventricle and pulmonary artery. Coarctation of the aorta and a patent ductus arteriosus may coexist. Although coarctation is nearly always juxtaductal anatomically, it may be pre or post ductal functionally. If functionally post ductal, it tends to increase left to right shunting; if pre ductal and severe, it may lead to right to left shunting through the ductus and is a rare cause of differential cyanosis. The effect of the ductus on more complex anomalies such as pulmonary atresia, aortic atresia, interrupted aortic arch, etc. is discussed separately under those specific headings.

Differential diagnosis

The differential diagnosis of a patent ductus arteriosus is essentially that of a continuous murmur or of increased peripheral arterial pulses. It includes the jugular venous hum, the mammary souffle of pregnancy, an aortico-pulmonary window, a persistent truncus arteriosus, systemic-pulmonary collateral arteries, a ruptured sinus of Valsalva aneurysm, a coronary-cardiac fistula, and aortic regurgitation in combination with a small ventricular septal defect.

Venous hum

A jugular venous hum is frequently confused with the continuous murmur of a patent ductus, especially if it is loud and well heard below the clavicles. Much is made of head turning or pressure over the jugular veins to alter a hum and differentiate it from a patent ductus arteriosus, but it is much simpler to listen with the patient recumbent. The murmur of a ductus is not greatly influenced by position while a jugular venous hum always disappears or markedly attenuates in the recumbent position.

Mammary souffle

The mammary souffle of late pregnancy or the early post partum period may also closely simulate a patent ductus arteriosus (Tabatznik et al, 1960). It is generated by large arterial blood flow to the breasts and is usually best heard along the upper left and/or right sternal borders. The murmur peaks during systole and may or may not spill into diastole. Unlike the murmur of a patent ductus or a venous hum, the mammary souffle of pregnancy is best heard with the patient supine. It disappears with local pressure.

Aortico-pulmonary window

An aortico-pulmonary window consists of a communication between the ascending aorta and the adjacent main pulmonary artery (Neufeld et al, 1963). Since a window is usually large, early congestive heart failure is common and arterial pulses are bounding. The murmur of an aortico-pulmonary window is most commonly systolic but may spill into diastole. There is no reliable way to distinguish a large window from a large patent ductus arteriosus clinically. (An occasional aortico-pulmonary window is small, and its loud continuous murmur and mildly to moderately increased peripheral pulses exactly mimic the findings of a small patent ductus arteriosus.) In the presence of advanced pulmonary vascular disease an aortico-pulmonary window and a ventricular septal defect are clinically indistinguishable, since in each entity unsaturated blood enters the ascending aorta and is distributed equally to the upper and lower body, producing generalized rather than differential cyanosis.

Truncus arteriosus

A persistent truncus arteriosus only occasionally produces a continuous murmur, but full arterial pulses may be present in the face of congestive heart failure with either a persistent truncus or a large patent ductus. Cyanosis may not be evident in an infant with a truncus if pulmonary blood flow is sufficiently large, further compounding the difficulty in differential diagnosis.

Systemic-pulmonary collateral arteries

Systemic-pulmonary collateral arteries may produce a continuous murmur which can be confused with that of a patent ductus. The murmur of collaterals is usually more widely heard anteriorly and posteriorly, however, and is rarely confined to the upper left chest as is the murmur of a patent ductus. (Large and audible collaterals most commonly accompany tetralogy of Fallot, with or without pulmonary atresia.)

Sinus of valsalva aneurysm

A ruptured sinus of Valsalva aneurysm generates a continuous murmur which must be differentiated from that of a patent ductus (Ch. 25). If rupture is into the right ventricle or right atrium, the murmur tends to be maximal lower along the sternum than with a patent ductus. Also, with rupture into the right ventricle the murmur typically is louder in diastole, since the aortico-right ventricular gradient is larger during that phase of the cardiac cycle. Sinus of Valsalva aneurysms almost never rupture in infancy, but the sudden onset of a loud continuous murmur during childhood or early adult life, with or without signs of congestive heart failure, is highly suggestive of the diagnosis.

Pulmonary artery stenosis

In the premature infant the murmur of a patent ductus arteriosus usually extends beyond the second heart sound but is occasionally only systolic and then must be differentiated from the systolic murmur of 'physiologic' pulmonary artery stenosis of the newborn (Ch. 10). A ductus is always louder at the high left sternal border than in the axillae or over the back, however, while the murmur of pulmonary artery stenosis is usually nearly equally loud anteriorly and posteriorly. Brisk arterial pulses are a clue to the presence of a patent ductus, but must be interpreted with caution, since pulses may be quite full in the 'normal' premature.

Other

The combination of a small ventricular septal defect and aortic regurgitation may produce a seemingly continuous mid left sternal border murmur which may be confused with a patent ductus (Ch. 13). However, separate systolic and diastolic murmurs can sometimes be appreciated at the low left and the high right sternal borders, respectively. The continuous murmur of a coronary-cardiac fistula is heard lower along the sternum than that of a ductus (Ch. 20). A continuous venous hum is sometimes heard in infants with total anomalous pulmonary venous return (Ch. 8). If return is to the left superior vena cava, the hum may closely simulate a ductal murmur but is more influenced by respiration or straining. A surgically created systemic-pulmonary anastomosis may exactly mimic a patent ductus arteriosus. Systemic arteriovenous fistulae in the thoracic wall or lower cervical region may produce a continuous murmur which can be confused with that of a patent ductus arteriosus.

Summary

In summary, most infants and children with a patent ductus arteriosus have a continuous murmur which is loudest under the left clavicle. Conversely, a continuous murmur which is maximal in that area is nearly always due to a patent ductus. A jugular venous hum is easily differentiated by its disappearance in the recumbent position. Symptoms rarely occur during the first month of life unless the infant is premature.

REFERENCES

Danilowicz D, Rudolph A M, Hoffman J I E 1966 Delayed closure of the ductus arteriosus in premature infants. Pediatrics 37:74

Gray I R 1956 Paradoxical splitting of the second heart sound. British Heart Journal 18:21

Neufeld H N, Lester R G, Adams P Jr, Anderson R C, Lillehei C W, Edwards J E 1962 Aorticopulmonary septal defect. American Journal of Cardiology 9:12

Tabatznik B, Randall T W, Hersch C 1960 The mammary souffle of pregnancy and lactation. Circulation 22:1069

Venables A W 1965 The syndrome of pulmonary stenosis complicating maternal rubella. British Heart Journal 27:49

7

Endocardial cushion defects

Endocardial cushion defects (atrioventricular canal defects, atrioventricular defects) may occur in otherwise normal children but are especially common in association with certain syndromes. They are the most common cardiac anomaly in Down's syndrome, occurring in 43 percent of cases with organic heart disease in a recent large series (Park et al, 1977) and are even more common with situs ambiguous (Moller et al, 1967; Ivemark, 1955).

There is a considerable spectrum of anatomic abnormalities and consequently a wide spectrum of hemodynamic and clinical findings. Although endocardial cushion defects can exist singly (e.g. ventricular septal defect of the atrioventricular canal type, isolated cleft of the mitral valve, isolated ostium primum atrial septal defect), in most patients there are identifiable abnormalities of the interatrial and interventricular septa and of the atrioventricular valve(s). The interatrial communication is almost always large and is located immediately proximal to the atrioventricular valves. It results from failure of the septum primum to anchor to the crest of the interventricular septum and is therefore referred to as a 'primum' defect. The portion of interventricular septum immediately distal to the atrioventricular valves is almost invariably deficient but there is not always an interventricular communication, since the atrioventricular valve tissue may be closely attached to the crest of the deficient interventricular septum, separating right and left ventricular cavities. If there are two separate atrioventricular valve orifices, the anterior leaflet of the mitral valve is almost always cleft (Fig. 7.1). An extension of this cleft across the interventricular septum and through the septal tricuspid leaflet results in a common atrioventricular orifice, which then has anterior and posterior bridging leaflets (Fig. 7.2). In either case, there may or may not be atrioventricular valvar regurgitation, since the edges of a cleft anterior mitral leaflet (or anterior and posterior bridging leaflets of a common atrioventricular valve) may coapt. The mitral valve is much more commonly regurgitant than the tricuspid valve.

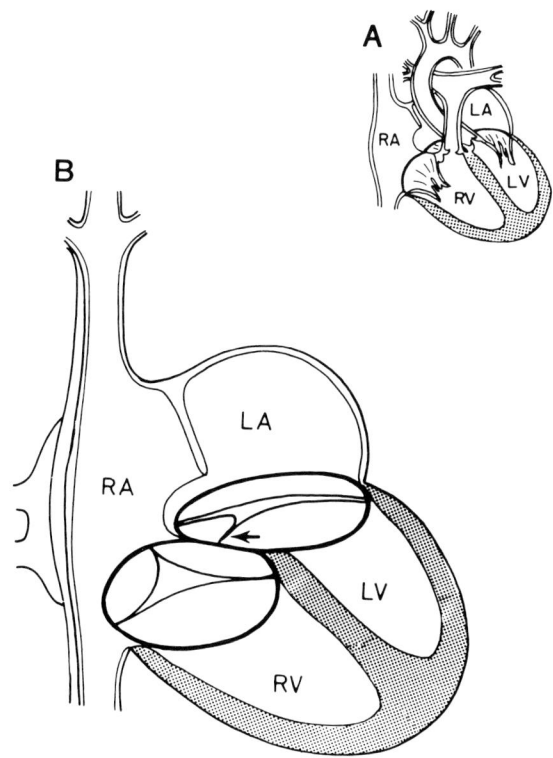

Fig. 7.1 A. Diagram of partial endocardial cushion defect. B. View without great arteries. There is no interventricular communication but the anterior leaflet of the mitral valve is cleft (arrow).

The two major determinants of the clinical course of an individual with an endocardial cushion defect are the size of the interventricular communication and the degree of mitral regurgitation. It is therefore useful to classify cases as 'complete' endocardial cushion defects, with a large interventricular communication, or as 'partial' endocardial cushion defects, without an interventricular communication. In transitional forms with a small interventricular communication the clinical course, surgical repair and prognosis are little altered by the small interventricular opening. Such cases will be considered a variant of partial endocardial cushion defect.

PARTIAL ENDOCARDIAL CUSHION DEFECT

The anomaly

'Partial endocardial cushion defect' and 'partial atrioventricular canal' are synonymous terms used to describe an ostium primum interatrial septal defect. The mitral and tricuspid orifices are separate but adjacent and no interatrial septum attaches to their common border. The common border does attach to the crest of the deficient interventricular septum, separating right and left ventricular cavities. The anterior mitral leaflet is almost always cleft, the septal leaflet of the tricuspid valve less frequently so (Fig. 7.1).

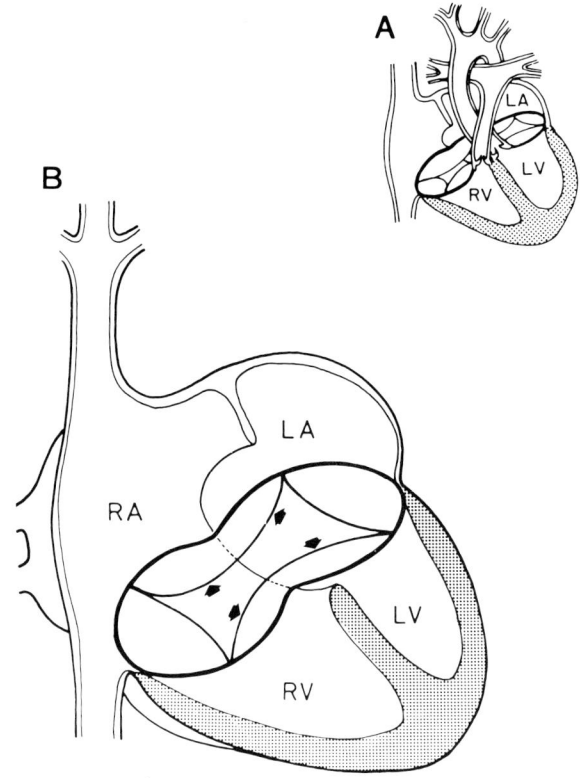

Fig. 7.2 A. Diagram of complete endocardial cushion defect. B. View without great arteries. There is a confluent communication at atrial and ventricular levels. The common atrioventricular valve has anterior and posterior bridging leaflets (arrows).

Clinical course

If the mitral valve is competent the clinical course and physical findings are identical to those of a secundum interatrial septal defect. Symptoms are rare in infancy and childhood and the onset of pulmonary hypertension and pulmonary vascular disease are long delayed. Mild mitral regurgitation is quite well tolerated but moderate or severe regurgitation increases the volume load of both ventricles; the left ventricle directly and the right ventricle because of the increased left to right atrial shunt occasioned by the mitral regurgitation. In this setting, exercise intolerance and even congestive heart failure occur more frequently and at an earlier age than expected with an interatrial septal defect alone.

Physical findings

General

Cyanosis does not occur with an uncomplicated partial endocardial cushion defect. The jugular venous pulse, arterial pulse and blood pressure are usually normal. (If there is major mitral regurgitation a 'V' wave may be transmitted from the left to the right atrium and to the jugular veins, simulating tricuspid regurgitation (Perloff, 1978). A poorly sustained left sternal border impulse is common and reflects the increased right ventricular stroke volume present with a large interatrial shunt. The left ventricular apical impulse is exaggerated in the presence of major mitral regurgitation.

Auscultation

A high left sternal border systolic murmur, a low left sternal border mid-diastolic murmur and a fixedly split second heart sound are characteristic of a large interatrial shunt, whether it be via a secundum or a primum interatrial defect. The first heart sound is commonly loud at the low left sternal border in a secundum defect, but the long PR interval which is usual with a primum defect tends to soften the first heart sound (Fig. 7.3). If a small interventricular communication is present a loud harsh pansystolic murmur is heard at the low left sternal border. This murmur may be soft and high-pitched if the defect is tiny (Fig. 7.3). The murmur of mitral regurgitation is usually pansystolic and maximal at the apex but may radiate more toward the sternum than toward the axilla, since the regurgitant jet through the cleft is directed more anteriorly and to the right than it is in other varieties of mitral insufficiency (Fig. 7.4). (It may

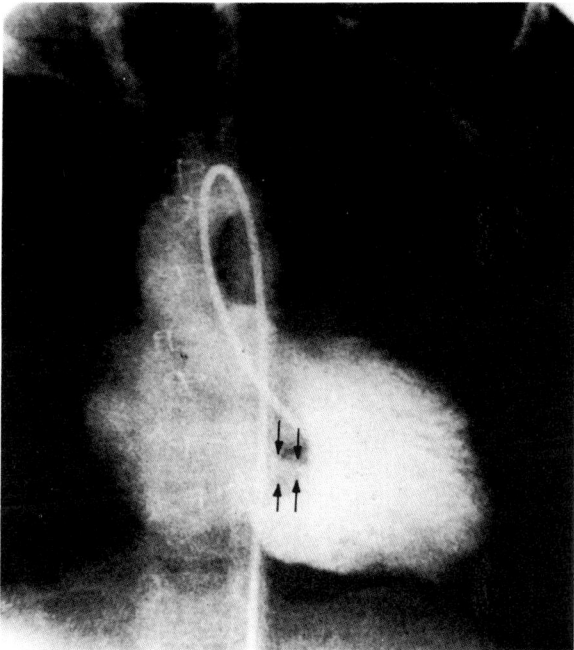

Fig. 7.4 Child with a partial endocardial cushion defect and mitral regurgitation. The left ventriculogram shows the rightwardly directed jet of the regurgitation (arrows).

be impossible to clinically distinguish mitral regurgitation from a small interventricular communication.) Although the mitral valve is abnormal in an endocardial cushion defect, it may be competent and there may be no murmur of mitral regurgitation.

COMPLETE ENDOCARDIAL CUSHION DEFECT

The anomaly

'Complete endocardial cushion defect' and 'complete atrioventricular canal' are terms which describe confluent interatrial and interventricular septal defects. As in a partial endocardial cushion

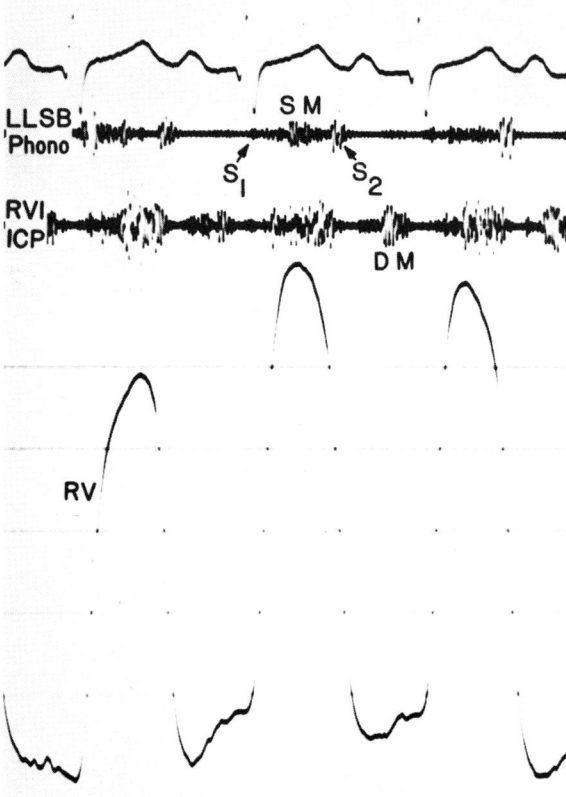

Fig. 7.3 Child with an ostium primum interatrial septal defect and tiny interventricular septal defect. The low left sternal border phonocardiogram (LLSB phono) shows a soft first heart sound (due to long PR interval) and a soft systolic murmur (SM). The phonocardiogram recorded in the right ventricle (RV ICP) shows the systolic murmur of the interventricular defect as well as the diastolic murmur of relative tricuspid stenosis.

defect, both the lower portion of the interatrial septum and the crest of the interventricular septum are deficient. Instead of separate tricuspid and mitral orifices, however, there is a common atrioventricular orifice, with anterior and posterior atrioventricular valve leaflets bridging across the interventricular septum (Fig. 7.2). Chordae tendinae may extend from the leaflet to the septum, or the leaflets may be 'free floating'.

Clinical course

The clinical course of a complete endocardial cushion defect is similar to that of a large interventricular septal defect. The onset of congestive heart failure occurs most commonly during the second or third month of life. If there is severe mitral regurgitation, failure may appear even earlier and may be severe and refractory to treatment.

Physical findings

General

Cyanosis is seen in some individuals with a complete endocardial cushion defect, even before severe pulmonary vascular disease develops. When present cyanosis is mild and intermittent, occurring only with crying, straining or with respiratory infections. It is due to mixing at atrial level and is more common if the interatrial defect is very large or if the atrial septum is absent. A precordial bulge is common. There is usually a prominent left sternal border systolic lift, and a vigorous apical impulse suggests major mitral regurgitation. Unless there is associated pulmonic stenosis, pulmonary artery pressure is always elevated in a complete endocardial cushion defect. In older children and adults systolic pulsations of the pulmonary artery may occasionally be palpated at the upper left sternal border.

Auscultation

The second heart sound at the high left sternal border may be single or split and the pulmonic component is accentuated. Even in a complete endocardial cushion defect the ventricular septal defect may be somewhat restrictive. The resulting interventricular pressure gradient results in a harsh pansystolic murmur at the low left sternal border. If the ventricular communication is larger and unrestrictive, the murmur may be only early systolic or the ventricular defect may be 'silent'. If there is good evidence of severe pulmonary hypertension, a prominent pansystolic murmur anywhere from the apex to the low left sternal border is more likely to represent mitral regurgitation than to emanate from a ventricular septal defect. If there is a sizeable left to right shunt, rapid systolic flow across the pulmonic valve and through the pulmonary arteries generates a soft systolic ejection murmur at the high left sternal border, in the axillae and across the back. If diastolic flow across the atrioventricular valve is sufficiently great a mid-diastolic murmur is generated. This murmur is usually heard better at the low left sternal border than at the apex but may be audible at both areas. A mid diastolic apical rumble is usually audible if there is important mitral regurgitation.

Pulmonary hypertension

Pulmonary vascular disease tends to develop early in patients with complete endocardial cushion defect and may be advanced and irreversible by the end of the first year or two of life. Its presence may be signaled by the appearance of cyanosis, a loud single second heart sound, or the diastolic murmur of hypertensive pulmonary regurgitation. It is also suggested by the disappearance of a low left sternal border mid diastolic murmur or a softening or disappearance of a low left sternal border systolic murmur. An occasional patient with a complete endocardial cushion defect and advanced pulmonary vascular disease has no murmur.

Associated anomalies

Pulmonary stenosis is occasionally associated with an endocardial cushion defect, more commonly with the complete variety. The obstruction may be valvar and/or infundibular and, if severe, causes right to left shunting. The cyanosis, mid or high left sternal border systolic murmur, and single second heart sound in such cases may exactly mimic the physical findings of a patient with tetralogy of Fallot.

COMMON ATRIUM

The anomaly

A common atrium may occur in an otherwise normal child but may also be seen in association with the Ellis-van Creveld syndrome (Giknis, 1963). In a common atrium the rightward and leftward portions of the common chamber have right and left atrial morphologic characteristics (or bilaterally right or left morphology in the presence of situs ambiguous). In some cases the atrioventricular valves are cleft, suggesting that the anomaly is a variety of endocardial cushion defect (Ellis, 1959). In other cases the atrioventricular valves are normal and the anomaly probably results from complete lack of development of the septum primum and the septum secundum rather than from defective development of the endocardial cushions (Munoz-Armas et al, 1968).

Clinical course

The clinical course and physical findings of a common atrium resemble those of a large interatrial septal defect, but with some important differences. The magnitude of the left to right shunt may be unusually great in infancy and early childhood, due chiefly to the size of the interatrial communication but also to the mitral regurgitation which may be present if the mitral valve is cleft. Symptoms of easy fatigue and even of congestive heart failure may thus occur earlier than expected with a simple interatrial septal defect. Also, complete lack of an interatrial septum leads to some mixing of pulmonary and systemic venous returns at atrial level and therefore results in a degree of arterial unsaturation.

Physical findings

The physical findings are very similar to those of a large interatrial septal defect, with a systolic ejection murmur at the high sternal border, a mid-diastolic murmur of relative tricuspid stenosis at the low left sternal border, a fixedly split second heart sound and a prominent left sternal border systolic impulse. In addition, the apical systolic murmur of mitral regurgitation may be heard. If cyanosis is present it is usually mild and intermittent. A firm diagnosis cannot be made clinically but the entity should be considered in a child who has signs of a large left to right shunt at atrial level and who either becomes symptomatic at an unusually early age or who shows evidence of arterial unsaturation.

Other endocardial cushion defect variants such as an isolated cleft in the mitral valve and an isolated ventricular septal defect of the atrioventricular canal type are dealt with in Chapters 15 and 4, respectively.

REFERENCES

Ellis F H Jr, Kirklin J W, Swan H J C, DuShane J W, Edwards J E 1959 Diagnosis and surgical treatment of common atrium (cor trilocularebiventriculare). Surgery 45: 160

Giknis F L 1963 Single atrium and the Ellis–van Creveld syndrome. Journal of Pediatrics 62: 558

Ivemark B I 1955 Implications of agenesis of the spleen on the pathogenesis of cono-truncus anomalies in childhood: Analysis of the heart malformations in the splenic agenesis syndrome, with fourteen new cases. Acta Pediatrica 44 (Suppl 104): 1

Moller J H, Nakib A, Anderson R C, Edwards J E 1967 Congenital cardiac disease associated with polysplenia. Circulation 36: 789

Munoz-Armas S, Gorrin J R D, Anselmi G, Hernandez P B Anselmi A 1968 Single atrium: embryologic, anatomic, electrocardiographic and other diagnostic features. American Journal of Cardiology 21: 639

Park S C, Mathews R A, Zuberbuhler J R, Rowe R D, Neches W H, Lenox C C 1977 Down syndrome with congenital heart malformation. American Journal of Diseases of Children 131: 29

Perloff J K 1978 The clinical recognition of congenital heart disease. Saunders, Philadelphia, p 354

8

Anomalous pulmonary venous connection

In anomalous pulmonary venous connection, one or more of the pulmonary veins drains to the right atrium or, more commonly, to a systemic venous tributary of the right atrium. If all of the pulmonary veins drain to the right atrium directly or indirectly, total anomalous pulmonary venous connection is present; if only part of the pulmonary venous return is so directed, partial anomalous pulmonary venous connection exists. Anomalous pulmonary venous connection may occur as an isolated anomaly or associated with other cardiovascular defects.

TOTAL ANOMALOUS PULMONARY VENOUS RETURN

The anomaly

In most cases of total anomalous pulmonary venous connection, pulmonary veins from both lungs join in a confluence which lies directly behind the left atrium but which does not connect to it. Drainage from the confluence may be to the left innominate vein, the right superior vena cava, the coronary sinus or to the portal vein or inferior vena cava (Fig. 8.1). In some cases drainage is mixed, some pulmonary venous return being via one anomalous channel and some via another. Rarely, pulmonary veins drain separately to the right atrium.

Clinical course

There is a spectrum of clinical presentation of total anomalous pulmonary venous connection which ranges from the dyspneic cyanotic newborn in congestive heart failure to the older child with little or no cyanosis or disability. Pulmonary venous obstruction is a major determinant of clinical course (Gathman & Nadas, 1970). If there is no such obstruction pulmonary blood flow tends to be large and cyanosis to be mild. Pulmonary hypertension may or may not be present. In cases without obstruction congestive heart failure may appear in infancy or may be delayed for several years. If there is severe pulmonary venous obstruction, pulmonary blood flow is reduced and pulmonary artery pressure is at or above systemic levels. Cyanosis is present at birth but the newborn's color may be

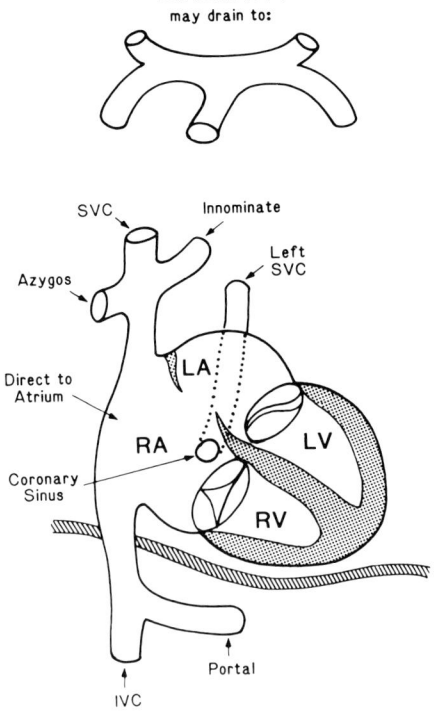

Fig. 8.1 Diagram showing possible drainage routes in anomalous pulmonary venous connection.

more gray than deep blue, probably reflecting a combination of arterial unsaturation and low systemic blood flow. If there is severe venous obstruction, tachypnea and congestive heart failure appear in the neonatal period and death during the first few days or weeks of life is the rule (Hastreiter et al, 1962). Pulmonary venous obstruction is the rule if drainage is below the diaphragm and is very common if it is to the right superior vena cava or azygos vein.

Physical findings

General

Although children with total anomalous pulmonary venous connection of any variety tend to have slow weight gain and poor development, the specific physical findings are strongly influenced by the presence or absence of pulmonary venous obstruction. Since there is always right to left flow across the interatrial septum, arterial unsaturation is inevitable. Cyanosis, however, is variable and tends to be inversely proportional to pulmonary blood flow, being severe if pulmonary venous obstruction leads to low pulmonary flow and mild if free pulmonary venous drainage permits high pulmonary flow. Since there is right ventricular volume overload in patients with total anomalous pulmonary venous return — and often pressure overload as well — the left parasternal impulse is usually quite prominent. Peripheral and jugular venous pulses are usually normal.

Auscultation

Heart sounds. The first heart sound is often accentuated at the low left sternal border. The second heart sound is split in most cases, sometimes widely, and splitting may or may not vary with

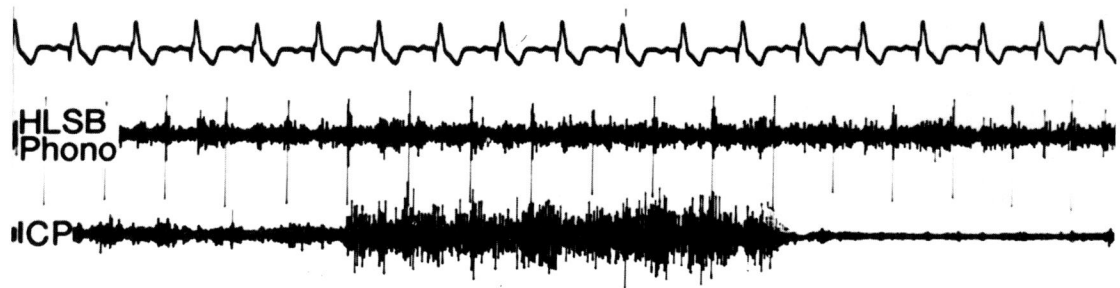

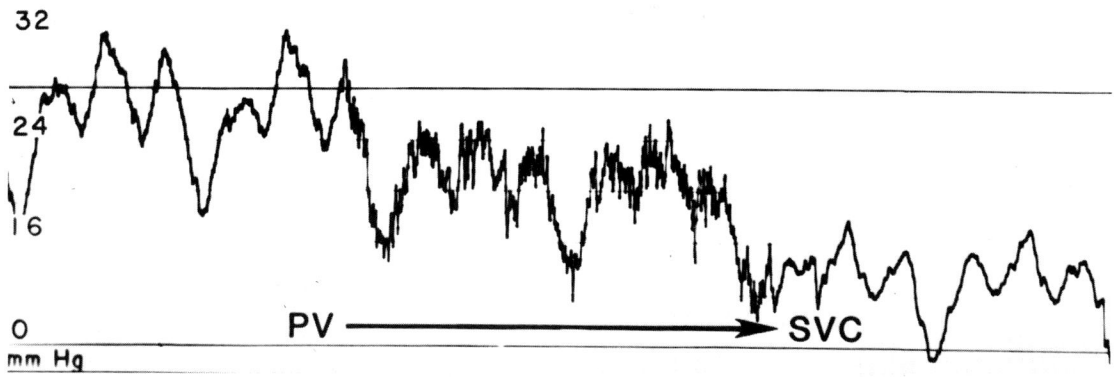

Fig. 8.2 Infant with total anomalous pulmonary venous return to a left superior vena cava. There is obstruction at the junction of pulmonary vein (PV) and superior vena cava (SVC) and a continuous murmur is recorded at that site (ICP) and in the high left sternal border phonocardiogram (HLSB Phono).

respiration. The pulmonic closure sound may be of normal intensity or be loud, depending on whether or not pulmonary hypertension is present. A third heart sound is common. A fourth heart sound has been reported in patients with pulmonary hypertension (Gathman & Nadas, 1970) but has been very rare in the author's experience.

Murmurs. A soft crescendo-decrescendo systolic murmur is usually present at the high left sternal border and there is usually a short medium pitched mid-diastolic murmur at the low left sternal border. These murmurs are caused by increased flow across the pulmonic and tricuspid valves, respectively, and may not be present in cases with severe pulmonary venous obstruction and low pulmonary blood flow. A continuous hum, almost always soft and subtle, may be heard over the anomalous channel; at the high left sternal border with return to the left innominate (Fig. 8.2), at the high right sternal border with return to the right superior vena cava and over the low left or right sternal border with return to the coronary sinus (Zuberbuhler et al, 1975). The hum indicates a gradient within the anomalous channel but not necessarily organic obstruction, since the gradient may be related to large flow with no discrete obstruction demonstrable by cineangiography or post mortem examination. The hum may have late systolic accentuation and tends to vary with the changes in intrathoracic pressure occasioned by straining. Rarely, the venous hum may be very loud and have an associated thrill (Chia et al, 1974).

Differential diagnosis

Total anomalous pulmonary venous connection should be suspected in any cyanotic infant with an audibly split second heart sound, especially if there is a low left sternal border diastolic murmur or a continuous hum over the precordium. In the occasional child who survives infancy without severe symptoms and who is not obviously cyanotic, a systolic murmur at the high left sternal border, a mid-diastolic murmur at the low left sternal border and a widely or even fixedly split second heart sound may mimic an uncomplicated interatrial septal defect. There is usually at least faint cyanosis, however, which suggests the correct diagnosis. A continuous venous hum or 'roar' over the anomalous channel is almost pathognomonic if recognized.

PARTIAL ANOMALOUS PULMONARY VENOUS RETURN

Partial anomalous pulmonary venous return is rarely isolated, usually accompanying an interatrial septal defect, and the physical findings are those of the interatrial communication.

REFERENCES

Chia B, Tan N, Tan L K A 1974 Total anomalous pulmonary venous drainage: case presenting with prominent right supraclavicular thrill and loud continuous murmur. American Journal of Cardiology 34: 850

Delisle G, Ando M, Calder A L, Zuberbuhler J R, Rochenmacher S, Alday L E, Mangini O, Van Praagh S, Van Praagh R 1976 Total anomalous pulmonary venous connection. American Heart Journal 91: 99

Gathman G E, Nadas A S 1970 Total anomalous pulmonary venous connection. Circulation 42: 143

Hastreiter A R, Paul M H, Molthan M E, Miller R A 1962 Total anomalous pulmonary venous connection with severe pulmonary venous obstruction. Circulation 25: 916

Zuberbuhler J R, Lenox C C, Park S C, Neches W H 1975 Continuous murmurs in the newborn. Physiologic principles of heart sounds and murmurs. American Heart Association Monograph 46. American Heart Association, New York, p 209

9

Coarctation of the aorta

The anomaly

In coarctation of the aorta the narrowing is usually at the junction of the aortic arch and the descending aorta, but may rarely be more distal in the thoracic or even in the abdominal aorta. In typical coarctation there is infolding of the posterior aortic wall at the site of obstruction, apparent internally as a well developed transverse ridge. Coarctation has been classified according to its supposed relationship to the ductus arteriosus, being either preductal, juxtaductal, or postductal. In reality, the maximal narrowing is almost always *at* the junction of the ductus arteriosus and the aorta (Fig. 9.1), although the aortic arch proximal to this point can display varying degrees of hypoplasia as well.

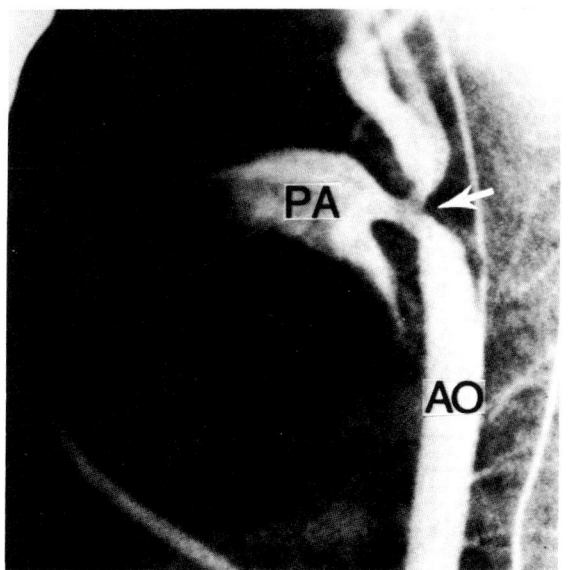

Fig. 9.1 Coarctation of the aorta. Cineangiogram showing the close proximity of the coarctation (arrow) and the ductus arteriosus.

Coarctation of the aorta may occur as an isolated entity, or there may be associated cardiac or vascular anomalies. The most common of these is a bicuspid aortic valve, variously estimated to be present in from 25 percent (Tawes et al, 1969) to 85 percent (Edwards et al, 1965) of cases of coarctation. Mitral valve anomalies, patent ductus arteriosus, ventricular septal defect and aortic stenosis are other relatively commonly associated anomalies. Coarctation is a frequent accompaniment to Turner's syndrome.

Clinical course

In some individuals coarctation of the aorta produces no symptoms in infancy or childhood and is diagnosed only when hypertension or pulse asymmetry is discovered on routine physical examination. In others, especially those with associated intracardiac anomalies, coarctation results in congestive heart failure in early infancy. Still others with coarctation suffer a cerebral vascular accident as a result of an associated intracranial aneurysm. Other complications include infectious endocarditis and rupture of the aorta.

Physical findings

General

The essence of coarctation of the aorta is obstruction, and the most important physical findings are related directly to that obstruction or to the collateral circulation which develops around it. The most common finding is a discrepancy in pulse amplitude and in blood pressure above and below the coarctation, and if lower pressure and weaker pulses are present in the legs than in the arms, a firm clinical diagnosis of coarctation is justified. Leg pulses may be delayed as well as attenuated (Fig. 9.2); this phenomenon is best appreciated by palpating the right brachial or axillary pulse and a femoral pulse simultaneously. Occasionally, femoral pulses are delayed but only slightly diminished, probably because unusually well developed collateral arteries transmit a relatively undamped but delayed pulse wave.

The right subclavian artery nearly always arises proximal to a coarctation of the aorta, but the origin of the left subclavian artery is more variable. If it arises proximal to the coarctation there will be symmetrical pulses and blood pressure in the two arms. If the left subclavian arises at the coarctation pulses and blood pressure will be lower in the left arm than in the right and may approximate those in the legs. The rare combination of a coarctation involving the left subclavian artery and a retroesophageal right subclavian artery arising distally beyond the coarctation results in decreased blood pressures in all four extremities, carotid pulses remaining strong. (Another rare anomaly which can produce this particular type of pulse asymmetry is a large intracranial arteriovenous fistula, discussed in Ch. 20.) Suprasternal notch pulsations are often quite strong in patients with coarctation and are transmitted from the aortic arch and brachiocephalic arteries. A suprasternal notch thrill is not uncommon.

Elevation of arm blood pressure is common in coarctation of the aorta, and blood pressure should always be measured in both arms and in a leg. Systolic pressure is usually elevated out of proportion to diastolic, resulting in a wide pulse pressure and full pulses in arteries arising above the obstruction. The upper extremity pulse pressure tends to widen with increasing age, and both pulse pressure and the difference in arm and leg blood pressure tends to increase with exercise (Dahlback et al, 1964).

The jugular venous pulse is normal. The apical impulse may be forceful and sustained if there is systemic arterial hypertension, and a prominent left sternal border systolic lift may be present in patients with right ventricular overload. Such overload may occur when left ventricular dysfunction causes a large left to right shunt across an interatrial communication.

Most of the collateral flow around a coarctation arises from the subclavian arteries, passes through periscapular and internal mammary arteries, and eventually rejoins the distal aorta via the intercostals. These collateral channels may be seen, felt and heard. In older children enlarged periscapular and intercostal arteries can often be palpated over the posterior thoracic wall. They may be located by lightly passing a hand over the interscapular and subscapular areas and then further defined using the tips of the fingers for palpation. Collaterals can often be seen in relief if viewed in an oblique light from behind and to one side. Enlarged epigastric arteries can occasionally be seen and felt running vertically down the abdominal wall near the lateral border of the rectus abdominis muscle.

Auscultation

Heart sounds. The first and second heart sounds are normal in a patient with an uncomplicated coarctation, but the aortic component of the second heart sound may be loud if there is severe systemic hypertension. A third heart sound is rarely prominent unless there is congestive heart failure. A fourth heart sound may be present if there is severe systemic hypertension. An apical early systolic ejection sound is very common (Fig. 9.3), usually originating at a bicuspid aortic valve and less commonly in a dilated ascending aorta.

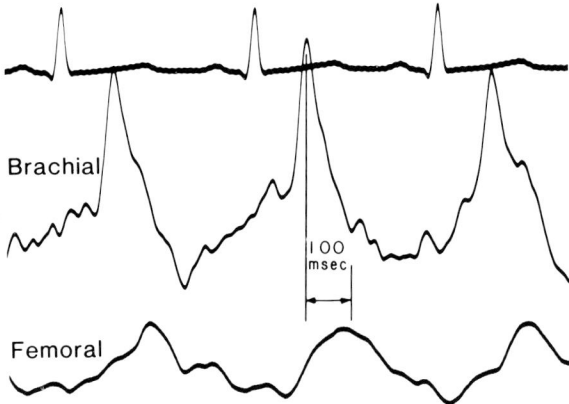

Fig. 9.2 Simultaneous brachial and femoral arterial pulse tracings of a child with coarctation. The femoral pulse is slow rising and delayed about 100 msec.

COARCTATION OF THE AORTA 61

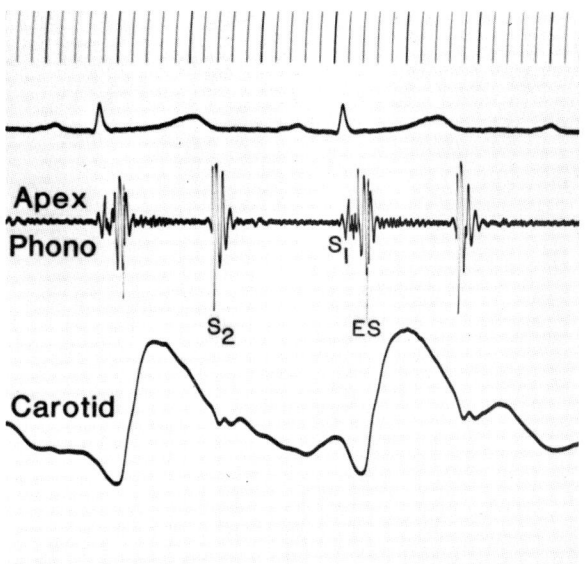

Fig. 9.3 Apex phonocardiogram showing prominent early systolic ejection sound in a child with coarctation of the aorta.

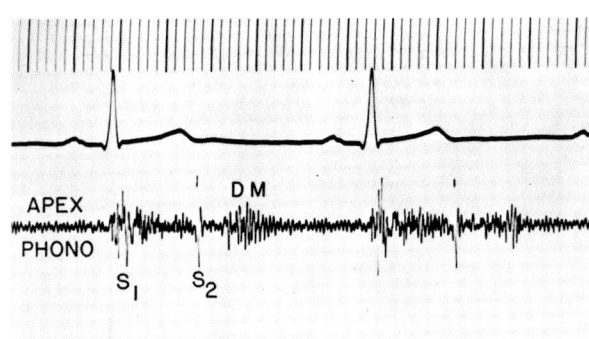

Fig. 9.5 Apex phonocardiogram in a child with coarctation of the aorta. There is a prominent mid diastolic murmur (DM) but no presystolic accentuation. (Pulmonary artery wedge pressure was normal in this child.)

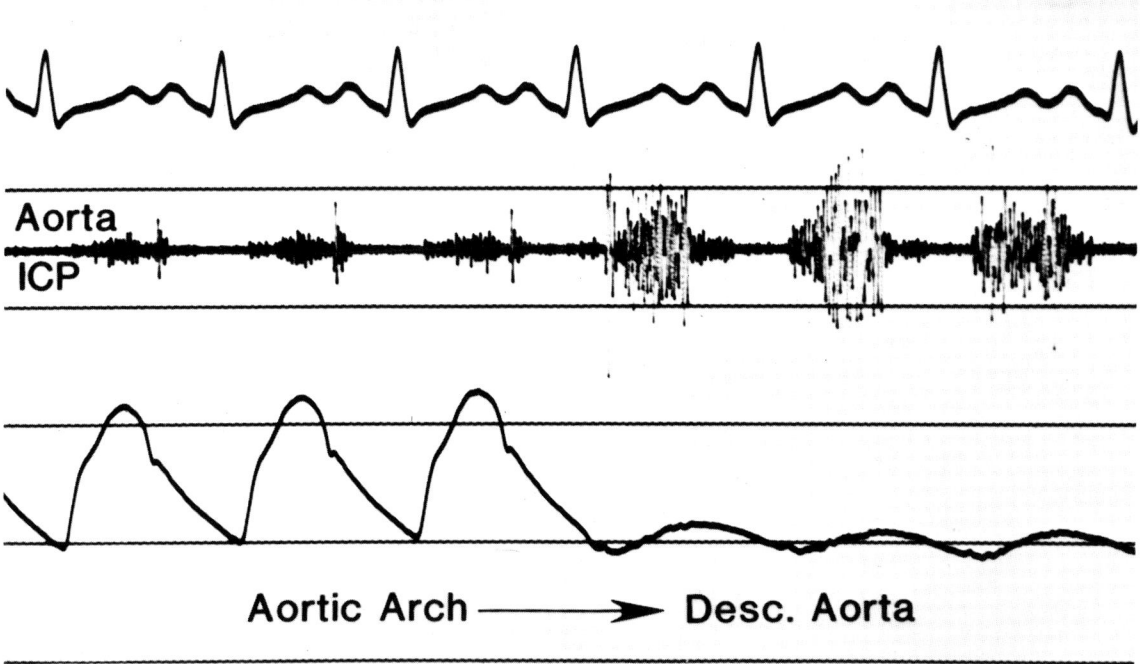

Fig. 9.4 Sound and pressure recording during pullback of a micromanometer tipped catheter from the aortic arch to the descending aorta. There is a loud murmur distal to the coarctation.

Murmurs. In an individual with coarctation of the aorta, a high right sternal border systolic murmur likely arises at a bicuspid aortic valve. The large subclavian arterial flow commonly present in coarctation may produce another systolic murmur, which is maximal under the clavicles and out toward the shoulders. Large internal mammary arterial flow may generate a systolic murmur heard down the sternal borders. Long systolic or even continuous murmurs over the back arise in collateral arteries, or, if localized to the left paraspinal area, may originate at the coarctation itself (Fig. 9.4) (Spencer et al, 1958). A continuous murmur localized to the high left sternal border suggests an associated patent ductus arteriosus.

Diastolic murmurs may be generated by the aortic and mitral valve anomalies which commonly accompany coarctation. Probably the most common diastolic murmur is a mid diastolic apical rumble (Fig. 9.5). It seems certain that this murmur originates at the mitral valve, since several reports have detailed anomalies of the mitral apparatus which might result in such a murmur (Becker et al, 1970; Easthope et al, 1969; Rosenquist, 1974). Demonstrable mitral stenosis is, however, less common than the murmur itself. A high pitched decrescendo diastolic murmur at the mid left sternal border indicates aortic regurgitation, usually associated with a bicuspid aortic valve.

Early infancy

In infancy, the physical findings associated with coarctation of the aorta may differ. Collateral arteries may be heard but are rarely visible or palpable. In an occasional newborn with coarctation the femoral pulses are normal at birth and then become attenuated or disappear. The explanation usually given is that the aortic end of the ductus, while patent, acts as a conduit around the coarctation, and when the ductus closes the coarctation seems more severe (Elseed et al, 1974; Rudolph et al, 1972). Alternatively, contraction of ductal tissue present in the wall of the aorta near the ductus may exaggerate the severity of the coarctation (Ho & Anderson, 1979). Contraction of aortic ductal tissue could also explain the variable femoral pulses which are occasionally noted in a newborn whose ductus has already closed.

Congestive heart failure is more common in the infant than the older child, especially if there are associated anomalies. The relatively high incidence of congestive heart failure in early infancy may be due to an exaggeration of the workload normally put on the left ventricle during the transition from fetal to adult circulatory patterns, as well as to the extra stress imposed by the associated anomalies. Congestive heart failure may improve as the left ventricle adapts to its work load and as more adequate collateral arteries develop.

Associated anomalies

Associated anomalies are common and alter the physical findings in various ways. If an associated patent ductus arteriosus communicates freely with the descending aorta beyond a severe coarctation, the direction of blood flow in the ductus will depend upon the degree of pulmonary hypertension. If pulmonary artery pressure is sufficiently high a right to left shunt will occur and may be large enough to produce differential cyanosis, with the right arm, the lips and upper trunk being pink and the legs and lower trunk blue. The skin color of the left arm is variable, depending upon the site of origin of the left subclavian artery. A pansystolic murmur at the mid or low left sternal border signals the presence of a ventricular septal defect, while a loud systolic ejection murmur at the high right sternal border indicates obstruction at the aortic valve. A long systolic murmur at the apex suggests mitral regurgitation but may also originate in collateral arteries. (If a similar murmur is present over the corresponding area of the right hemithorax, collateral arterial origin of the murmur is more likely.) An interatrial septal defect is uncommon in older children with coarctation of the aorta, but a left to right shunt at atrial level may complicate coarctation in early infancy. Atrial shunting can be of large magnitude, being exaggerated by the elevated left ventricular diastolic pressure commonly present in a neonate with severe coarctation. Atrial shunting should be suspected if the second heart sound is prominently split, especially if there is a mid-diastolic murmur at the low left sternal border.

REFERENCES

Becker A E, Becker M J, Edwards J E 1970 Anomalies associated with coarctation of the aorta. Circulation 41: 1067

Dahlback O, Dahn I, Westling H 1964 Hemodynamic observation in coarctation of the aorta with special reference to the blood pressure above and below the stenosis at rest and during exercise. Scandinavian Journal of Clinical Laboratory Investigation 16: 339

Easthope R N, Tawes R L, Bonham-Carter R E, Aberdeen E, Waterston D J 1969 Congenital mitral valve disease associated with coarctation of the aorta. American Heart Journal 77: 743

Edwards J E, Carey L S, Newfeld H N, Lester R G 1965 Congenital heart disease, vol. 2. Saunders, Philadelphia, p 684

Elseed A M, Shinebourne E A, Paneth M 1974 Manifestation of juxtaductal coarctation after surgical ligation of persistent ductus arteriosus in infancy. British Heart Journal 36: 687

Ho S Y, Anderson R H 1978 Coarctation, tubular hypoplasia, and the ductus arteriosus: histological study of 35 specimens. British Heart Journal 41: 268

Rosenquist G C 1974 Congenital mitral valve disease associated with coarctation of the aorta: a spectrum that includes parachute deformity of the mitral valve. Circulation 49: 985

Rudolph A M, Heymann M A, Spitznas U 1972 Hemodynamic considerations in the development of narrowing of the aorta. American Journal of Cardiology 30: 514

Spencer M P, Johnston F R, Meredith J H 1958 The origin and interpretation of murmurs in coarctation of the aorta. American Heart Journal 56: 722

Tawes R L Jr, Berry C L, Aberdeen E 1969 Congenital bicuspid aortic valves associated with coarctation of the aorta in children. British Heart Journal 31: 127

10

Pulmonic stenosis with intact ventricular septum

General

Obstruction to right ventricular outflow may be complete or incomplete, may be isolated or associated with a ventricular septal defect, and may be valvar, supravalvar or subvalvar in location. Only isolated incomplete obstruction will be considered here; isolated complete obstruction (pulmonary atresia with intact ventricular septum) is dealt with in Chapter 17 and complete and incomplete obstruction associated with a ventricular septal defect (tetralogy of Fallot) in Chapter 18.

Clinical course

The clinical course of patients with pulmonic stenosis is determined by the severity of obstruction. Unless stenosis is very severe, symptoms are absent in infancy and childhood, exercise tolerance is good and congestive failure is a very late event. Cyanosis may occur in patients with pulmonic stenosis and an intact ventricular septum, but only if there is an interatrial communication and if the right ventricle becomes sufficiently hypertrophic and 'stiff' to impede right atrial emptying. This usually occurs only when right ventricular pressure is suprasystemic — and not necessarily even then. It must be emphasized that right ventricular *diastolic* pressure is the prime determinant of right to left atrial shunting since the right atrium 'sees' the right ventricle only in diastole. Relative *systolic* pressures in the two ventricles determine ventricular shunting if there is an interventricular communication, as in tetralogy of Fallot.

Physical findings

Certain physical findings are common to all varieties of pulmonic stenosis while others differ with the locus of the obstruction. A systolic murmur, for instance, is present in virtually all patients with right ventricular outflow obstruction but its characteristics vary with the location of the obstruction and even more importantly, with its severity. The loudness, duration, and shape of the murmur of pulmonic stenosis are, in fact, very useful clinical indicators of the degree of obstruction, as is the intensity of the pulmonic component of the second heart sound. Signs of right ventricular hyperactivity should be sought in patients with pulmonic stenosis, but a prominent right ventricular lift is the exception in infants and children with 'isolated' right ventricular outflow obstruction, even if it is quite severe. (A lift is more likely to be prominent if there is both pressure *and* volume overload of the right ventricle.) If right ventricular hypertrophy becomes sufficiently marked, diastolic compliance lessens and right atrial contractions become more vigorous and may be evident as presystolic jugular venous or hepatic pulsations. Clinical evidence of forceful right atrial contractions are very uncommon in infants or children with pulmonic stenosis, however.

Associated anomalies

Right ventricular outflow tract obstruction may be associated with certain syndromes with distinctive extracardiac physical findings. Valvar pulmonic stenosis with dysplastic cusps is the most common cardiac defect found in Noonan's syndrome (Noonan, 1968). In this syndrome short stature, a relatively short neck, shield chest with wide spaced nipples, hypertelorism, ptosis and mental retardation are characteristic findings. Pulmonary artery stenosis may be part of the maternal rubella syndrome, along with deafness, cataracts and mental retardation (Venables, 1965). Pulmonary artery stenosis is also found in association with supravalvar aortic stenosis (Beuren et al, 1964).

VALVAR PULMONIC STENOSIS

The anomaly

Valvar pulmonic stenosis is by far the most common variety of right ventricular outflow tract obstruction. It usually consists of partial and symmetrical fusion of all three valve commissures, with variable thickening of the pulmonary cusps. The valve is usually mobile and forms a convex dome into the main pulmonary artery during systole (Fig. 10.1). Less commonly, the valve is dysplastic with little or no commissural fusion, the obstruction resulting from the marked thickening and immobility of the cusps.

Physical findings

Heart sounds. The pulmonic component of the second heart sound is of normal intensity with mild valvar pulmonic stenosis. With progressively more severe obstruction pulmonary artery pressure falls, and since pulmonary artery pressure is a major determinant of the intensity of the pulmonic closure sound one expects a progressive attenuation of this sound as obstruction increases. In patients with very severe obstruction, right ventricular mechanical systole becomes prolonged. With lower pulmonary artery pressure pulmonic closure occurs later on the descending limb of the right ventricular pressure curve. Both phenomena cause the closure sound to occur later in the cardiac cycle and, as a consequence, width of splitting of the second heart sound increases. It must be noted, however, that some patients with mild to moderate pulmonic stenosis have rather wide splitting of the second heart sound (Vogelpoel & Schrire, 1960) (Fig. 10.2). In such patients the delay in the pulmonic closure sound is due not to prolonged right ventricular mechanical systole but to increased capacitance of the pulmonary vascular bed. In such a 'loose' system, the momentum of the right ventricular stroke output causes forward flow into the pulmonary artery to continue even after right ventricular pressure has begun to fall, and in the face of a negative pressure gradient. Simultaneous high fidelity pressure recordings in the right ventricle and pulmonary artery show a separation of the descending limbs of the two pressure curves. The dicrotic notch of the pulmonary artery pressure curve 'hangs out' beyond the right ventricular pressure curve and accounts for the delay in the pulmonic closure sound (Shaver et al, 1975).

In general the loudness of the pulmonic closure sound is a better indicator of severity than is the width of splitting. If the second heart sound is widely split but the second component is well preserved, pulmonic stenosis is almost certainly mild. If the second sound is soft and single or inaudible at the high left sternal border, pulmonic stenosis is likely to be quite severe.

A prominent third heart sound is not a feature of valvar pulmonic stenosis. An audible fourth heart sound may be present in an adult with severe stenosis (Vogelpoel & Schrire, 1960) but is a very unusual finding in an infant or child with any degree of severity of pulmonic stenosis.

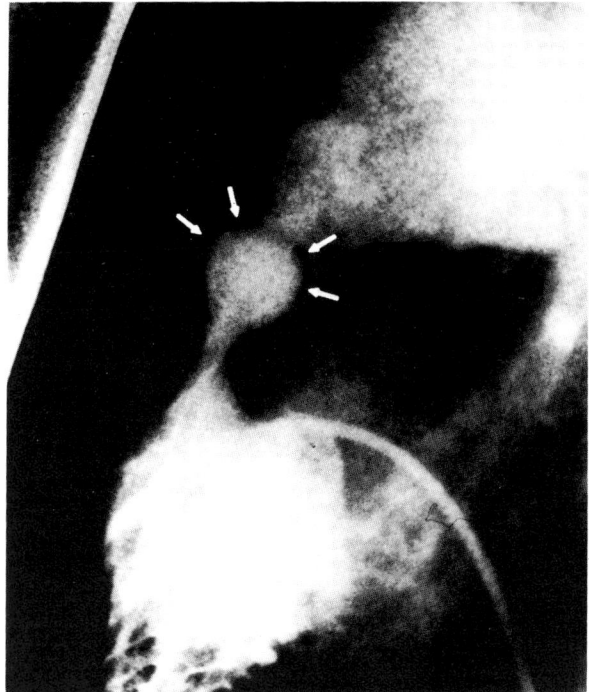

Fig. 10.1 Cineangiogram showing doming of the pulmonic valve (arrows) in a child with valvar pulmonic stenosis.

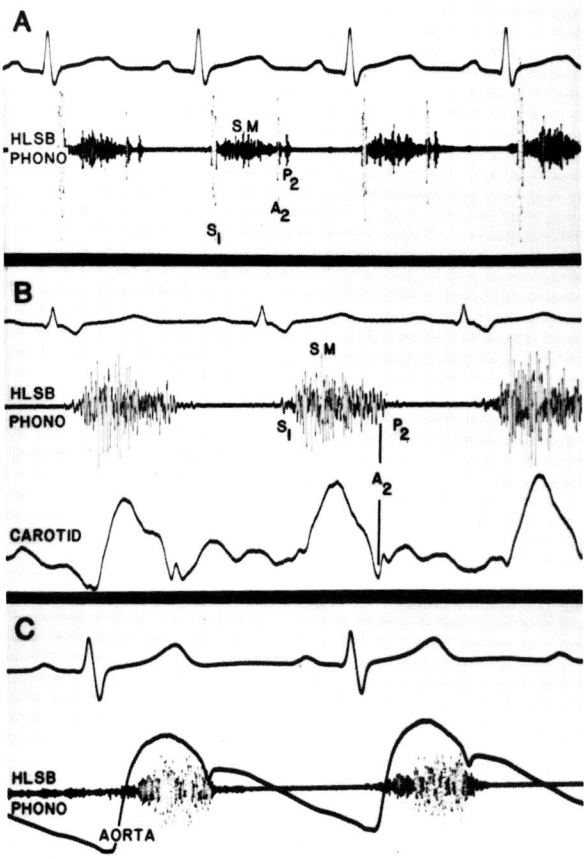

Fig. 10.2 High left sternal border phonocardiograms in children with valvar pulmonic stenosis of varying severity. A. Mild stenosis. The murmur is soft, peaks early and ends before aortic closure (A_2). The second sound is widely split and the pulmonic component well preserved. B. Moderately severe stenosis. The murmur is loud and extends to aortic closure. The pulmonic closure sound is soft. C. Severe stenosis. The murmur is 'kite shaped' and extends beyond aortic closure. Pulmonic closure is not audible or recordable.

An early systolic ejection sound (click) is heard in all but the most severe valvar stenosis and occurs as the doming pulmonic valve reaches the zenith of its incursion into the pulmonary artery (Figs. 10.1, 10.3). The sound is high pitched and clicking and is maximal at the high left sternal border. It varies strikingly with respiration, being louder with expiration and softer or even inaudible with inspiration (Fig. 10.4). The respiratory variability of the ejection sound is usually explained by its dependence on the position of the valve at the beginning of mechanical systole (Hultgren et al, 1969). Systemic venous return increases with inspiration and during end diastole right ventricular pressure may equal or exceed pulmonary artery pressure, causing the pulmonic valve to float up into the pulmonary artery before ventricular systole commences (Weyman et al, 1974). There is then no sudden tensing or 'doming' of the pulmonic valve with right ventricular systole and no ejection sound is generated. In contrast, systemic venous return decreases with expiration and the pulmonic valve does not open until the onset of ventricular systole. The sudden doming of the pulmonic valve with the rapid rise in right ventricular pressure then produces an early systolic ejection sound.

It may be somewhat difficult to distinguish an ejection sound from the first heart sound. With the very low pulmonary artery pressure of severe pulmonic stenosis, for example, the ejection sound occurs early in systole and may blend with the first heart sound (Gamboa et al, 1964). If the first heart sound is not audible at the high left sternal border in a patient with valvar pulmonic stenosis, only the ejection sound may be heard near the onset of ventricular systole. The high pitch of the sound and its respiratory variation serve to identify it, however, and simultaneous high left sternal border and apex phonocardiograms usually show the ejection sound occurring slightly later than the apical first heart sound. With very severe pulmonic stenosis there is often no ejection sound, since transmission of a large right atrial 'A' wave to the right ventricle causes presystolic opening of the pulmonic valve and little further doming occurs during ventricular systole. A pulmonic ejection sound is not present with the dysplastic variety of valvar stenosis.

Murmurs. The systolic murmur of valvar pulmonic stenosis is maximal in the second intercostal space at the left sternal border. The murmur varies in shape, duration and, to a lesser degree, intensity as one traverses the spectrum of severity of obstruction (Fig. 10.2). The murmur is soft with very mild obstruction and loud with moderate or severe stenosis. The murmur of mild obstruction is short and peaks before mid systole. With increasing obstruction the murmur lengthens and peaks later in systole. With very severe obstruction the murmur is 'kite' shaped, peaking in late systole,

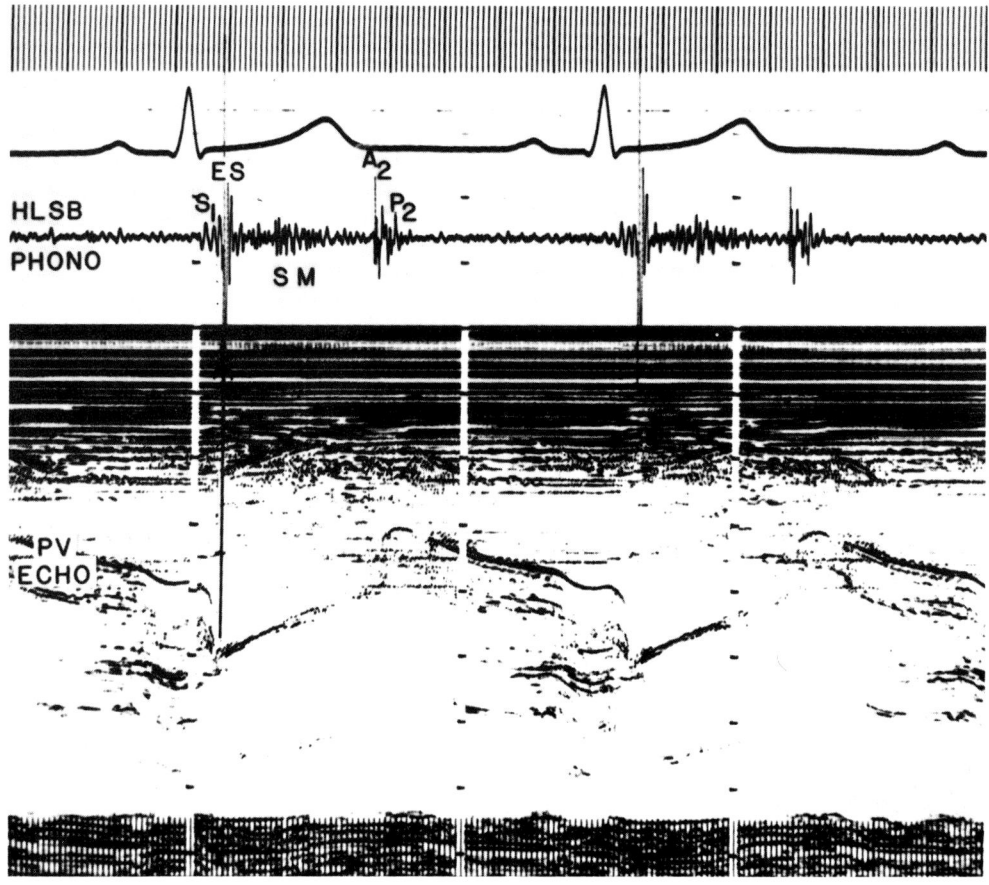

Fig. 10.3. High left sternal border phonocardiogram and pulmonic valve echocardiogram in a child with valvar pulmonic stenosis. The prominent early systolic ejection sound (ES) occurs as the pulmonic valve leaflet opens maximally.

and so prolonged that it extends beyond and often obscures the aortic closure sound (Vogelpoel & Schrire, 1960). This lengthening of the murmur can be related both to an increased duration of right ventricular mechanical systole and to prolongation of the ejection phase until near the end of systole, with late crossover of right ventricular and pulmonary arterial pressures.

The neonate

In the neonate, critical pulmonic stenosis presents a very different clinical picture. If obstruction is extreme the entity closely resembles pulmonary atresia with intact ventricular septum. Cyanosis is the rule and results from right to left shunting at atrial level. Congestive heart failure may also occur.

The high left sternal border systolic murmur of critical pulmonic stenosis is soft and high pitched, since flow across the pulmonic valve is quite reduced. The continuous murmur of a patent ductus arteriosus may be present, and a high pitched blowing systolic murmur at the low left sternal border indicates associated tricuspid regurgitation. The prognosis of this variety of stenosis is nil unless the obstruction can be surgically relieved.

SUBVALVAR PULMONIC STENOSIS

The anomaly

Subvalvar pulmonic stenosis is less common than valvar obstruction. Infundibular stenosis usually is associated with a ventricular septal defect

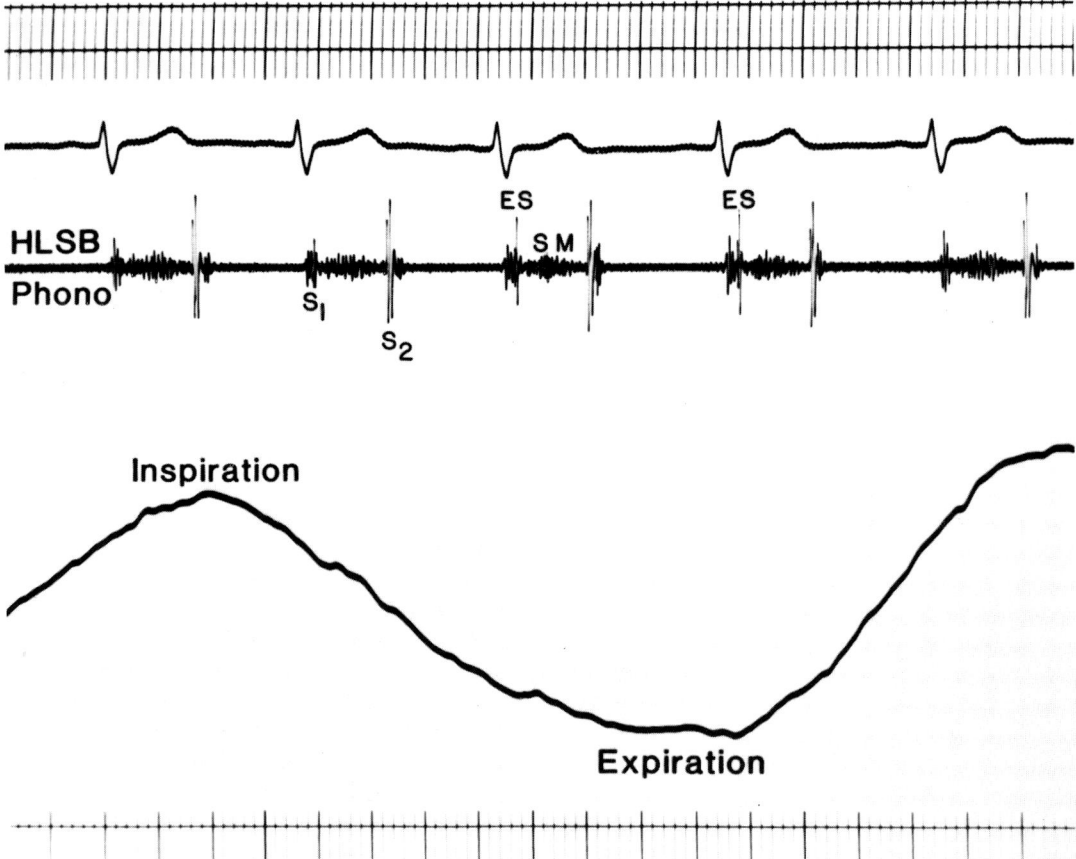

Fig. 10.4 High left sternal border phonocardiogram showing variation of an early systolic ejection sound (ES) with respiration.

(tetralogy of Fallot); isolated infundibular obstruction is not common. Subvalvar pulmonic stenosis may also be proximal to the infundibulum and is then caused by an enlarged moderator band or an anomalous muscle bundle. The obstructing muscle mass sometimes forms a muscular partition which partially divides the right ventricle (double chamber right ventricle).

Physical findings

An early systolic ejection sound is not present with subvalvar pulmonic stenosis and its absence helps to distinguish the subvalvar from the valvar variety of obstruction. The pulmonic closure sound may be normal, soft, or inaudible, depending upon the severity of the obstruction. The systolic murmur and thrill of subvalvar pulmonic stenosis are lower along the left sternal border than those of valvar obstruction and in the infundibular variety are maximal in the third or even fourth left intercostal space. The murmur of subinfundibular stenosis is usually very loud, sometimes Grade VI, and both the thrill and murmur have a 'superficial' quality, seeming to be just beneath the skin. This murmur may be crescendo–descrescendo (Fig. 10.5), or may be holosystolic and plateau shaped and be indistinguishable from the murmur of a ventricular septal defect (Fig. 10.6). The clinical resemblance of subinfundibular pulmonic stenosis to a ventricular septal defect is heightened by the location of the murmur (usually in the fourth or fifth intercostal space) and cardiac catheterization may be required to differentiate the two entities.

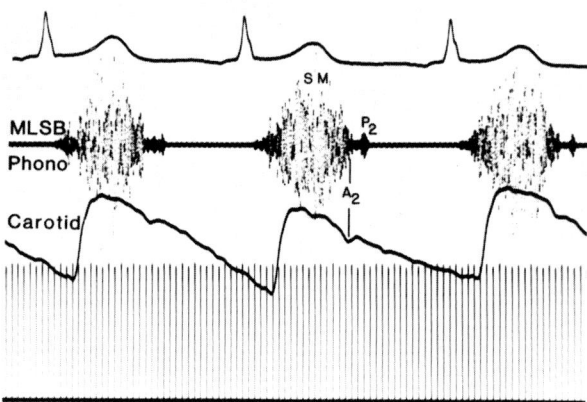

Fig. 10.5 Phonocardiogram and carotid pulse tracing in a child with sub-infundibular pulmonic stenosis. The murmur is crescendo–decrescendo and extends to aortic closure, as indicated by the dicrotic notch of the pulse tracing.

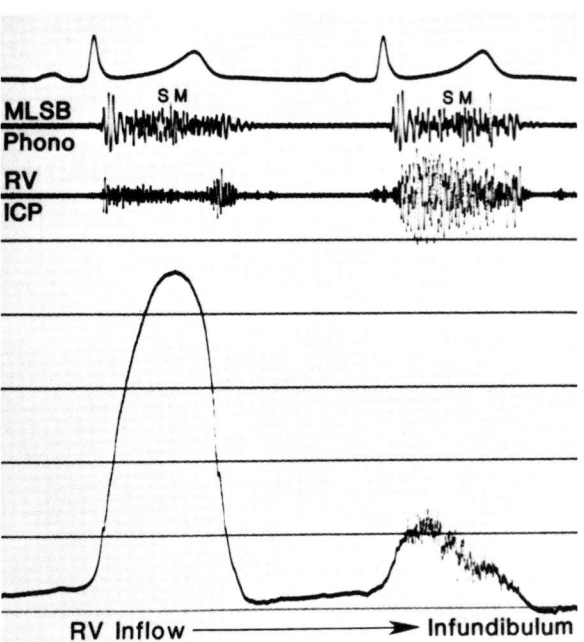

Fig. 10.6 Child with subinfundibular pulmonic stenosis. The mid left sternal border phonocardiogram shows a plateau shaped holosystolic murmur. The intracardiac phonocardiogram (RV ICP) shows the murmur to be louder beyond the obstruction.

SUPRAVALVAR PULMONIC STENOSIS

The anomaly

Supravalvar pulmonic stenosis most commonly consists of multiple areas of narrowing in the pulmonary arterial tree. Occasionally the obstruction is localized in the proximal right and/or left pulmonary arteries (Franch & Gay, 1963). A membranous stenosis in the main pulmonary artery has been described but is quite rare.

Physical findings

The pulmonic closure sound is usually normal and does not consistently correlate with the severity of supravalvar obstruction. There is normal respiratory variation of splitting of the second heart sound (Perloff & Lebauer, 1969). An ejection sound is not present with pure supravalvar pulmonic stenosis. If there are multiple areas of stenosis the resulting murmur is systolic and well heard at the base, in the axillae and across the back, being nearly as loud over the posterior thorax as the anterior. The lack of a diastolic component is explained by the characteristically low diastolic pressure in the main pulmonary artery (Fig. 10.7). In this entity the main pulmonary artery is small and its wall relatively inelastic; both features contribute to a rapid diastolic fall in main pulmonary artery pressure. Only when arterial stenosis is localized and the remainder of the pulmonary arterial tree normal is diastolic pressure in the proximal pulmonary artery high enough to cause a continuous murmur. The systolic murmur of pulmonary artery stenosis is not uncommon in newborns, particularly prematures, and probably results from relative hypoplasia of the right and left pulmonary arteries and from their more acute angle of origin from the main pulmonary artery in this age group (Danilowicz et al, 1972).

Surgical banding of the pulmonary artery results in iatrogenic pulmonary artery stenosis. The resulting systolic murmur is maximal at the high left sternal border and there is good radiation to the axillae and back. The loudness of the murmur, width of splitting of the second heart sound and the intensity of the pulmonic closure sound are variable and are not reliable guides to the effectiveness of the pulmonary band.

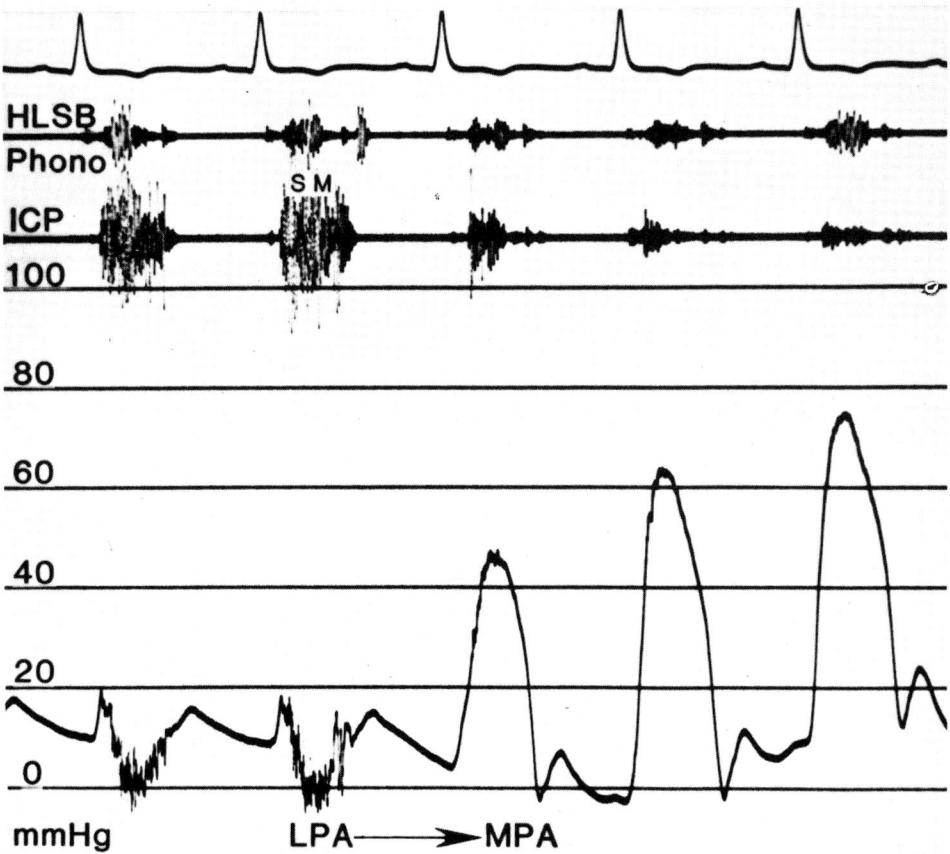

Fig. 10.7 Child with pulmonary artery stenosis. The murmur is only systolic and is louder distal to the obstruction (ICP). Note the low diastolic pressure and wide pulse pressure in the main pulmonary artery.

REFERENCES

Beuren A J, Schulze C, Eberle P, Harmjanz D, Apitz J 1964 The syndrome of supravalvar aortic stenosis, peripheral pulmonary stenosis, mental retardation and similar facial appearance. American Journal of Cardiology 13: 471

Danilowicz D A, Rudolph A M, Hoffman J I E, Heymann M 1972 Physiologic pressure differences between main and branch pulmonary arteries in infants. Circulation 45: 410

Franch R H, Gay B B Jr 1963 Congenital stenosis of the pulmonary artery branches. American Journal of Medicine 35: 512

Gamboa R, Hugenholtz P G 1964 Accuracy of the phonocardiogram in assessing severity of aortic and pulmonic stenosis. Circulation 30: 35

Hultgren H N, Reeve R, Cohn K, McLeod R 1969 The ejection click of valvular pulmonic stenosis. Circulation 40: 631

Noonan J A 1968 Hypertelorism with Turner phenotype: a new syndrome with associated congenital heart disease. American Journal of Diseases of Children 116: 373

Perloff J K, Lebauer E J 1969 Auscultatory and phonocardiographic manifestations of isolated stenosis of the pulmonary artery and its branches. British Heart Journal 31: 314

Shaver J A, O'Toole J D, Curtiss E I, Thompson M E, Reddy P S, Leon D F 1975 Second heart sound: the role of altered greater and lesser circulation. Physiologic principles of heart sounds and murmurs. American Heart Association Monograph 46. The American Heart Association, New York, p 58

Venables A W 1965 The syndrome of pulmonary stenosis complicating maternal rubella. British Heart Journal 27: 49

Vogelpoel L, Schrire V 1960 Auscultatory and phonocardiographic assessment of pulmonary stenosis with intact ventricular septum. Circulation 22: 55

Weyman A E, Dillon J C, Feigenbaum H, Chang S 1974 Echocardiographic patterns of pulmonary valve motion in valvular pulmonary stenosis. American Journal of Cardiology 35: 644

11

Congenital pulmonic regurgitation

The anomaly

Congenital pulmonic regurgitation may be associated with idiopathic dilatation of the pulmonary artery (Brayshaw & Perloff, 1962) or can be due to a variety of anatomic abnormalities of one or more pulmonary valve cusps, ranging from dysplasia to complete absence. It may be isolated or associated with other cardiac anomalies, the most common combination being absence of the pulmonic valve, a stenotic pulmonary annulus and a ventricular septal defect (tetralogy of Fallot with absent pulmonic valve). Congenital pulmonic regurgitation is usually associated with normal or lower than normal pressure in the pulmonary artery. Acquired pulmonic regurgitation, on the other hand, is usually secondary to long standing elevation of pulmonary artery pressure although occasionally it is caused by infectious endocarditis, most commonly due to 'main-line' drug abuse.

Clinical course

The clinical course and physical findings in individuals with pulmonic regurgitation are quite variable, depending on whether the regurgitation is due to pulmonary hypertension or is congenital, and whether it is isolated or occurs in combination with other hemodynamically significant cardiac anomalies. Only the congenital variety will be considered here, acquired hypertensive pulmonic regurgitation being dealt with in Chapter 22.

Isolated pulmonic regurgitation is usually a benign lesion (Holmes et al, 1968). Even patients with severe regurgitation may never develop cardiac symptoms since the right ventricle seems able to tolerate a volume overload for an extended period of time (Rushmer, 1958). The high pulmonary artery pressure present in utero and for a short while after birth increases the severity of regurgitation (Smith et al, 1959), and an occasional patient with isolated pulmonic regurgitation shows signs of failure at birth or in the neonatal period. Symptoms then abate as pulmonary artery pressure falls. Congestive heart failure occurs later in life in some patients with isolated congenital pulmonic regurgitation. In such patients failure may be related either to chronic pulmonary disease or to left ventricular dysfunction, either of which tends to raise pulmonary artery pressure and to increase the severity of regurgitation.

The usual benign course of patients with isolated pulmonic regurgitation is in striking contrast to that of patients with an absent valve and tetralogy of Fallot, who frequently develop congestive heart failure or signs of bronchial obstruction in early infancy (Lakier et al, 1974). In the latter entity the bronchial obstruction, which may be severe and life threatening, is due to the huge proximal right and left pulmonary arteries which are a characteristic finding. Although the narrow annulus constitutes pulmonic stenosis, the obstruction is usually mild in infancy and most such infants are not cyanotic. Cyanosis may develop in childhood or adolescence as the stenosis becomes more severe.

Physical findings

General
Unless there is congestive heart failure, the jugular venous pulse, arterial pulse and blood pressure are normal in patients with congenital pulmonic regurgitation. The abnormal physical findings which do occur are related to the regurgitation

itself or to the consequent increase in right ventricular stroke volume. If the regurgitation is marked, the increase in right ventricular stroke volume causes a left parasternal lift. The lift may be striking in the newborn period, when elevated pulmonary artery pressure increases the severity of the regurgitation and also adds a pressure load to the already volume overloaded right ventricle (Fig. 11.1A). The right ventricular lift becomes less prominent over the first few days of life as pulmonary artery pressure falls (Fig. 11.1B). Since the right ventricle tends to be quite large in patients with congenital pulmonic regurgitation, the lift may extend well out toward the apex.

Auscultation

Heart sounds. The first heart sound is normal in patients with congenital pulmonic regurgitation. The aortic component of the second heart sound is also normal but the pulmonic component is variable. It may be absent if the valve cusps themselves are absent or badly deformed. If the pulmonic component is present, it tends to be delayed and the second heart sound to be widely split. Although the delay could be due to prolongation of right ventricular mechanical systole secondary to increased right ventricular stroke volume, it is more likely due to low impedance in

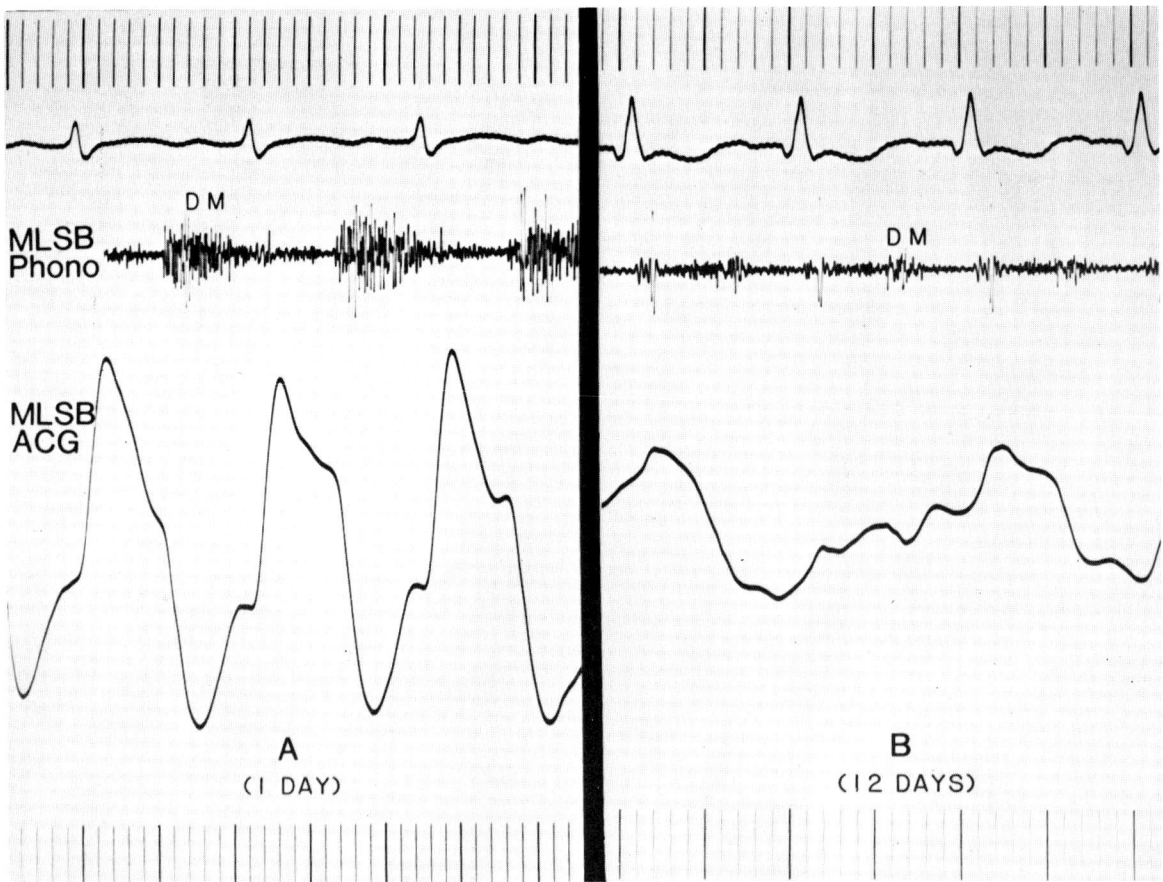

Fig. 11.1 Mid left sternal border phonocardiogram and pulse tracing (MLSB ACG) of an infant with isolated pulmonic regurgitation. A. At one day of age, there is a loud diastolic murmur and a prominent systolic lift. B. At twelve days of age, the diastolic murmur is much softer and the lift is less evident.

the dilated pulmonary artery with resultant 'hang out' of the pulmonary incisura (Ch. 3). In some patients with congenital pulmonic regurgitation there is persistent expiratory splitting, or even fixed splitting of the second heart sound. A third sound may be present but a fourth heart sound is not expected.

Murmurs. The auscultatory hallmark of normotensive pulmonic regurgitation is a medium to low pitched diastolic murmur which is loudest along the high and mid left sternal border (Holmes et al, 1968). The murmur is usually of Grade II or III intensity but may be louder and have an associated thrill. The murmur may begin with the second component of a split second heart sound but in most patients with congenital pulmonic regurgitation the pulmonic valve is either absent or so deformed as to be 'silent'. The murmur then begins at an interval after aortic valve closure. The murmur of normotensive pulmonic regurgitation is typically crescendo-decrescendo and ends well before the first heart sound (Fig. 11.2). It is characteristically louder in the recumbent than in the sitting or standing position and may show respiratory variation, being louder during inspiration. Since low pulmonary artery pressure ensures a low velocity of the regurgitant stream, the murmur is medium to low pitched. (The murmur is higher pitched in an occasional patient with congenital pulmonic regurgitation, and such patients usually have elevated pulmonary artery pressure (Nemickas et al, 1964). The shortness of the diastolic murmur of normotensive pulmonic regurgitation is a result of equalization of right ventricular and pulmonary arterial pressures well before the end of diastole. The late onset of the murmur, like the delayed pulmonic closure sound, is likely due to the capacious pulmonary artery and the consequent low impedance to right ventricular ejection.

The murmur of low pressure pulmonic regurgitation should not be confused with the murmur of aortic regurgitation. The latter is much higher pitched, begins with the aortic closure sound and tends to be longer. Unlike the murmur of pulmonic regurgitation, the diastolic murmur of aortic regurgitation is usually louder in the sitting than in the recumbent position. (The diastolic murmur of hypertensive pulmonic regurgitation cannot clinically be distinguished from the diastolic murmur of aortic regurgitation.)

Patients with isolated pulmonic regurgitation usually have a mid or high left sternal border crescendo-decrescendo systolic murmur, generated by rapid flow across the right ventricular outflow tract. The murmur is usually soft (Fig. 11.1) but may be Grade III or IV if the pulmonic regurgitation is severe and the right ventricular stroke volume sufficiently great. The systolic murmur is loud and usually has an accompanying thrill in patients with tetralogy of Fallot and absent pulmonic valve. The left sternal border to and fro murmur of pulmonic regurgitation and relative or organic pulmonic stenosis is quite distinctive and should suggest the diagnosis of congenital pulmonic regurgitation.

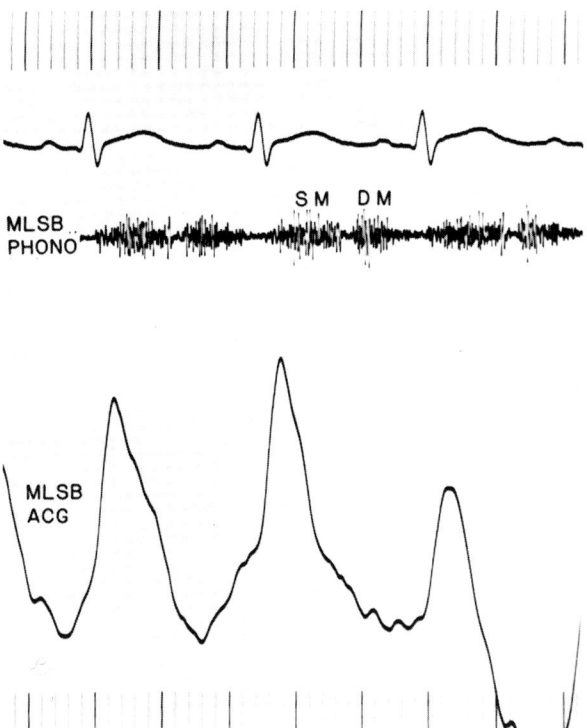

Fig. 11.2 Infant with absent pulmonic valve and tetralogy of Fallot. The mid left sternal border phonocardiogram shows a to and fro murmur. Both systolic and diastolic components are crescendo-decrescendo. The mid left sternal border pulse tracing (MLSB ACG) shows a prominent systolic lift.

REFERENCES

Brayshaw J R, Perloff J K 1962 Congenital pulmonary insufficiency complicating idiopathic dilatation of the pulmonary artery. American Journal of Cardiology 10: 282

Holmes J C, Fowler N O, and Kaplan S 1968 Pulmonary valvular insufficiency. American Journal of Medicine 44: 851

Lakier J B, Stangler P, Heymann M A, Hoffman J I E, Rudolph A M 1974 Tetralogy of Fallot with absent pulmonic valve: natural history and hemodynamic considerations. Circulation 50: 167

Nemickas R, Roberts J, Gunnar R M, Tobin J R Jr 1964 Isolated congenital pulmonic insufficiency. American Journal of Cardiology 14: 456

Rushmer R F 1958 Work of the heart. Modern Concepts of Cardiovascular Disease 27: 473

Smith R D. DuShane W, Edwards J E 1959 Congenital insufficiency of the pulmonary valve. Circulation 20: 554

12

Aortic stenosis

Aortic stenosis is an important and relatively common variety of congenital heart disease. It may be valvar, supravalvar or subvalvar. Since a murmur is present in the neonatal period, early diagnosis should be the rule.

Certain hemodynamic consequences of left ventricular outflow obstruction are common to all varieties of aortic stenosis. They are mirrored in the physical examination, indicating the presence of obstruction and providing evidence of its severity. Other physical findings differ in the various types and serve to identify the site of obstruction. Valvar aortic stenosis, the most common variety, will be discussed in detail as the prototype.

VALVAR AORTIC STENOSIS

The anomaly

In valvar aortic stenosis the valve is usually essentially bicuspid; one part of the valve being the noncoronary cusp and the other a combined right and left coronary cusp, partially subdivided by rudimentary commissure or raphe. There is usually some fusion of the commissures on either side of the noncoronary cusp as well. During ventricular systole the cusps cannot fold back against the aortic wall, remaining in the lumen and forming the dome shaped structure which is a typical angiographic feature of this variety of aortic stenosis.

Physical findings

General

The general physical examination is normal. There is no cyanosis and the jugular venous pulse is unremarkable. Most children with valvar aortic stenosis have normal arterial pulses. With severe obstruction, some patients have a typical parvus et tardus pulse, but for a given degree of obstruction pulses are less likely to be abnormal in children than in adults. Precordial motion is normal in mild aortic stenosis. With more severe obstruction the systolic apical impulse is forceful and sustained, reflecting a greater degree of ventricular hypertrophy. With very severe stenosis there may be a presystolic impulse at the apex, mirroring forceful atrial contraction against an hypertrophied and poorly compliant left ventricle (Fig. 12.1).

Auscultation

Heart sounds. The first heart sound is normal. The aortic component of the second heart sound is well preserved in children and young adults, even with severe obstruction, in striking contrast to the attenuation of the pulmonic closure sound which occurs with severe pulmonic stenosis. (This is because aortic pressure, a major determinant of the intensity of the aortic closure sound, cannot fall to the low levels seen in the pulmonary artery with pulmonary stenosis.) Beyond young adulthood, scarring and calcification may decrease mobility of the valve and thus attentuate the aortic closure sound. In most children with aortic stenosis the second sound is physiologically split. But if the left ventricular ejection time is prolonged the aortic component of the second heart sound will be delayed and splitting of the second sound will be narrow, absent or even paradoxical, depending upon the degree of delay (Gray, 1956). Children with aortic stenosis, like normal children, may have a prominent third heart sound. An audible fourth heart sound (Fig. 12.1) is evidence of severe obstruction and has the same genesis as the presystolic impulse described above (Caulfield et al, 1971).

An early systolic ejection sound is present in almost all children and young adults with valvar aortic stenosis (Hancock, 1966), being generated as the aortic valve domes and reaches the peak of its incursion into the aorta (Fig. 12.2). The sound is dependent upon mobility of the valve and may be absent in an infant with thick myxomatous cusps or in an older individual whose valve has become calcified. An aortic ejection sound is usually maximal at the apex and is often louder with the patient sitting or standing than supine. The sound is of nearly the same pitch as the first heart sound and cannot accurately be described as a 'click'. An aortic ejection sound does not vary with respiration. It can usually be distinguished from the ejection sound of valvar pulmonic stenosis, which is high pitched, maximal at the high left sternal border and audibly diminishes with inspiration. It may be more difficult to distinguish a first sound–ejection sound sequence from a split first heart sound or from a fourth sound–first sound sequence unless phonocardiography is employed, with either a carotid pulse tracing or an echocardiogram (Fig. 12.2).

Murmurs. The most constant physical finding of valvar aortic stenosis is a harsh crescendo-decrescendo systolic murmur. The murmur is almost always maximal at the high right sternal border and radiates well to both carotids. (In an occasional infant the murmur is loudest at the mid left sternal border.) With very mild aortic stenosis the systolic murmur tends to be soft and short and to end in mid systole, while the murmur of moderate or severe aortic stenosis tends to be loud and to extend almost to the aortic closure sound. Regardless of the severity the murmur peaks midway in its course. Severe aortic stenosis does not show the late systolic peak and 'kite' configuration of the

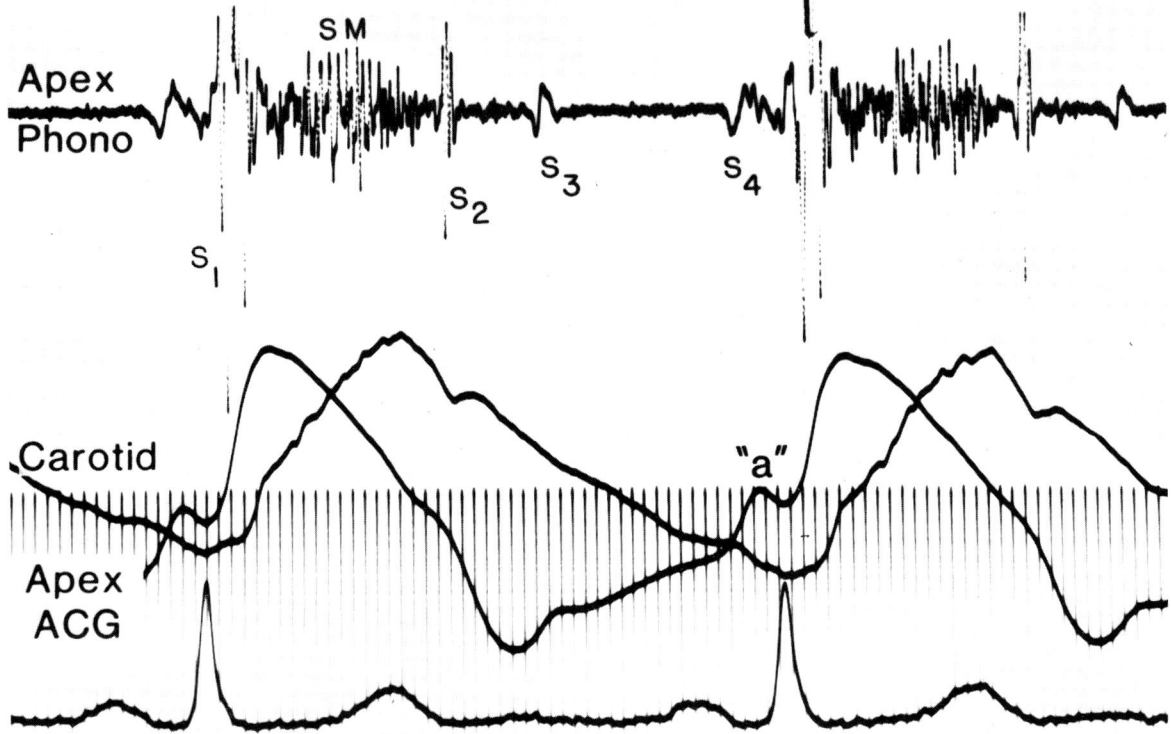

Fig. 12.1 Apexcardiogram (ACG), phonocardiogram and carotid pulse tracing of a patient with severe valvar aortic stenosis. The carotid upstroke is slow. There is a prominent fourth heart sound (S4) and an accompanying presystolic wave ('a') on the ACG. The systolic murmur is crescendo-decrescendo and ends just before the second heart sound (S_2).

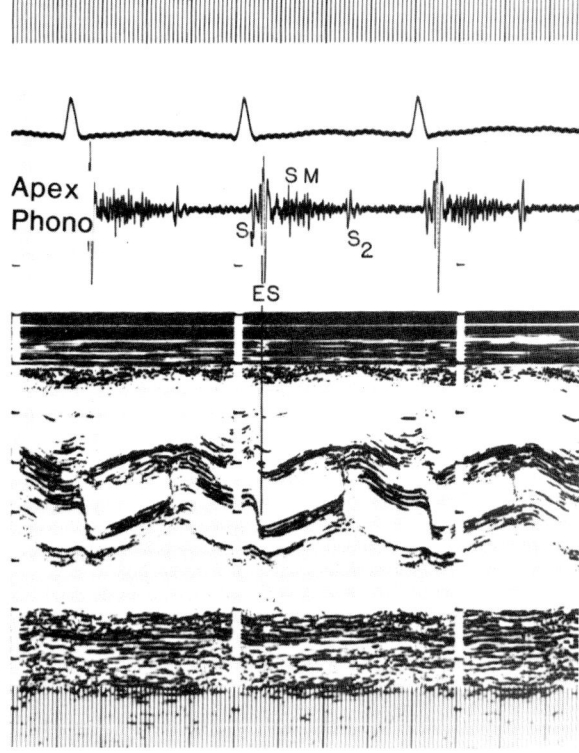

Fig. 12.2 Simultaneous apex phonocardiogram and echocardiogram of a child with valvar aortic stenosis. The early systolic ejection sound (ES) occurs as the aortic cusps reach the limit of their excursion.

or chest roentgenogram. Even with moderately severe stenosis there may be no thrill in a very very obese child with a thick chest wall. In spite of the above exceptions, the presence or absence of a thrill has proven to be very useful in selecting children for cardiac catheterization. If a child with typical findings of valvar aortic stenosis is apparently healthy, if there is no resting thrill and if the electrocardiogram and chest roentgenogram are normal, catheterization can safely be deferred. If there is a thrill, catheterization should be performed, even if there are no symptoms or electrocardiographic or roentgenographic signs of severe obstruction. Cardiac catheterization remains the only reliable means of assessing the severity of obstruction in such a patient, since a large gradient may be present with a relatively short systolic murmur and a normal electrocardiogram and chest roentgenogram (Fig. 11.3). It should be noted that the loudness of a murmur and prominence of a thrill are augmented by increased cardiac output. Both murmur and thrill thus become much more prominent with exercise and, to a lesser degree, with fever.

murmur of severe valvar pulmonic stenosis. Although there is a tendency for the murmur to be louder and longer with severe obstruction, the characteristics of the systolic murmur of aortic stenosis — loudness, duration and shape — are not as reliable a guide to severity of obstruction as they are with pulmonic stenosis (Fig. 12.3).

A high right sternal border systolic thrill is common with valvar aortic stenosis and is nearly always present if obstruction is moderate or severe. Stated another way, if no thrill is present obstruction is almost always mild. This general rule does not apply if cardiac output is low, since the aortic gradient is dependent on flow as well as on the size of the aortic orifice. In a patient with very severe aortic stenosis and low output, however, there is always other clinical evidence of severe left ventricular outflow obstruction: symptoms, poor pulses, or an abnormal electrocardiogram

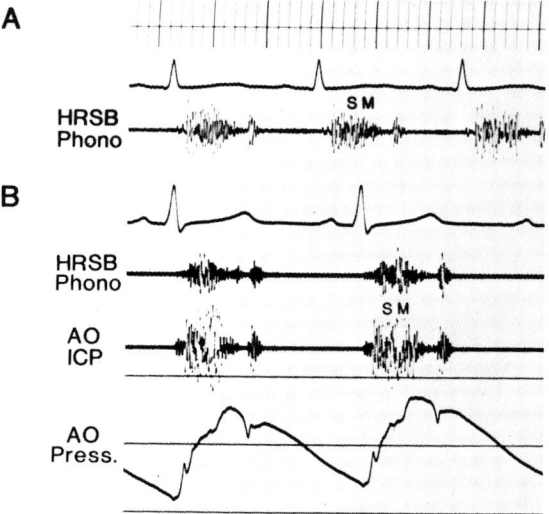

Fig. 12.3 Phonocardiograms of two children with aortic stenosis. Both have crescendo-decrescendo murmurs which end well before the aortic closure sound (A_2). Patient B has mild valvar aortic stenosis with a 30 mmHg peak systolic gradient. The systolic murmur is of similar duration and configuration in the surface phonocardiogram (HRSB) and in the aortic root (AO ICP). Patient A has a 90 mmHg peak systolic gradient in spite of a short murmur.

Critical aortic stenosis

The infant with critical aortic stenosis typically develops symptoms very early in life. Respiratory distress and hepatomegaly are common, as are signs of decreased cardiac output such as cool, pale extremities and decreased or even imperceptible peripheral pulses. If the infant is seen early enough in life the evidence of severity may be confined to generally decreased peripheral pulses. The remainder of the physical examination and the chest roentgenogram and electrocardiogram may give no clue that the obstruction is very severe. There may be peripheral cyanosis if output is sufficiently low. The apical impulse is usually quiet in infants with critical aortic stenosis but a prominent left parasternal impulse may be present and reflect right ventricular overload. (Pulmonary hypertension may result from left ventricular failure. If there is left to right shunting through a stretched patent foramen ovale, a volume overload of the right ventricle is present as well.) An early systolic ejection sound may or may not be present. The systolic murmur of the aortic stenosis may be short, soft and without a thrill (Lakier et al, 1974). There may be associated mitral regurgitation and an apical pansystolic murmur (Fig. 12.4). In the newborn, critical aortic stenosis may be difficult to distinguish from aortic atresia or myocarditis, especially if there is no ejection sound.

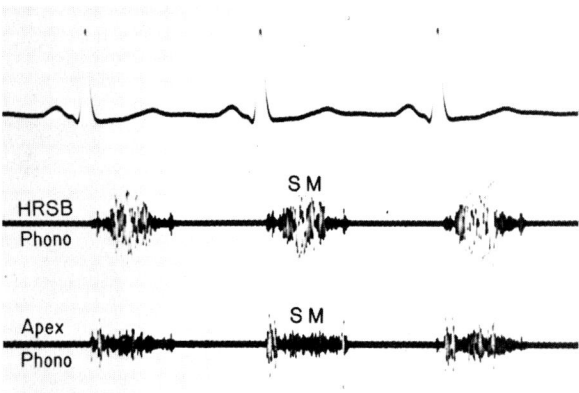

Fig. 12.4 Apical and high right sternal border (HRSB) phonocardiogram of an infant with critical aortic stenosis. The HRSB systolic murmur is crescendo-decrescendo, while the apical murmur, representing mitral regurgitation, is plateau-shaped.

Associated aortic regurgitation

Aortic regurgitation may accompany aortic stenosis and is discussed in Chapter 13. Its presence is signaled by a high pitched decrescendo diastolic murmur which begins with the aortic closure sound and which is typically loudest at the mid left sternal border.

SUBVALVAR AORTIC STENOSIS

There are several varieties of subvalvar aortic stenosis. The most useful subdivision is into one group with fixed and more or less localized fibrous or fibromuscular obstruction, and another group with variable obstruction due to myocardial hypertrophy.

FIXED OBSTRUCTION

The anomaly

Fixed subaortic stenosis may be due to a band of fibrous tissue which encircles the muscular portion of the left ventricular outflow tract and extends on to the anterior leaflet of the mitral valve. The aortic valve is often abnormal as well, and aortic regurgitation is relatively common. Fixed obstruction may be more diffuse, and the left ventricular outflow tract may show fibromuscular tunnel-like narrowing. Obstruction may also be due to abnormal mitral valve leaflets or to abnormal chordal insertion into the left ventricular outflow tract. In univentricular hearts with rudimentary outlet chamber and ventriculoarterial discordance, a restrictive communication between the ventricle and the outlet chamber constitutes subaortic stenosis.

Physical findings

The hemodynamic consequences of fixed subaortic stenosis resemble those of valvar aortic stenosis. The pattern of precordial motion is similar in the two varieties, but in discrete subaortic stenosis the arterial pulse is less likely to be slow rising and small than in valvar stenosis. Unlike the valvar variety, an ejection sound is not present with subaortic stenosis (Hancock, 1966). The characteristics of the systolic murmur are similar, except that it may be louder at the mid left than the high right sternal border, especially with the 'tunnel' variety of subaortic stenosis (Maron et al, 1976). Since the obstruction is fixed, the response to exercise and pharmacologic intervention is similar to that in valvar stenosis.

HYPERTROPHIC OBSTRUCTION

The anomaly

The muscular variety of subaortic stenosis has several appellations, including asymmetric septal hypertrophy (ASH), idiopathic hypertrophic subaortic stenosis (IHSS) and hypertrophic obstructive cardiomyopathy (HOCM). Hypertrophic subaortic stenosis is often familial and the incidence of sudden death is distressingly high (Frank & Braunwald, 1968), much higher than with fixed aortic obstruction. In the author's personal experience only a single patient with valvar aortic stenosis has died suddenly (a 15 year old boy with a 50 mmHg gradient at catheterization two years before death). In contrast, five patients with hypertrophic subaortic obstruction have died without warning — even though valvar stenosis is many times more common than the hypertrophic variety. Syncope, angina and paroxysmal arryhthmias are also more common with hypertrophic subaortic stenosis.

Physical findings

General

A sustained systolic apical impulse is common in patients with hypertrophic subaortic stenosis and is due to the unusual degree of left ventricular hypertrophy characteristic of this entity. A presystolic apical impulse is also frequent and is related to a vigorous left atrial contraction against the decreased diastolic compliance of the hypertrophied ventricle. Pulses are typically quick-rising, even with severe obstruction, since the obstruction occurs only after ejection has begun. Such late onset obstruction causes a characteristic bifid systolic pulse (Fig. 12.5) (Frank & Braunwald, 1968).

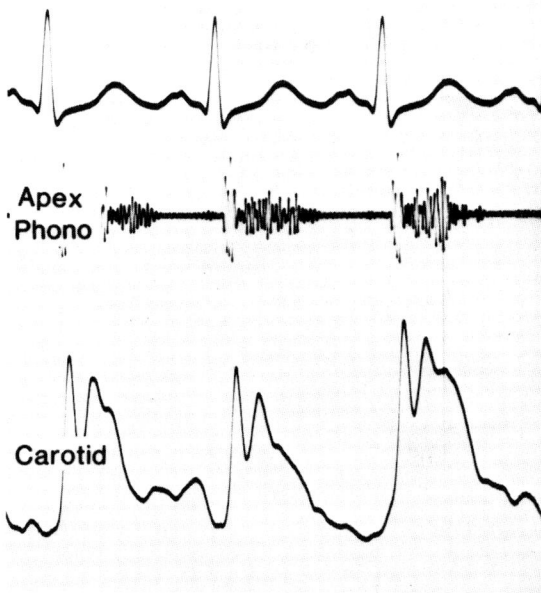

Fig. 12.5 Apex phonocardiogram and carotid pulse tracing of a three year old child with hypertrophic subaortic stenosis. The systolic murmur is crescendo-decrescendo and the pulse is bifid.

Auscultation

Heart sounds. The first heart sound is normal and the aortic component of the second heart sound is well preserved with hypertrophic subaortic stenosis. The second heart sound is probably more often paradoxically split than with valvar aortic stenosis (Fig. 12.7), but is usually single or physiologically split. A fourth heart sound is common in this entity and has the same genesis as the presystolic impulse. An early systolic ejection sound is not present.

Murmurs. The systolic murmur of hypertrophic subaortic stenosis is typically maximal in the third or fourth intercostal space at the left sternal border but may be as loud or louder at the apex. Mitral regurgitation occurs, and it may be difficult to distinguish its murmur from that of the obstruction. An apical mid-diastolic murmur may be heard with hypertrophic subaortic stenosis. It can be recorded in the left ventricle near the mitral orifice (Fig. 12.6) and is probably related to distortion of the mitral apparatus by the asymmetric myocardial hypertrophy.

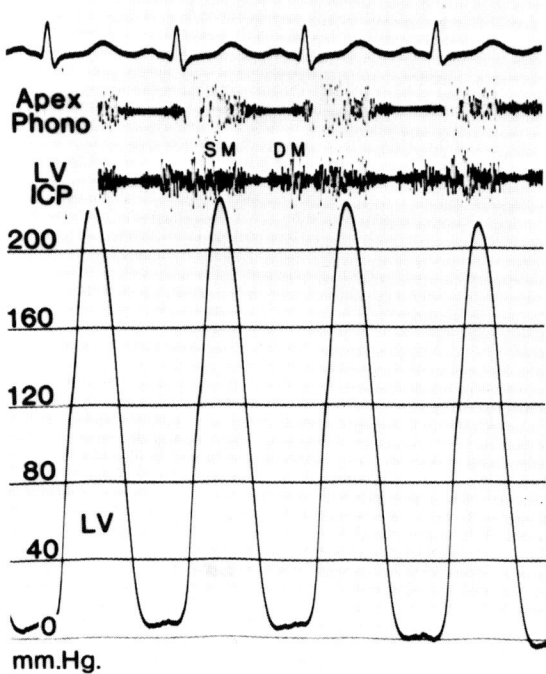

Fig. 12.6 Apex phonocardiogram and high fidelity sound (LV ICP) and pressure recording in the same child as in Figure 12.5. An audible mid diastolic murmur is poorly recorded on the external phonocardiogram but is well demonstrated on the left ventricular phonocardiogram recorded near the mitral orifice.

Both the degree of obstruction and the resultant systolic murmur may vary spontaneously and are easily manipulated by physical maneuvers or pharmacologic agents. The obstruction varies with left ventricular volume; the smaller the left ventricular cavity the more closely the hypertrophied interventricular septum and the anterior leaflet of the mitral valve approximate during systole. This results in greater obstruction and a louder murmur. Conversely, dilatation of the left ventricular cavity reduces obstruction and attenuates the murmur. Squatting increases both systemic venous return and arterial resistance, enlarging the left ventricular cavity and decreasing the systolic murmur. Sudden rising to a standing position has the opposite effect: the left ventricular cavity becomes smaller, obstruction increases and the systolic murmur accentuates. The strain phase of the Valsalva maneuver also reduces venous return and accentuates the murmur of hypertrophic subaortic stenosis. During the release phase venous return and cardiac output increase, the left ventricular cavity enlarges, obstruction lessens and the murmur softens. (Response to the Valsalva maneuver is thus opposite to the expected response with fixed aortic obstruction.)

Pharmacologic agents which decrease afterload (amyl nitrite) or increase myocardial contractility (isoproterinol) increase obstruction and enhance the murmur. Agents which increase afterload (phenylephrine) or reduce myocardial contractility (propranolol) decrease obstruction and attenuate the murmur (Fig. 12.7). (Manipulation of afterload has little effect on the murmur of fixed obstruction.) Maneuvers which increase left ventricular outflow tract obstruction may bring out a latent fourth heart sound and bifid arterial pulse.

SUPRAVALVAR AORTIC STENOSIS

The anomaly

Supravalvar aortic stenosis is the least common variety of left ventricular outflow tract obstruction. Obstruction may be localized, resulting in an 'hour-glass' deformity of the aorta, or there may be generalized hypoplasia of the ascending aorta. Supravalvar stenosis has been described as part of a syndrome which includes mental retardation and peculiar 'elfin facies' (Williams et al, 1961), and in some children with this syndrome there is a history of infantile hypercalcemia. Familial supravalvar aortic stenosis with normal facies and without mental retardation has also been reported (Martin & Moseley, 1973).

Physical findings

The cardiac physical findings differ in some respects from those of other forms of aortic stenosis. Although systolic blood pressure may normally be slightly higher in the right arm than in the left, in supravalvar aortic stenosis the difference may exceed 20 mmHg (Fig. 12.8). The asymmetry has been attributed to the Coanda effect, or tendency for a fluid jet to adhere to a wall (French & Guntheroth, 1970). The supravalvar obstruction supposedly directs the jet toward the right aortic

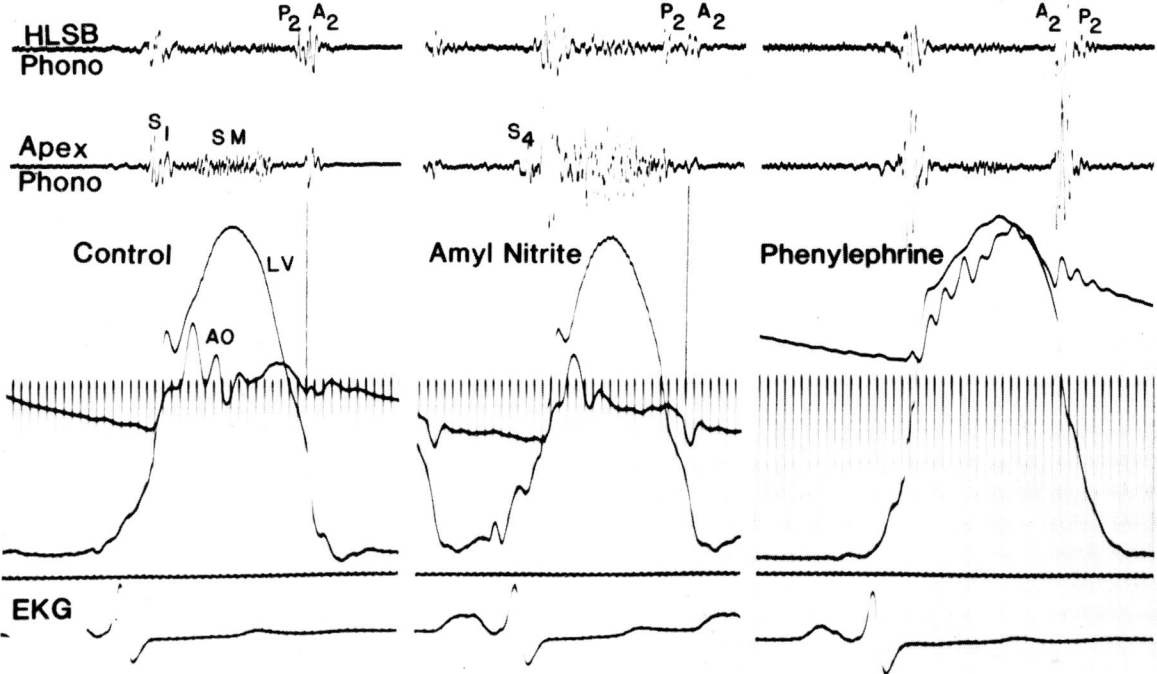

Fig. 12.7 Response to pharmacologic intervention in hypertrophic subaortic stenosis. In the control panel there is a modest gradient. The systolic murmur is soft and the second heart sound is physiologically split. With inhalation of amyl nitrite the gradient increases, the murmur intensifies and the second sound splits paradoxically (A_2 follows P_2). Phenylephrine eliminates the gradient and the systolic murmur.

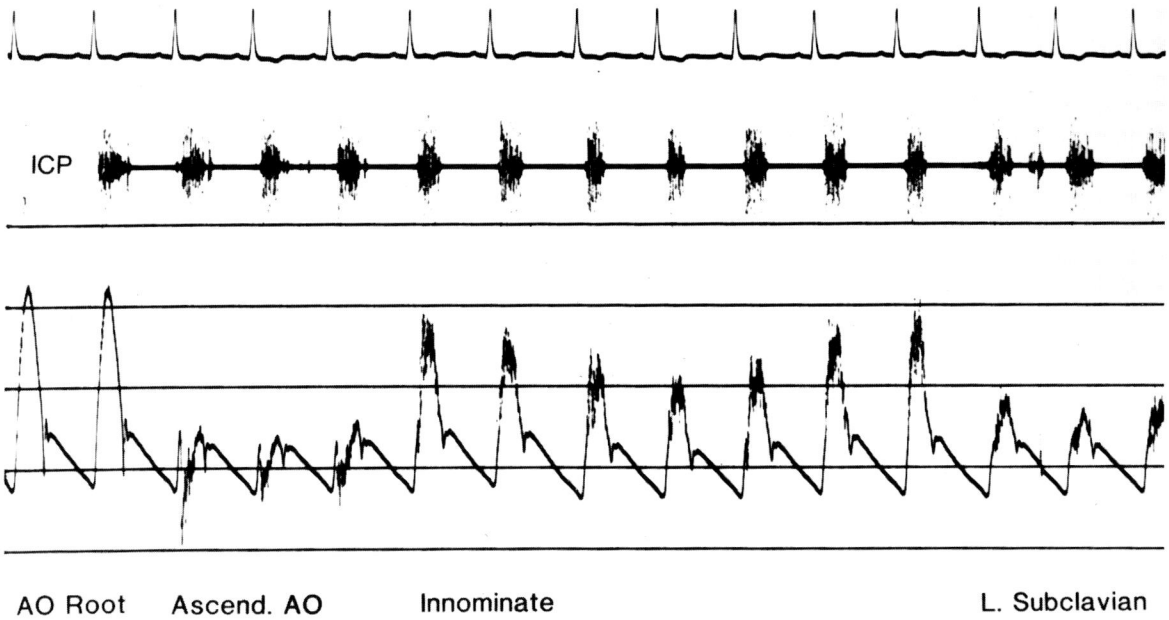

Fig. 12.8 Intra-aortic pressure and sound recording in a boy with supravalvar aortic stenosis. A gradient is present between the aortic root and the ascending aorta (site of the supravalvar obstruction) and pressure is higher in the innominate artery (and in the right subclavian — not shown) than in the left subclavian.

wall and the Coanda effect 'leads' the jet into the innominate artery. As the stream slows in the innominate, the kinetic energy of the high velocity stream is converted to potential energy, which is measurable as blood pressure. In the presence of normal pulse and blood pressure in the legs, asymmetry of arm blood pressure should suggest the diagnosis of supravalvar aortic obstruction. It must be noted, however, that some patients with this entity have symmetrical pulse and blood pressure.

The systolic murmur of supravalvar aortic stenosis is similar to that of the valvar variety but may radiate more to the right than the left carotid. If the systolic murmur is heard well in the axillae and across the back, pulmonary artery stenosis is a likely accompaniment to the supravalvar obstruction.

REFERENCES

Caulfield W H, de Leon A C, Perloff J K, Steelman B 1971 The clinical significance of the fourth heart sound in aortic stenosis. American Journal of Cardiology 28: 179

Frank S, Braunwald E 1968 Idiopathic hypertrophic subaortic stenosis. Circulation 37: 759

French J W, Guntheroth W G 1970 An explanation of asymmetric upper extremity blood pressures in supravalvular aortic stenosis: the Coanda effect. Circulation 42: 31

Gray I R 1956 Paradoxical splitting of the second heart sound. British Heart Journal 18: 21

Hancock E W 1966 The ejection sound in aortic stenosis. American Journal of Medicine 40: 569

Lakier J B, Lewis A B, Heymann M A, Stanger P, Hoffman J I E, Rudolph A M 1974 Isolated aortic stenosis in the neonate: natural history and hemodynamic considerations. Circulation 50: 801

Maron B J, Redwood D R, Roberts W.C, Henry W.L, Morrow A G, Epstein S E 1976 Tunnel subaortic stenosis: left ventricular outflow tract obstruction produced by fibromuscular tubular narrowing. Circulation 54: 404

Martin E C, Moseley I F 1973 Supravalvar aortic stenosis. British Heart Journal 35: 758

Williams J C P, Barratt-Boyes B G, Lowe J B 1961 Supravalvular aortic stenosis. Circulation 24: 1311

13

Aortic regurgitation

The anomaly

Aortic regurgitation most commonly occurs with a bicuspid aortic valve (Roberts, 1970), which may or may not be significantly stenotic. It may also accompany discrete subaortic stenosis (Newfeld et al, 1976), a supracristal or perimembranous ventricular septal defect (Dimich et al, 1973), tetralogy of Fallot (Zuberbuhler et al, 1975), or persistent truncus arteriosus. Aortic regurgitation not associated with a congenital cardiac anomaly is most commonly a result of acute rheumatic fever, but may also be caused by infectious endocarditis or accompany rheumatoid arthritis. Aortic regurgitation may also result from the aortic root dilatation seen in patients with Marfan's syndrome.

Clinical course

The clinical course of aortic regurgitation depends both on its severity and on the acuteness of its onset. Mild aortic regurgitation is well tolerated indefinitely and the only evidence of its presence is the characteristic diastolic murmur. Severe chronic aortic regurgitation may cause surprisingly few symptoms for several years, but eventually leads to left ventricular failure. Severe acute aortic regurgitation, on the other hand, is not well tolerated, since left ventricular stroke volume cannot increase sufficiently to maintain a normal cardiac output (vide infra). A clinical picture of shock may rapidly develop and the patient will not survive unless the regurgitation can be surgically repaired.

Physical findings
General

If aortic regurgitation is mild, the sole abnormal physical finding is the diastolic murmur of the regurgitation itself. With more severe chronic aortic regurgitation the reflux of blood from the aortic root to the left ventricle in diastole causes a decrease in aortic diastolic pressure, with a resultant increase in aortic pulse pressure and in the magnitude of peripheral pulses. The velocity of left ventricular ejection also increases and systolic pressure rises, accentuating the width of the pulse pressure. With progressively more severe regurgitation pulses have been described as 'full', 'bounding' and 'water hammer'; Corrigan described visible pulsations of major arteries in patients with very severe regurgitation (quoted by Willius & Keys, 1941a). Pulses can be appreciated more peripherally with severe regurgitation, being palpable in the palms, along the sides of the digits and even in the finger tips themselves. The capillary pulse of Quincke, another consequence of widened pulse pressure, consists of an alternate systolic flushing and diastolic blanching of the fingernails as light pressure is applied to them (quoted by Willius & Keys, 1941b). A very wide pulse pressure can also result in a sudden systolic tensing of medium and large size systemic arteries which generates an early systolic sound over the artery (Traube's pistol shot sound) (Fig. 13.4). A double or 'bifid' arterial pulse (pulses bisfiriens) is sometimes present with aortic regurgitation (Fig. 13.3). A carotid thrill or 'shudder' is common. The jugular venous pulse is normal. The left ventricular apical systolic impulse is prominent and may impart a rocking motion to the precordium.

Auscultation

Heart sounds. With chronic aortic regurgitation

the first heart sound is of normal intensity and the second sound is physiologically split. A third heart sound is rarely prominent and there is no fourth heart sound. If there is a bicuspid aortic valve or valvar aortic stenosis, an early systolic ejection sound is expected, but may disappear with very severe regurgitation.

Murmurs. The most common and characteristic physical finding in patients with aortic regurgitation is a decrescendo diastolic murmur which begins with the aortic component of the second sound and which is usually maximal at the mid left sternal border (Fig. 13.1). This murmur is high

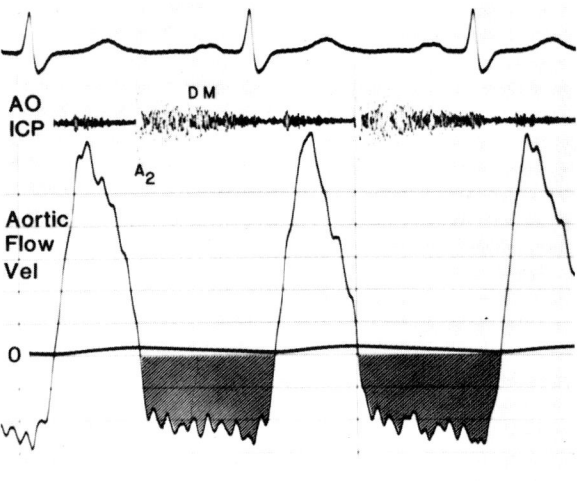

Fig. 13.1 Simultaneously recorded sound (AO ICP) and flow velocity in the aortic root of a child with aortic regurgitation. The diastolic murmur begins with the aortic closure sound and is decrescendo. There is retrograde diastolic aortic flow (hatched area).

pitched and may be quite soft, being best heard with the diaphragm of the stethoscope. The murmur should be listened for with the patient sitting and leaning forward with the breath held in expiration, or during squatting. (The increase in systemic vascular resistance and aortic pressure which accompanies squatting tends to increase the degree of aortic regurgitation and the murmur may be heard only during this maneuver.) The murmur of aortic regurgitation occasionally has a musical or 'cooing' quality. This variety of murmur is likely to be louder at the right than the left sternal border (Hurst & Logue, 1966) and is more common if the aortic regurgitation is due to eversion, perforation, or tearing of an aortic cusp, rather than to the more usual central or intercommissural leak.

Another diastolic murmur, described by Austin Flint, is common with severe aortic regurgitation (quoted by Willius & Keys, 1941c). This murmur is maximal at the apex and is low pitched and rumbling (Fig. 13.2). There is often a pre-systolic accentuation, and early and mid-diastolic peaks may also occur, lending a triple cadence to the murmur. The location and characteristics of an Austin Flint murmur easily distinguish it from the diastolic murmur of aortic regurgitation itself. An Austin Flint murmur is probably generated by movement of the anterior mitral valve leaflet. In diastole this leaflet hangs like a curtain between the aortic and mitral orifices, and in the presence of significant aortic regurgitation it may move to and fro between the incoming streams of blood from the aorta and the left atrium. Such 'fluttering' of the anterior mitral leaflet can be demonstrated by echocardiography (Gray & Barritt, 1975; Morganroth et al, 1977) (Fig. 13.2). A slightly different view of the genesis of an Austin Flint murmur postulates actual narrowing of the mitral orifice as the anterior leaflet is displaced posteriorly by the aortic regurgitant stream. Because of its location, low pitch, and presystolic accentuation, an Austin Flint murmur may bear considerable resemblance to the murmur of mitral stenosis. The two may be differentiated by inhalation of amyl nitrite. This drug acutely reduces systemic resistance and therefore lowers aortic pressure. As aortic pressure falls, regurgitation diminishes and an Austin Flint murmur attenuates. Amyl nitrite also increases cardiac output and therefore increases the flow and the gradient across a stenosed mitral valve, accentuating the diastolic murmur of mitral stenosis. Thus, an apical diastolic murmur which becomes softer with amyl nitrite is related to aortic regurgitation and one which becomes louder is caused by mitral stenosis.

With mild aortic regurgitation the volume of diastolic reflux from aorta to left ventricle is provided by the elastic recoil of the ascending aorta. When regurgitation is severe there is retrograde diastolic flow from more peripheral sites.

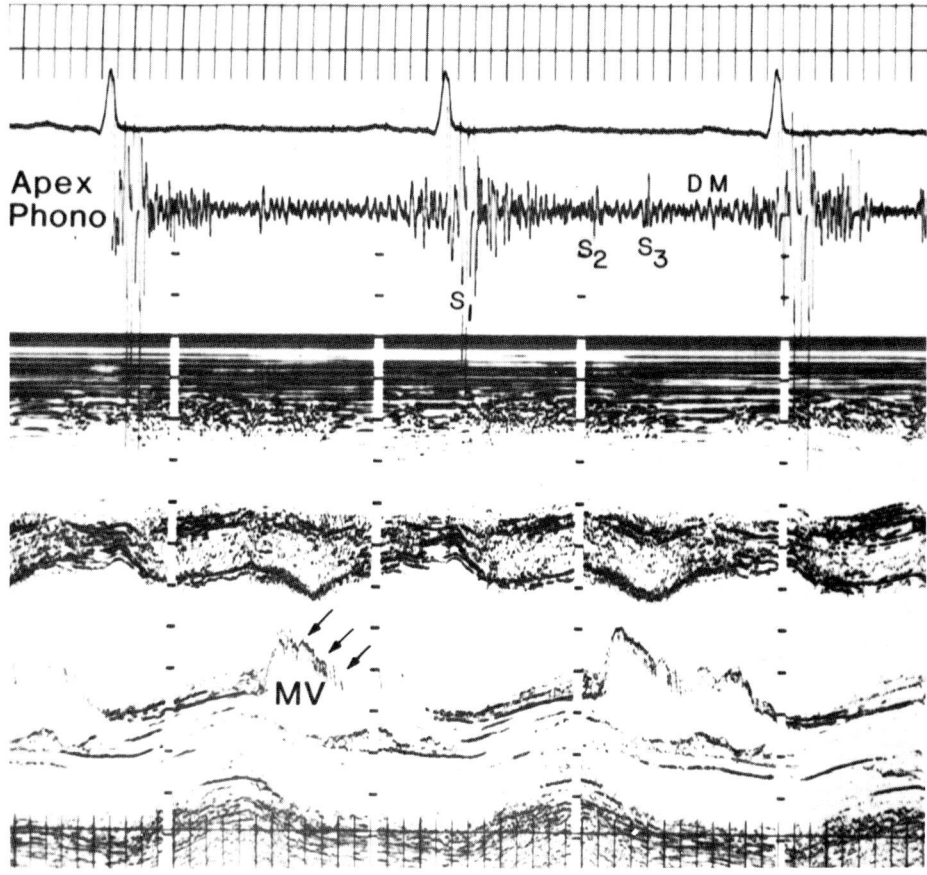

Fig. 13.2 Austin Flint murmur (DM) in an adolescent with severe aortic regurgitation. There is presystolic accentuation of the murmur. The echocardiogram shows fluttering of the anterior mitral leaflet (arrows).

This phenomenon can be documented cineangiographically by injecting contrast medium into the aortic arch or distal aorta, and can also be demonstrated by an electromagnetic flow probe catheter (Fig. 13.3). Such diastolic retrograde arterial flow is the genesis of the Duroziez sign, a to and fro murmur heard over a femoral artery when it is manually compressed (quoted by Willius & Keys 1941d). In the normal individual, external compression of a femoral artery produces a systolic murmur, a consequence of systolic flow through the iatrogenic arterial stenosis. A diastolic murmur will be present as well if there is sufficient retrograde flow during diastole (Fig. 13.4). (The to and fro murmur can best be appreciated if the artery is compressed by the distal edge of the tilted diaphragm head of the stethoscope (Fig. 13.5).) A Duroziez sign is indicative of very severe aortic regurgitation.

Acute aortic regurgitation

Acute severe aortic regurgitation may be caused by infectious endocarditis, by trauma, by spontaneous eversion of a congenitally abnormal cusp, or by acute rheumatic fever. The abrupt onset of severe regurgitation has certain hemodynamic consequences which alter the clinical picture described above. If aortic incompetence worsens gradually an increase in left ventricular end diastolic volume is accomplished with little increase in end diastolic pressure. The velocity of ejection and magnitude of stroke volume both increase, and normal cardiac output is maintained, even in the presence of

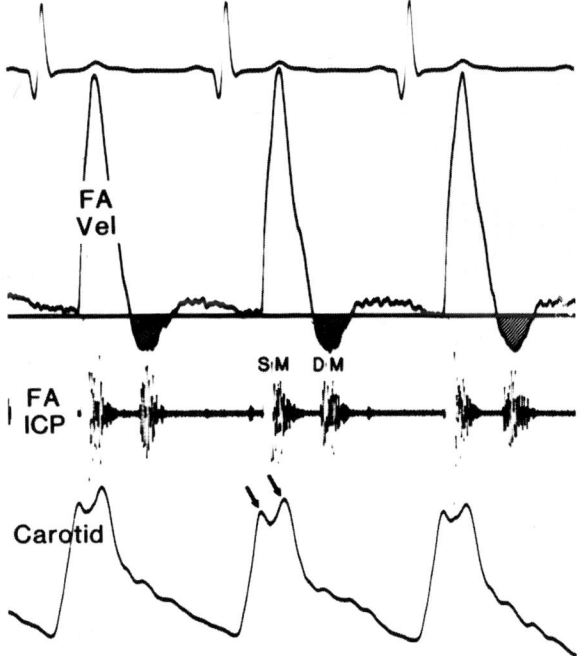

Fig. 13.3 Simultaneously recorded sound (FA ICP) and flow velocity (FA VEL) in the femoral artery of a child with chronic severe aortic regurgitation. The systolic and diastolic murmurs in the femoral artery are related to forward and retrograde (hatched area) flow, respectively. The carotid pulse tracing is bifid (pulsus bisferiens).

marked regurgitation. If severe regurgitation develops acutely, however, stroke volume cannot increase sufficiently to maintain a normal cardiac output, since the left ventricle has not yet dilated. Poor peripheral perfusion and even shock may result. Severe acute aortic regurgitation necessarily results in a considerable increase in ventricular end diastolic pressure with consequent shortening of the diastolic murmur of aortic regurgitation — since aortic and left ventricular pressures tend to equalize during the latter part of diastole (Fig. 13.6). High left ventricular end diastolic pressure also prevents aortic diastolic pressure from falling to very low levels, and pulse pressure and peripheral pulse magnitude are not as great as they are with severe regurgitation which is chronic. High left ventricular diastolic pressure may also result in premature closure of the mitral valve, causing the first heart sound at the apex to be soft or even inaudible (Fig. 13.6) (Morganroth et al, 1977).

Associated anomalies

Except for a bicuspid aortic valve, a ventricular septal defect, either perimembranous or supracristal in location (Tatsuno et al, 1973; Van Praagh & McNamara, 1968), is the cardiac anomaly found

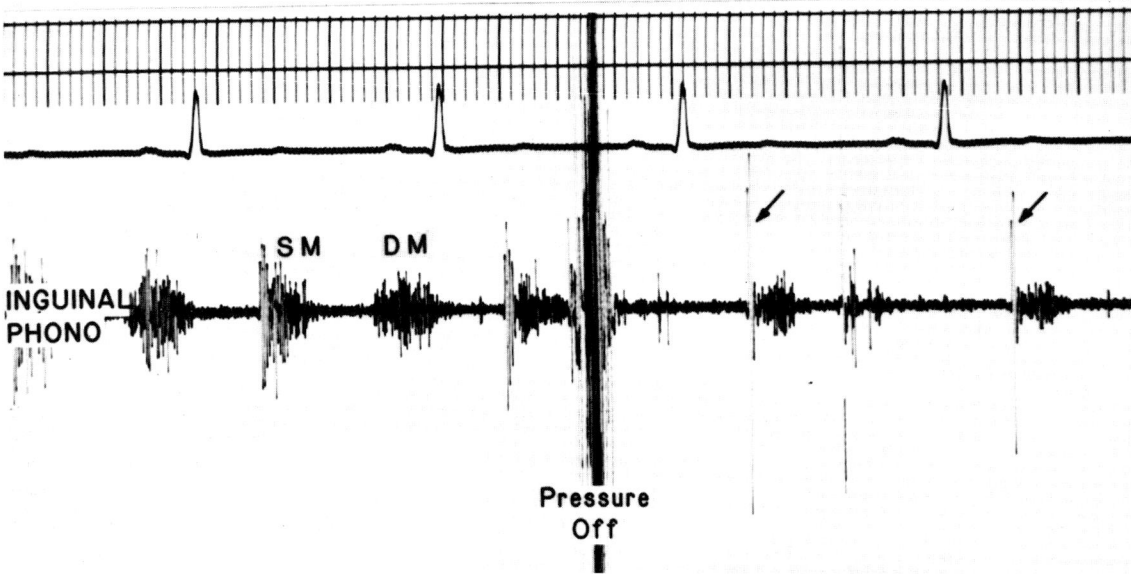

Fig. 13.4 Phonocardiogram over the femoral artery in a child with severe aortic regurgitation. Prominent systolic and diastolic murmurs are present during application of pressure over the artery (Duroziez sign), but only a soft systolic murmur persists when pressure is removed. There is a loud early systolic sound (arrow) over the artery.

AORTIC REGURGITATION 87

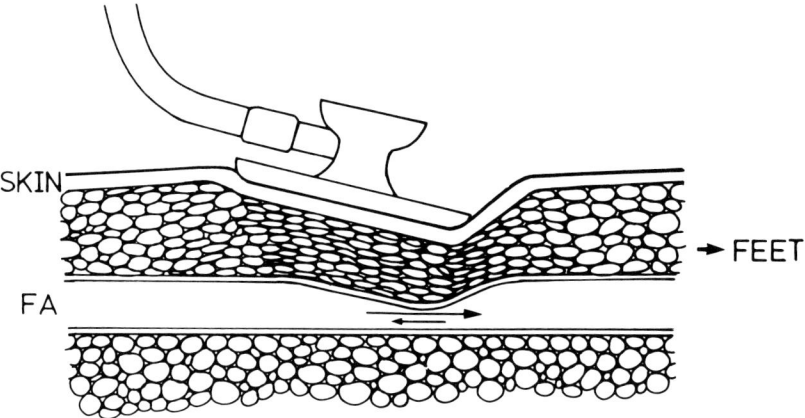

Fig. 13.5 Diagram of femoral artery compression by the tilted stethoscope head to elicit a Duroziez sign.

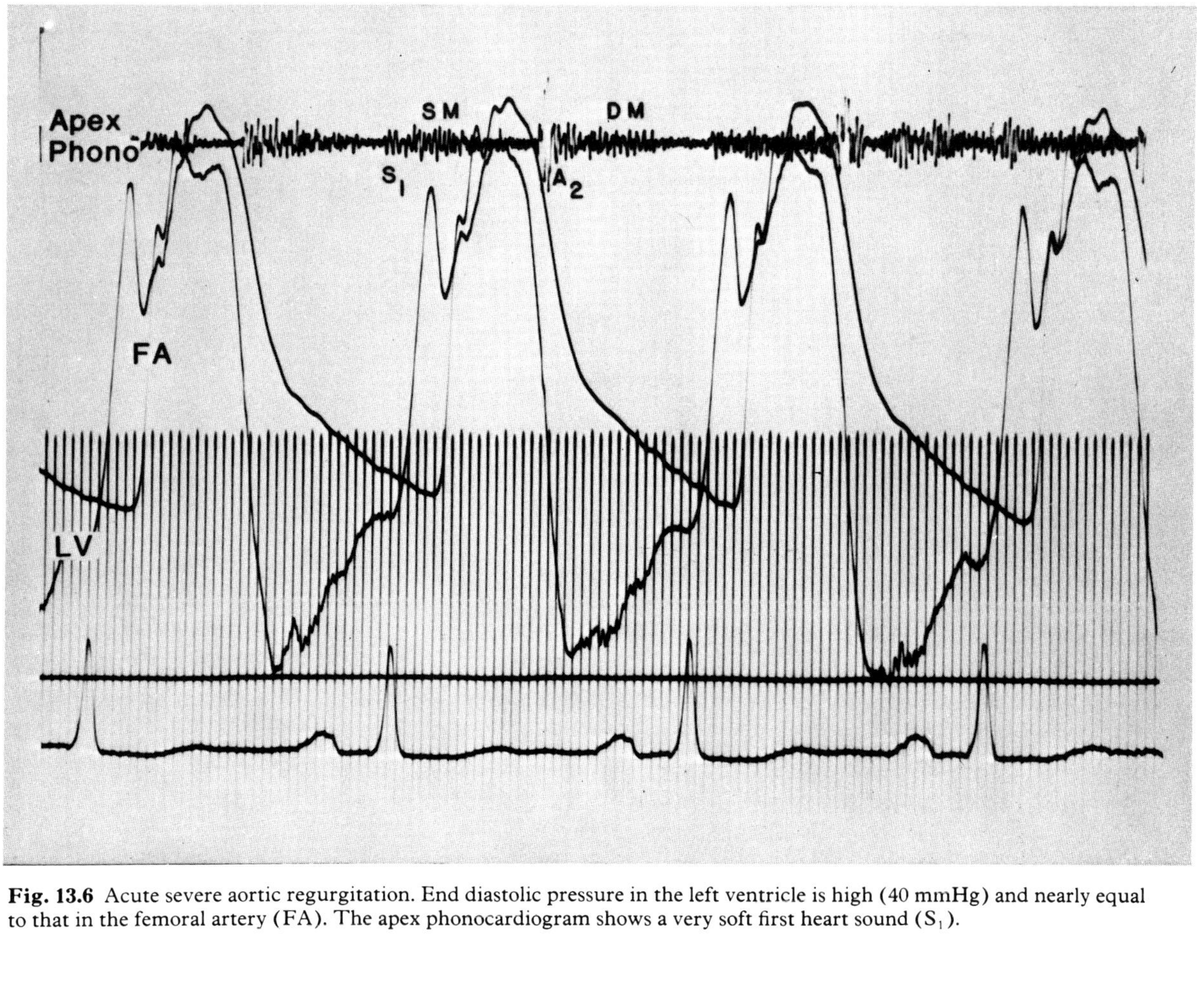

Fig. 13.6 Acute severe aortic regurgitation. End diastolic pressure in the left ventricle is high (40 mmHg) and nearly equal to that in the femoral artery (FA). The apex phonocardiogram shows a very soft first heart sound (S_1).

most commonly with congenital aortic regurgitation. A perimembranous defect is more commonly associated, although the incidence is much higher with the less common supracristal type. If the defect is perimembranous the aortic valve tends to be intrinsically abnormal. In contrast, if the defect is supracristal the aortic valve is usually normal but is poorly supported and tends to prolapse as the right coronary cusp progressively enlarges. The aortic regurgitation associated with a supracristal defect is not present at birth, usually appearing between 2 and 10 years of age. There is a strong tendency for progression.

A patient with aortic regurgitation who also has a ventricular septal defect will have both a systolic and diastolic murmur. The murmur may seem continuous at the mid left sternal border if the ventricular septal defect is very small and generates a murmur similar in pitch to the murmur of the aortic regurgitation. The systolic murmur of a small ventricular septal defect extends to the aortic closure sound and the diastolic murmur of aortic regurgitation begins with the same sound, with no audible gap between the murmurs — hence, a 'continuous' murmur. Listening higher and lower along the left sternal border may identify the separate systolic and diastolic murmurs but the auscultatory resemblance to a coronary-cardiac fistula may be striking.

Aortic regurgitation is less common than pulmonic regurgitation in patients with tetralogy of Fallot (Zuberbuhler et al, 1975). The clinical distinction between aortic regurgitation and low pressure pulmonic regurgitation is usually not difficult, the murmur of aortic regurgitation being long, high pitched and decrescendo, while that of pulmonic regurgitation is short and of medium pitch.

AORTICO-LEFT VENTRICULAR TUNNEL

Aortico-left ventricular tunnel, a rare congenital cardiac anomaly, will be discussed in this chapter, although it is not, per se, an example of aortic regurgitation (Levy, 1963; Perez-Martinez, 1973). Anatomically, the anomaly consists of a 'tunnel' in the wall of the left ventricle. This tunnel opens distally into the aorta and proximally into the left ventricular cavity. During systole blood flows from the left ventricle to the aorta both through the aortic valve and through the tunnel. During diastole there is reflux to the left ventricle through the tunnel, and sometimes also through an incompetent aortic valve. The resulting to and fro murmur is present at birth and is similar to that heard with massive aortic regurgitation, with or without mild associated aortic stenosis. The runoff through the tunnel is usually severe and the peripheral signs described above for aortic regurgitation are present. The entity should be considered in any infant presenting with signs of severe aortic regurgitation. Diagnosis is by selective aortography.

REFERENCES

Dimich I, Steinfeld L, Litwak R S, Park S, and Silvers N 1973 Subpulmonic ventricular septal defect associated with aortic insufficiency. American Journal of Cardiology 32: 325

Gray K E, Barritt D W 1975 Echocardiographic assessment of severity of aortic regurgitation. British Heart Journal 37: 691

Hurst J W, Logue R B 1966 The heart, arteries and veins, 2nd edn. McGraw-Hill, New York, p 852

Levy M J, Lillehei C W, Anderson R C, Amplatz K, Edwards J E 1963 Aortico-left ventricular tunnel. Circulation 27: 841

Morganroth J, Perloff J K, Zeldis S M, Dunkman W B 1977 Acute severe aortic regurgitation. Annals of Internal Medicine 87: 223

Newfeld E A, Muster A J, Paul M H, Idriss F S, Riker W L 1976 Discrete subvalvular aortic stenosis in childhood. American Journal of Cardiology 38: 53

Perez-Martinez V, Quero M, Castro C, Moreno F, Brito J M, Merino G 1973 Aortico-left ventricular tunnel. A clinical and pathologic review of this uncommon entity. American Heart Journal 85: 237

Roberts W C 1970 The congenitally bicuspid aortic valve. American Journal of Cardiology 26: 72

Tatsuno K, Konno S, Ando M, Sakakibara S 1973 Pathogenetic mechanisms of prolapsing aortic valve and aortic regurgitation associated with ventricular septal defect. Circulation 48: 1028

Van Praagh R, McNamara J J 1968 Anatomic types of ventricular septal defects with aortic insufficiency. American Heart Journal 75: 604

Willius F A, Keys T E 1914a Cardiac classics. A collection of classic works on the heart and circulation with comprehensive biographic accounts of the authors. Mosby St. Louis, p 422
  1941b p 569
  1941c p 502
  1941d p 492

Zuberbuhler J R, Lenox C C, Neches W H, Park S C, Shaver J A 1975 Auscultatory spectrum of the tetralogy of Fallot. Physiologic principles of heart sounds and murmurs. American Heart Association Monograph 46 American Heart Association, New York, p 187

14

Mitral stenosis

The anomaly

The mitral valve apparatus consists of leaflets, chordae tendineae, papillary muscles and an annulus. Abnormalities of any of these components can lead to obstruction. If stenosis is secondary to rheumatic fever there is thickening of valve leaflets, fusion of commissures and shortening and thickening of chordae tendineae. Although congenital mitral stenosis may be morphologically similar to rheumatic, it has a wider range of pathology, especially if it is associated with other congenital cardiac anomalies. When mitral stenosis is part of the complex described by Schone et al (1963) (mitral stenosis, supravalvar stenosing ring, subvalvar aortic stenosis and coarctation of the aorta) the mitral obstruction is due to a 'parachute' arrangement of the valve, with chordae from both anterior and posterior leaflets inserting into a single papillary muscle. In other patients with congenital mitral stenosis, obstruction to left atrial inflow may be due to accessory mitral valve tissue, to unusually large papillary muscles or short thick chordae, or to a mitral arcade with attachment of the anterior leaflet directly to the anterior and posterior papillary muscles (Davachi et al, 1971).

Mitral valve abnormalities, often constituting mild mitral stenosis, are common in patients with coarctation of the aorta (Rosenquist, 1974), although hemodynamically significant mitral stenosis is less common. Mitral stenosis can also coexist with left ventricular outflow tract obstruction, a double outlet right ventricle (Sondheimer et al, 1977), a single ventricle (De La Cruz & Miller, 1968), an interatrial septal defect (Lutembacher's syndrome) (Steinbrunn et al, 1970), and occasionally with other cardiac anomalies.

Significant mitral stenosis implies a considerable diastolic gradient between the left atrium and left ventricle and therefore an elevation of left atrial pressure. If left atrial and pulmonary venous pressures are more than mildly elevated there will be 'passive' elevation of pulmonary arterial and right ventricular pressure. If pulmonary venous hypertension is severe an element of active pulmonary arteriolar vasoconstriction is added, further raising pulmonary artery pressure. The mitral valve gradient, pulmonary venous hypertension and secondary pulmonary hypertension are responsible for most of the signs and symptoms of mitral stenosis.

Clinical course and physical findings

General

In older children and adults the earliest and most common symptom of mitral stenosis is dyspnea on exertion. Orthopnea and paroxysmal nocturnal dyspnea appear if stenosis becomes severe. In infancy the earliest sign of mitral obstruction is usually tachypnea. If stenosis is severe and long-standing there may be poor growth and development. Cyanosis may occur, either episodically because of pulmonary edema or more chronically because of decreased cardiac output and increased oxygen extraction in the skin. A precordial bulge is common with severe congenital mitral stenosis and a prominent left sternal border impulse may occur if there is pulmonary hypertension. The apical impulse is inconspicuous or absent, although an apical diastolic thrill may be present.

Auscultation

Heart sounds. The auscultatory picture is usually quite characteristic. The first heart sound is loud (Fig. 14.1), especially with moderate or severe mitral stenosis. Since mitral valve closure occurs only when left ventricular pressure exceeds left atrial pressure, the high left atrial pressure of mitral stenosis delays closure somewhat, causing it to occur at a time when left ventricular pressure is rapidly rising. Coaptation of the leaflets is thus abrupt and the closure sound loud (Shah et al, 1970). It has been stated that the first heart sound is often of normal intensity with congenital mitral stenosis, because of relative immobility of the valve (Perloff, 1978a). But in the author's experience a loud first heart sound has been the rule, no matter what the etiology of the stenosis. The second heart sound is physiologically split but the split may be narrow. The pulmonic component is loud if there is secondary pulmonary hypertension. Since rapid left ventricular filling is impossible with tight mitral stenosis, third and fourth heart sounds are not present unless they are of right ventricular origin. An opening snap is common if the valve is relatively mobile but is less common with congenital than with rheumatic mitral stenosis (Perloff, 1978b). This early diastolic sound is high pitched and is maximal between the low left sternal border and the apex. The interval between the aortic closure sound and the opening snap tends to be short when stenosis is severe, since high left atrial pressure opens the mitral valve earlier in diastole (Tavel, 1978). An opening snap is not influenced

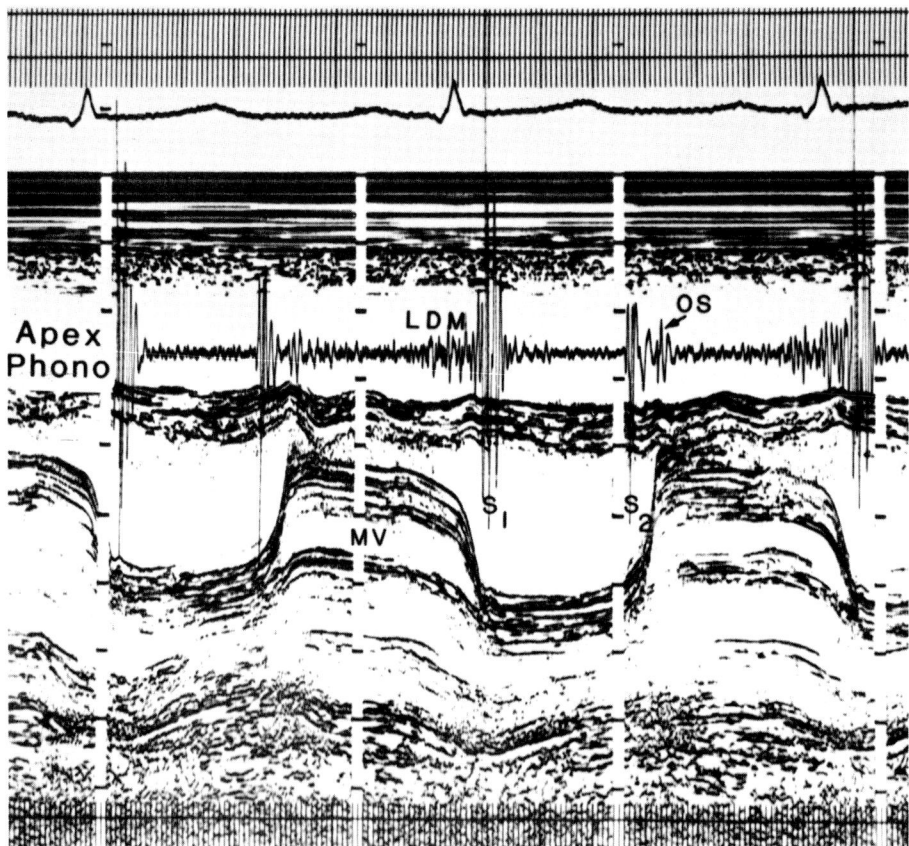

Fig. 14.1 Apex phonocardiogram and echocardiogram of an adolescent with mitral stenosis. The first heart sound (S_1) is loud and there is an opening snap (OS). There is late diastolic accentuation of the murmur (LDM). The mitral valve is thickened and moves abnormally.

by respiration. It may occasionally be difficult to differentiate a snap from a third heart sound but its more medial location, higher pitch and relative closeness to the aortic closure sound usually serve to identify the snap.

Murmurs. The most common and characteristic auscultatory feature of mitral stenosis is a low pitched apical diastolic murmur. When obstruction is mild a significant gradient is present only in early and late diastole (rapid passive filling phase and filling due to atrial contraction, respectively). With mild stenosis, therefore, the diastolic murmur begins after the second heart sound, fades and then reappears before the first heart sound (Fig. 14.1). With more severe stenosis a sizable gradient persists throughout diastole and the murmur then extends from shortly after the second heart sound to the first heart sound (Fig. 14.2). There is commonly a presystolic accentuation due to left atrial systole, but this is lost if there is atrial fibrillation. Occasionally, if obstruction is extremely severe and cardiac output very low, no diastolic murmur is audible ('silent mitral stenosis'). A loud first heart sound, an opening snap, and signs of pulmonary hypertension may then be the only evidence of obstruction to left atrial emptying.

A high pitched decrescendo diastolic murmur of hypertensive pulmonic regurgitation may be present in patients with severe mitral stenosis. Clinically, it is impossible to distinguish this murmur from the murmur of mild aortic regurgitation which may also accompany rheumatic mitral stenosis. A low left sternal border pansystolic murmur of tricuspid regurgitation may appear in patients with severe pulmonary hypertension secondary to mitral stenosis. If the right ventricle is large and the left ventricle relatively small, this murmur may be heard well at the apex and may closely simulate mitral regurgitation. (It should be noted that pulmonic regurgitation and tricuspid regurgitation secondary to mitral stenosis occur only with severe and longstanding obstruction and are therefore very rare in childhood.)

Associated anomalies

Associated lesions may produce other physical findings, such as the decreased femoral pulses of coarctation of the aorta or the cyanosis of double outlet right ventricle or of single ventricle. If mitral stenosis and a small interatrial communication coexist, a continuous murmur may be generated at the restrictive interatrial septal defect, since left atrial pressure exceeds right atrial pressure throughout the cardiac cycle (Aykent et al, 1965). This continuous murmur is maximal at the low right sternal border and tends to accentuate with inspiration and to decrease with the Valsalva maneuver.

Differential diagnosis

Mitral stenosis must be differentiated from other anomalies which produce an apical diastolic murmur. In children, the most common cause of such a murmur is 'relative' mitral stenosis, where the mitral gradient is related not to organic stenosis but to increased diastolic flow, most commonly due

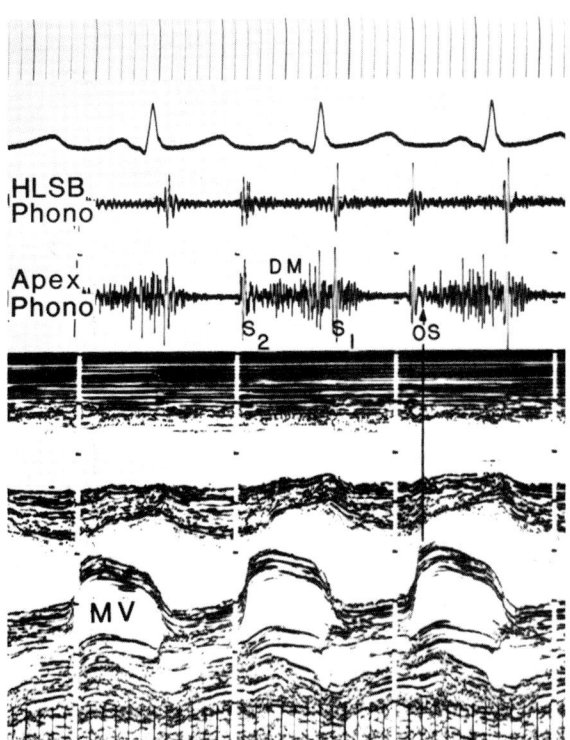

Fig. 14.2 Phonocardiogram and echocardiogram of an infant with congenital mitral stenosis. There is a pandiastolic murmur with presystolic accentuation. An early opening snap (OS) coincides with mitral valve opening. The mitral valve echo is abnormal.

to a ventricular septal defect, a patent ductus arteriosus or severe mitral regurgitation (Fig. 14.3). The murmur of relative mitral stenosis has no presystolic accentuation, since diastasis is reached by late diastole. With relative mitral stenosis, the first heart sound is of normal intensity, a third heart sound commonly introduces the murmur and an opening snap is not present. All these features help to distinguish relative from organic mitral obstruction. The apical diastolic rumble commonly heard in patients with severe aortic regurgitation (Austin Flint murmur; Fig. 13.2) may be quite similar to the murmur of organic mitral stenosis but the two can be differentiated by the administration of amyl nitrite (Nasser et al, 1966). As the amyl nitrite is inhaled, cardiac output increases and aortic pressure decreases. The increased cardiac output augments the intensity of the murmur of mitral stenosis while the lowered aortic pressure reduces aortic regurgitation and softens an Austin Flint murmur.

Summary

In summary, mitral stenosis may be congenital or acquired and may be isolated or associated with other congenital cardiac abnormalities. The auscultatory hallmark of mitral stenosis is a rumbling apical diastolic murmur. Other useful auscultatory signs are a loud first heart sound and/or an opening snap. If mitral stenosis is severe the physical findings of pulmonary hypertension are added.

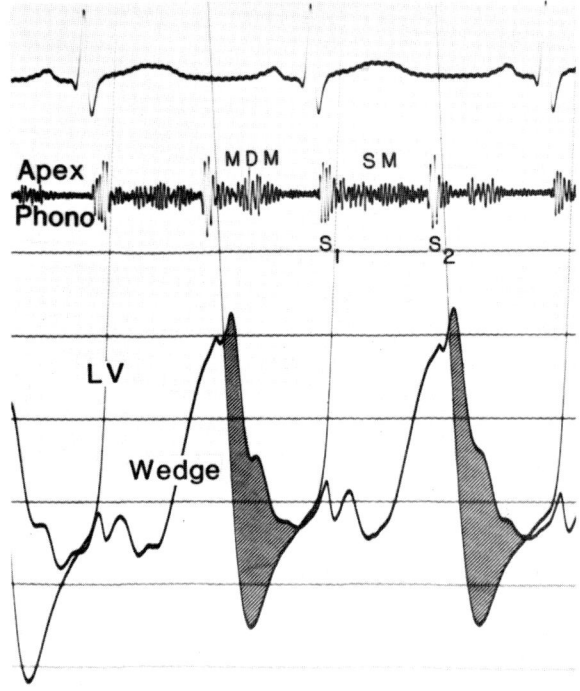

Fig. 14.3 Child with a large ventricular septal defect. Simultaneous pulmonary arterial wedge and left ventricular pressures show a diastolic mitral gradient (hatched area) which corresponds temporally to an apical mid diastolic murmur (relative mitral stenosis).

REFERENCES

Aykent Y, Thurmann M, Bussmann D W 1965 Continuous murmur in mitral stenosis. American Journal of Cardiology 15: 715

Davachi F, Moller J H, Edwards J E 1971 Diseases of the mitral valve in infancy: an anatomic analysis of 55 cases. Circulation 43: 565

De La Cruz M V, Miller B L 1968 Double-inlet left ventricle: two pathological specimens with comments on the embryology and on its relation to single ventricle. Circulation 37: 249

Nasser W, Tavel M E, Feigenbaum H, Fisch C 1966 Austin-Flint murmur versus the murmur of organic mitral stenosis. New England Journal of Medicine 275: 1007

Perloff J K 1978a The clinical recognition of congenital heart disease, 2nd edn. Saunders, Philadelphia, p 159

Perloff J K 1978b The clinical recognition of congenital heart disease, 2nd edn. Saunders, Philadelphia, p 160

Rosenquist G C 1974 Congenital mitral valve disease associated with coarctation of the aorta: a spectrum that includes parachute deformity of the mitral valve. Circulation 49: 985

Shah P M, Kramer D H, Gramiak R 1970 Influence of the timing of atrial systole on mitral valve closure and on the first heart sound in man. American Journal of Cardiology 26: 231

Shone J D, Sellers R D, Anderson R C, Adams P Jr, Lillehei C W. Edwards J E 1963 The developmental complex of 'parachute mitral valve', supravalvular ring of left atrium, subaortic stenosis, and coarctation of the aorta. American Journal of Cardiology 11: 714

Sondheimer H M, Freedom R M, Olley P M 1977 Double outlet right ventricle: clinical spectrum and prognosis. American Journal of Cardiology 39: 709

Steinbrunn W, Cohn K E, Selzer A 1970 Atrial septal defect associated with mitral stenosis: the Lutembacher syndrome revisited. American Journal of Medicine 48: 295

Tavel M E 1978 Clinical phonocardiography and external pulse recording, 3rd edn. Year Book Medical Publisher, Chicago, p 52

15

Mitral regurgitation

The anomaly

Mitral regurgitation is most frequently due to rheumatic fever and is by far the most common valvar consequence of that disease. Other less common causes of acquired mitral regurgitation include non-rheumatic myocarditis, rheumatoid arthritis and infectious endocarditis.

'Isolated' congenital mitral regurgitation is uncommon but when it occurs is usually due to a cleft or to abnormal chordae tendineae. More commonly, mitral regurgitation accompanies some other congenital cardiac anomaly such as an endocardial cushion defect or anomalous origin of the left coronary artery. In these entities the regurgitation may be trivial or may dominate the clinical picture.

Clinical course

The clinical course of mitral regurgitation depends both on the severity of the regurgitation and on the rapidity of onset. Mild mitral regurgitation produces no symptoms and chronic regurgitation of moderate or even severe degree may be well tolerated for a number of years before congestive heart failure appears. Severe mitral regurgitation of abrupt onset (e.g. infectious endocarditis, traumatic rupture of a papillary muscle, occasionally acute rheumatic fever) is less well tolerated, largely because the left atrium has not had time to dilate. With chronic regurgitation the left atrium may enlarge enormously and in such a 'lax' system even large regurgitant flow can be 'soaked up' and there is little systolic rise in left atrial pressure. In the 'tight' system of acute mitral regurgitation the left atrial pressure rises markedly in the latter part of systole, sometimes approximating left ventricular pressure. This rise in left atrial and pulmonary venous pressure results in tachypnea and dyspnea. (Pulmonary edema and death may occur if the regurgitation is sufficiently severe.)

Physical findings

Mitral regurgitation virtually always produces an apical systolic murmur and, conversely, a systolic murmur which is *maximal* at the apex almost always represents mitral regurgitation. (A defect in the apical portion of the interventricular septum constitutes a rare exception.) The murmur of mitral regurgitation is typically high pitched and is pansystolic and plateau shaped (Fig. 15.1). It usually radiates well to the left axilla. Variations do occur, however. For example, the murmur of mitral regurgitation may end well before the second heart sound, especially if the regurgitation is very mild or if it is severe and of recent onset (Fig. 15.2). In the latter situation the late systolic rise in left atrial pressure reduces or even eliminates the gradient responsible for the murmur (Fig. 15.3) (Sutton & Craige, 1967). As another example, the murmur of mitral regurgitation may radiate well to the base and may simulate aortic stenosis. This unusual radiation may occur if the regurgitation is due to an abnormality of the posterior leaflet; the regurgitant jet then is directed anteriorly, where it may strike the atrial septum near the aortic valve. If the regurgitation is acute and severe, the less than holosystolic duration of the murmur may heighten the resemblance to aortic stenosis. In another variation, the murmur of mitral regurgitation is late systolic, indicating onset of regurgitation well after closure of the mitral valve. The usual etiology of a late systolic murmur is late systolic prolapse of one or both of

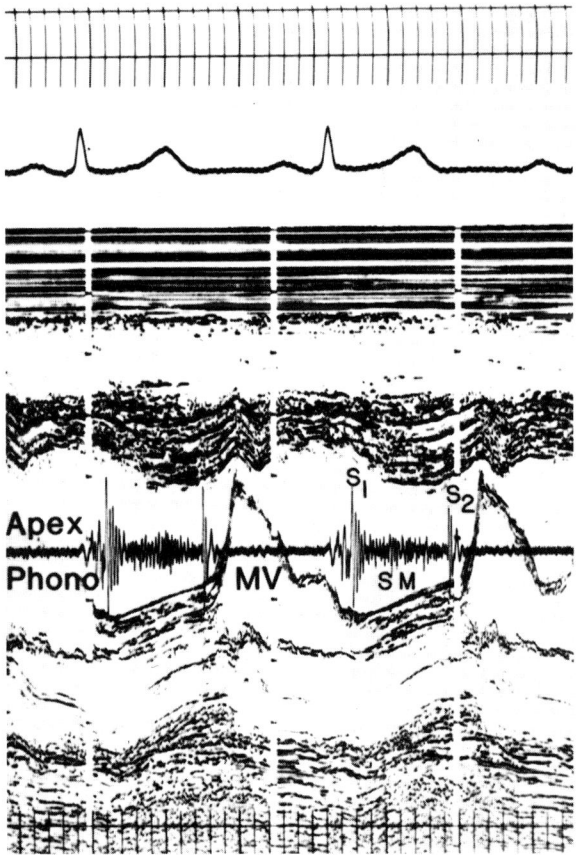

Fig. 15.1 Apex phonocardiogram and echocardiogram of a child with congenital mitral regurgitation. The murmur is holosystolic and plateau shaped.

the mitral leaflets into the left atrium. Papillary muscle dysfunction, in adults usually a consequence of arteriosclerotic coronary artery disease, is one cause of late systolic mitral regurgitation (Phillips et al, 1963). (Normally, contraction of the papillary muscles keeps tension on the chordae tendineae as the long axis of the ventricle shortens during systole, ensuring continued coaptation of the anterior and posterior leaflets.) Even if the papillary muscles are normal, prolapse can occur if a leaflet is large and 'billowing'. Such a 'floppy' mitral valve is the most common source of a late systolic murmur (Barlow et al, 1967) (Fig. 15.4). The underlying cause is usually obscure but prolapse may occur with Marfan's syndrome and may occasionally be a consequence of rheumatic fever.

The late systolic murmur of mitral prolapse is usually introduced by a mid systolic click, presumably generated as the redundant leaflet reaches the extent of its incursion into the left atrium (Fig. 15.4). The murmur is notoriously variable, at times disappearing and at other times becoming extremely loud. The click also varies and may occur without a murmur. An occasional patient is aware of an intermittent 'buzzing' or 'purring' in the chest and the murmur is sometimes audible to others several feet away. These phenomena do not necessarily indicate severe valvar disease and some patients require considerable reassurance.

It is usually difficult to assess the severity of mitral regurgitation solely on the basis of the intensity, duration and timing of the systolic murmur. However, other physical findings can be helpful. Mild mitral regurgitation produces no physical findings other than the systolic murmur, but large volume regurgitation into the left atrium has hemodynamic consequences which are reflected in the physical examination. Systolic reflux to the left atrium of a significant portion of the left ventricular stroke volume implies a large diastolic return across the mitral valve. If there is no associated mitral stenosis, most of this return is in early and mid diastole. This rapid protodiastolic flow to the left ventricle produces a prominent third heart sound, followed directly by a mid diastolic murmur (Fig. 15.5). There is no presystolic accentuation since left ventricular filling has largely been accomplished before atrial systole occurs. Further, the large left ventricular stroke volume implicit in major mitral regurgitation causes an active apical impulse. The apical impulse is usually rather poorly sustained (Sutton & Craige, 1967), but may be prolonged, especially if the regurgitation is associated with acute rheumatic fever (Fig. 15.5). As a corollary, a normal apical impulse very nearly rules out severe mitral regurgitation. A left parasternal lift may be evident in patients with severe mitral regurgitation and when present suggests secondary pulmonary hypertension (Fig. 15.6). A patient with a greatly enlarged left atrium and left ventricle may also have a prominent left sternal border impulse, even in the absence of pulmonary hypertension. Anterior displacement of the left ventricle by a posteriorly directed mitral regurgitant jet may also contribute to left sternal border motion (Tavel, 1978). A

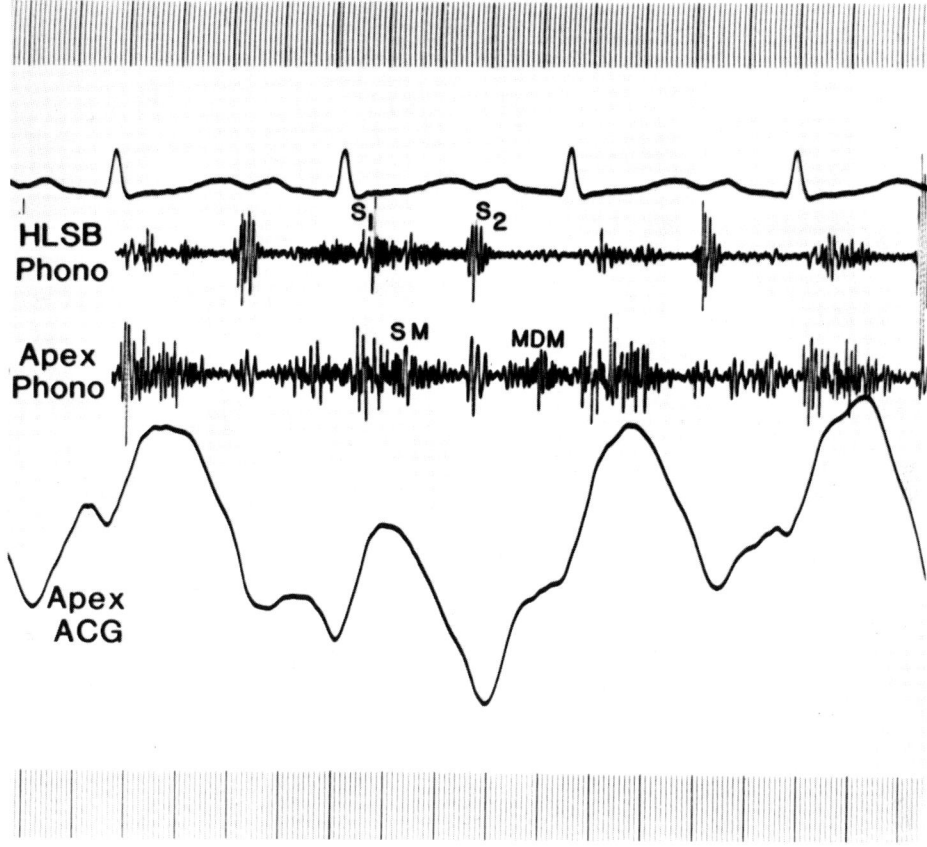

Fig. 15.2 Phonocardiogram and apex pulse tracing (Apex ACG) of a child with severe mitral regurgitation. The systolic murmur is decrescendo and ends before the second sound (S_2). There is a mid diastolic murmur (MDM) of relative mitral stenosis. The apical impulse is prominent and sustained.

'quick' and poorly sustained arterial pulse often accompanies very severe mitral regurgitation, since the left ventricle cannot sustain prolonged ejection into the aorta in the presence of another lower resistance exit (Gould et al, 1968).

The heart sounds may be abnormal in the presence of moderate to severe regurgitation. The first heart sound is often soft in adults with severe regurgitation but in the author's experience is usually of normal intensity in children. The second heart sound is physiologically split but the split may be wide (Bridgen & Leatham, 1953), since the shortened left ventricular ejection period of important mitral regurgitation causes the aortic component to be early. The pulmonic closure sound is of normal intensity unless the regurgitation has produced pulmonary hypertension (Fig. 15.6). (Secondary pulmonary hypertension is rare with long-standing incompetence since the left atrium becomes dilated and the regurgitant volume can be accommodated without much rise in left atrial pressure. With acute regurgitation high left atrial pressure results in elevation of pulmonary artery pressure and the physical signs of pulmonary hypertension may be evident.) As mentioned above, a prominent third heart sound is common with moderate to severe mitral regurgitation. A fourth heart sound may be heard if regurgitation is both severe and acute (Sutton & Craige, 1967).

Differential diagnosis

The systolic murmur of chronic mitral regurgitation may radiate to the high left sternal border and be crescendo–decrescendo, and if the second heart sound is prominently split an atrial septal defect

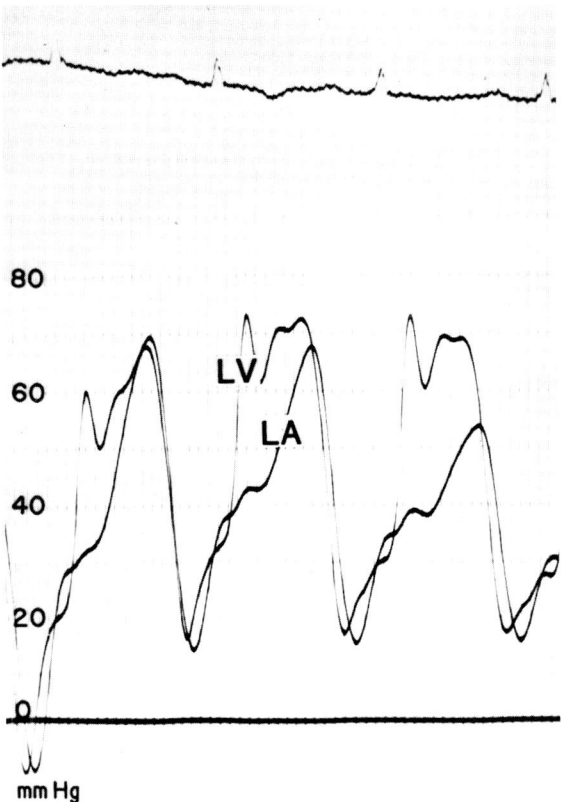

Fig. 15.3 Simultaneous left atrial and left ventricular pressures in a newborn with massive mitral regurgitation. In some cycles pressure in the left atrium (LA) and left ventricle (LV) are nearly equal in late systole.

may be suggested. With mitral regurgitation, however, the second sound is not fixedly split and there is no low left sternal border murmur of relative tricuspid stenosis. Lack of these findings makes an atrial defect unlikely. Differentiating mitral regurgitation and a ventricular septal defect is occasionally difficult, especially if a high pitched pansystolic murmur is maximal somewhere between the apex and the low left sternal border. In this situation, a comparison of the intensity of the murmur at the low *right* sternal border and at the apex can be useful; greater intensity at the low right sternal border favors a diagnosis of ventricular septal defect while greater intensity at the apex makes mitral regurgitation more likely. (A defect in the apical portion of the interventricular septum can exactly mimic mitral regurgitation clinically.) In general, an early systolic murmur points to a tiny ventricular septal defect while mitral regurgitation is more likely if the murmur is pan or late systolic.

The apical diastolic rumble of severe mitral regurgitation should not be confused with organic mitral stenosis, since there is no presystolic accentuation, the first heart sound is not loud and there is no opening snap. If both congestive failure and mitral regurgitation are present, the absence of physical signs of massive mitral regurgitation suggests that myocardial dysfunction is the cause rather than the effect of the regurgitation.

Physical maneuvers

Maneuvers which alter left ventricular volume or pressure can be useful in differential diagnosis. Sudden squatting tends to increase left ventricular pressure and usually intensifies the murmur of mitral regurgitation. The murmur may soften, however, if the regurgitation is on the basis of an obstructive cardiomyopathy. The systolic murmur and mid systolic click of a 'floppy' mitral valve may be strikingly influenced by physical maneuvers. For example, sudden standing or the strain phase of the Valsalva maneuver decreases left ventricular cavity size and this exaggerates the laxity of the mitral support apparatus. The click then occurs earlier in systole and the murmur becomes longer (Barlow et al, 1967). Conversely, the murmur shortens and the click is delayed as left ventricular volume increases with squatting or with the release phase of the Valsalva maneuver. The murmur may intensify as left ventricular pressure increases with squatting, or it may soften if the mitral regurgitation becomes trivial.

Pharmacologic maneuvers

Pharmacologic agents which increase systemic resistance and left ventricular pressure (phenylephrine, methoxamine, mephenteramine) tend to increase the intensity of the murmur of mitral regurgitation. These agents are not useful in differentiating mitral regurgitation and a ventricular septal defect, however.

Associated anomalies

The physical examination can be quite helpful in identifying accompanying malformations. In the

MITRAL REGURGITATION

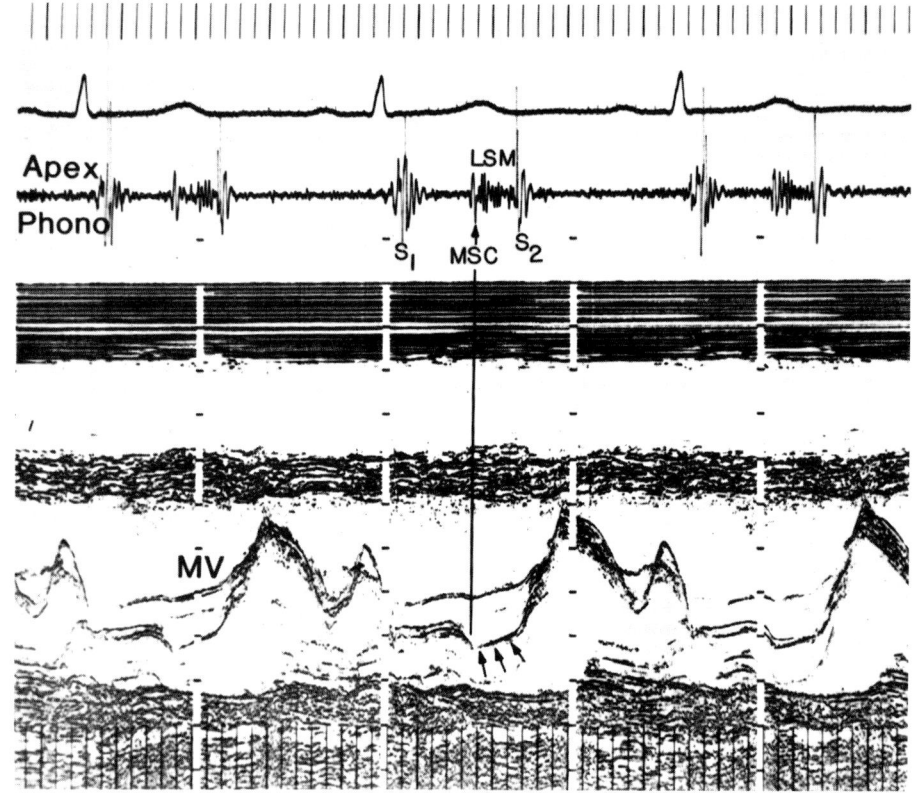

Fig. 15.4 Apex phonocardiogram and echocardiogram of a child with a prolapsing mitral leaflet. There is a late systolic murmur (LSM) which occurs during prolapse of a mitral leaflet (arrows). A mid systolic click (MSC) introduced the murmur.

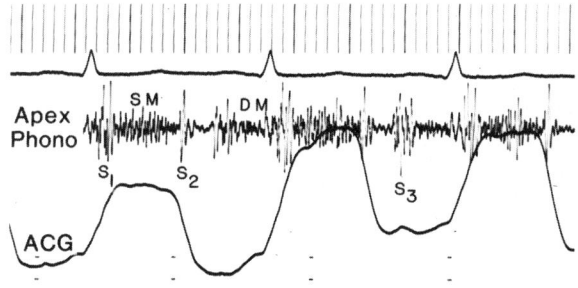

Fig. 15.5 Apex phonocardiogram and apical pulse tracing (ACG) of an adolescent girl with severe rheumatic mitral regurgitation. There are systolic and diastolic apical murmurs as well as a prominent sustained apical impulse.

Fig. 15.6 (*right*) Phonocardiogram and mid left sternal border pulse tracing (MLSB ACG) in a child with acute rheumatic fever. There is a systolic murmur (SM) of mitral regurgitation as well as an apical diastolic murmur introduced by a prominent third heart sound (S_3). The left sternal border lift and the loud second heart sound at the HLSB suggest the presence of pulmonary hypertension.

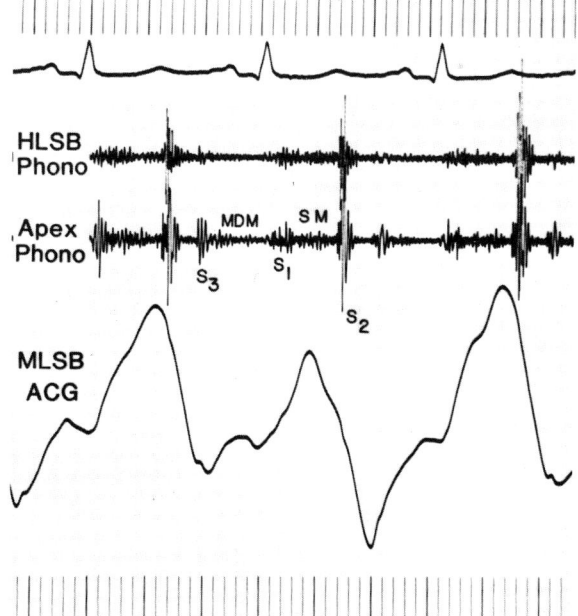

presence of mitral regurgitation, a fixedly split second heart sound suggests an interatrial septal defect, especially if a murmur of relative tricuspid stenosis is present. A fourth heart sound is very rare with the usual chronic mitral regurgitation, and if one is heard it suggests that the mitral regurgitation is on the basis of a hypertrophic cardiomyopathy. If the murmur of aortic regurgitation accompanies that of mitral regurgitation, the valvar abnormalities are almost certainly rheumatic.

REFERENCES

Barlow J B, Bosman C K, Pocock W A, Marchand P 1967 Late systolic murmurs and non-ejection (mid-late) systolic clicks. British Heart Journal 30: 203

Bridgen W, Leatham A 1953 Mitral insufficiency. British Heart Journal 15: 55

Gould L, Ettinger S J, Lyon A F 1968 Intensity of the first heart sound and arterial pulse in mitral insufficiency. Diseases of the Chest 53: 545

Phillips J E, Burch G E, De Pasquale N P 1963 The syndrome of papillary muscle dysfunction. Annals of Internal Medicine 59: 508

Sutton G C, Craige E 1967 Clinical signs of severe acute mitral regurgitation. American Journal of Cardiology 20: 141

Tavel M E 1978 Clinical phonocardiography and external pulse recording, 3rd edn. Year Book Medical Publishers, Chicago, p 248

16

Tricuspid valve anomalies

TRICUSPID REGURGITATION

The anomaly

Isolated tricuspid regurgitation is rare (Antia & Osunkoya, 1969); it more commonly accompanies other cardiac anomalies such as pulmonary atresia with intact ventricular septum, Ebstein's anomaly, or endocardial cushion defect. Regurgitation may be due to a cleft in a leaflet, dysplasia of one or more leaflets (Becker et al, 1971), or to absence of part or all of a leaflet or even of the entire valve (Kanjuh et al, 1964). Dilatation of the tricuspid annulus may result in 'functional' tricuspid regurgitation in patients with long-standing elevation of right ventricular pressure (e.g. pulmonary hypertension, transposition of the great arteries). Transient tricuspid regurgitation, possibly related to myocardial ischemia, may occur in a newborn in the absence of structural abnormality of the tricuspid valve (Freymann & Kallfelz, 1975). Tricuspid regurgitation may also be a complication of surgical repair of tetralogy of Fallot, ventricular septal defect, endocardial cushion defect, complete transposition of the great arteries or subpulmonic stenosis due to an anomalous muscle bundle. The tricuspid valve may also be damaged during attempted balloon septostomy if the inflated balloon is inadvertently pulled from the right ventricle to the right atrium.

Clinical course

Tricuspid regurgitation may have disastrous hemodynamic consequences in the newborn period, when high right ventricular pressure increases the severity of the regurgitation. Forward flow from the right ventricle may then be very low and there may be massive right to left shunting across a patent foramen ovale, resulting in severe arterial unsaturation and intense cyanosis. Death may occur, but, if the infant survives the newborn period, the severity of the regurgitation decreases as pulmonary vascular resistance and right ventricular pressure fall. Cyanosis and congestive heart failure may then diminish or disappear. Severe tricuspid regurgitation may be surprisingly well tolerated if pulmonary vascular resistance is low and there are no other cardiac anomalies — as illustrated by the young adult with endocarditis who does well after surgical excision of an infected tricuspid valve.

Physical findings

General

Cyanosis will likely occur in a patient with severe tricuspid regurgitation if there is an interatrial communication. Arterial pulses are normal in patients with tricuspid regurgitation unless there is severe congestive heart failure. Jugular venous 'V' waves and systolic hepatic pulsations may be present if tricuspid regurgitation is severe, especially if the regurgitation is acute and the right atrium is of normal size (Fig. 16.1). (If the tricuspid regurgitation is of long-standing and the right atrium has become quite dilated, the right ventricular systolic impulse is 'soaked up' by the capacious right atrium and is not transmitted to the jugular veins or liver.) A prominent left parasternal impulse is usually present with tricuspid regurgitation and is a result of the large right

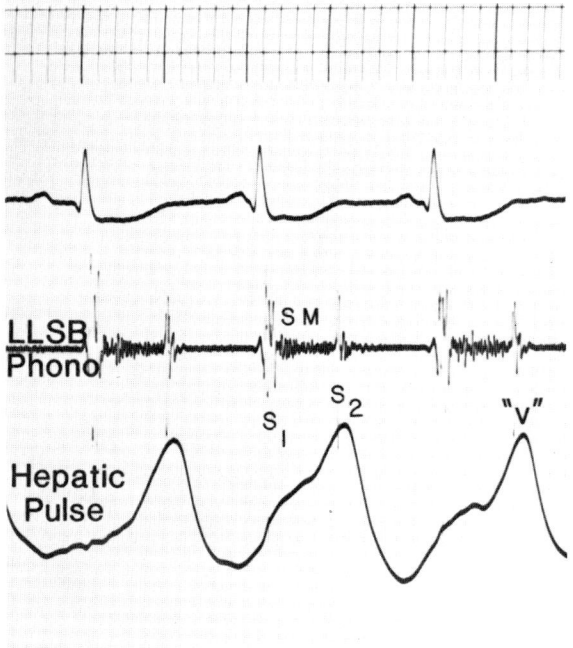

Fig. 16.1 Phonocardiogram and hepatic pulse tracing of an infant with complete transposition of the great arteries and tricuspid regurgitation. There is a low left sternal border systolic murmur and systolic hepatic pulsation.

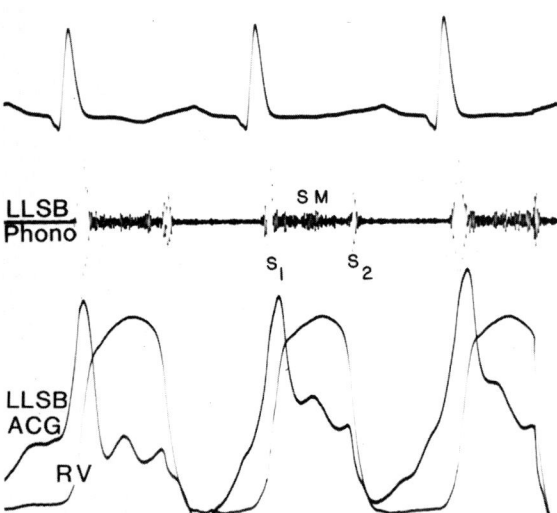

Fig. 16.2 Phonocardiogram, low left sternal border pulse tracing (LLSB ACG) and right ventricular pressure in an infant with congenital tricuspid regurgitation. There is a holosystolic systolic murmur and a poorly sustained left sternal border lift.

ventricular stroke volume (Fig. 16.2). The jet effect of severe regurgitation may cause a leftward shift of the entire precordium with ventricular systole, which is best appreciated by viewing the supine patient from the foot of the bed.

Auscultation

The first heart sound is usually normal in patients with tricuspid regurgitation. (If regurgitation is due to Ebstein's anomaly the first sound characteristically is widely split — see Figure 16.10 (Fontana & Wooley, 1972).) The second heart sound is normal. A third heart sound is common but a fourth sound is not part of the auscultatory picture of tricuspid regurgitation.

The systolic murmur of tricuspid regurgitation is typically maximal at the low left sternal border. It is usually soft, high pitched, plateau shaped and holosystolic (Figs 16.1, 16.2), but exceptions occur. If the tricuspid closure sound is delayed, as in Ebstein's anomaly, the systolic murmur begins with the second component of the first heart sound and is therefore not holosystolic (Fig. 16.3). In some patients the systolic murmur is descrescendo and may end well before the second heart sound (Fig. 16.10). The systolic murmur may have a musical quality, or in an occasional patient may be loud, harsh and accompanied by a thrill. The murmur of tricuspid regurgitation may be well heard near the apex if there is marked right

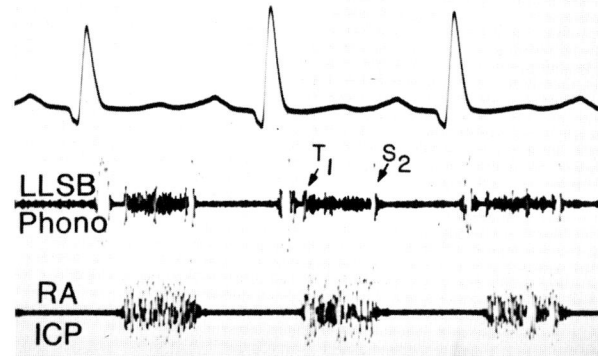

Fig. 16.3 The systolic murmur is not holosystolic in this child with congenital tricuspid regurgitation. It begins after an early systolic sound which probably represents delayed closure of the tricuspid valve (T_1). The late onset of the murmur is confirmed in the right atrial sound tracing (RA ICP).

ventricular enlargement and in such a patient may be mistaken for the murmur of mitral regurgitation. The systolic murmur of tricuspid regurgitation usually increases with inspiration and fades or even disappears with expiration (Rivero–Carvallo, 1946). Such inspiratory accentuation is thought to be due to an inspiratory increase in systemic venous return and right ventricular filling, with a consequent increase in the vigor of right ventricular contraction. It must be remembered, however, that an apparent respiratory change in intensity of a murmur may actually be due to a shift in the point of maximal intensity of the murmur. The systolic murmur of subvalvar pulmonic stenosis, for instance, may become louder at the low left sternal border during inspiration, but also become softer at the mid left sternal border (Fig. 16.4). (This phenomenon is especially common if the obstruction is low in the right ventricle and due to an anomalous muscle bundle.) An increase in intensity of a systolic murmur at the low left sternal border does not, therefore, imply tricuspid regurgitation if there is a reciprocal change in the intensity of the murmur higher along the left sternal border. The murmur of relative tricuspid stenosis is common if tricuspid regurgitation is severe (Fig. 16.5). This murmur is medium pitched and mid diastolic and is also maximal at the low left sternal border.

TRICUSPID STENOSIS

The anomaly

Tricuspid stenosis is rare in childhood and is almost always congenital. A small tricuspid orifice is usually associated with hypoplasia of the right ventricle; in some cases the tricuspid valve is diminutive but in proportion to the right ventricular cavity size, while in others the leaflets are dysplastic, with or without commissural fusion, and the tricuspid orifice is disproportionally small (Zuberbuhler & Anderson, 1979). Tricuspid stenosis is usually associated with other cardiac anomalies, such as severe pulmonic stenosis, pulmonic atresia (Zuberbuhler & Anderson, 1979), or Ebstein's anomaly of the tricuspid valve (Zuberbuhler et al, 1979). In such patients the clinical picture is dominated by the associated anomalies, the tricuspid stenosis itself being difficult to diagnose during

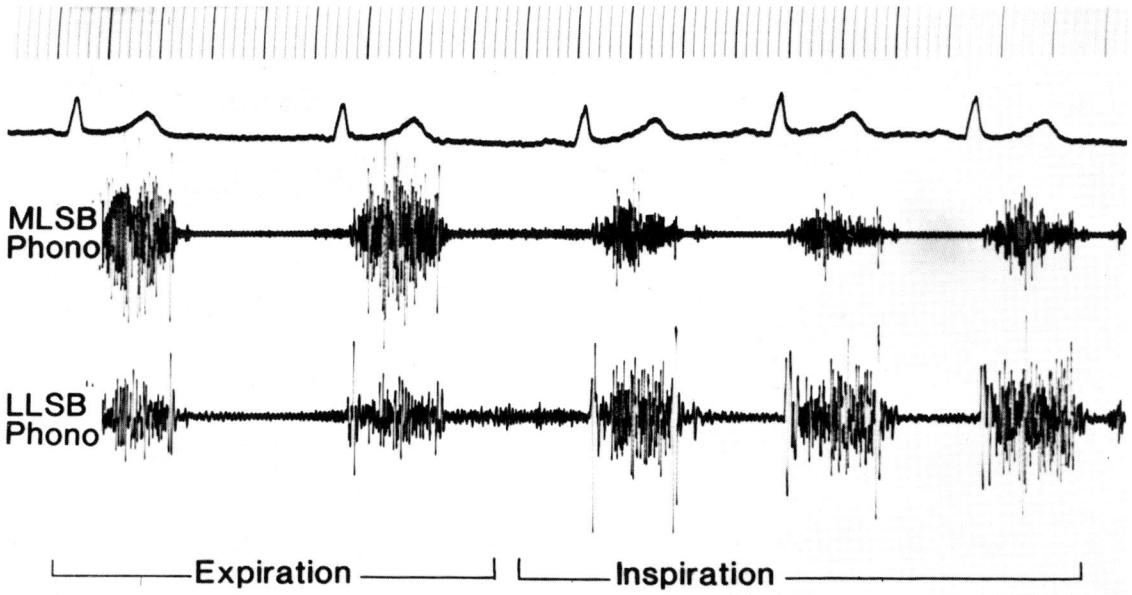

Fig. 16.4 'Pseudo' Carvallo's sign in a child with subinfundibular pulmonic stenosis. Although there is an inspiratory augmentation of the low left sternal border there is a reciprocal softening of the murmur at the mid left sternal border.

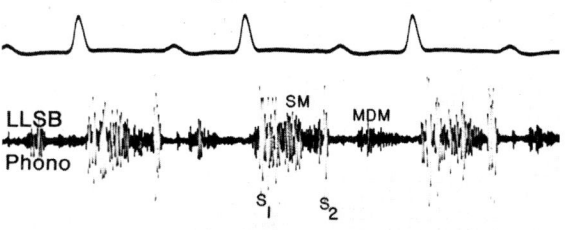

Fig. 16.5 Infant with single ventricle and severe tricuspid regurgitation. There is a decrescendo systolic murmur as well as a mid diastolic murmur of relative tricuspid stenosis.

life. 'Isolated' tricuspid stenosis is exceedingly rare but does occur. Tricuspid stenosis also may be rheumatic and is then virtually always associated with severe mitral valve disease.

Physical findings

General

Elevation of right atrial pressure is the major hemodynamic consequence of tricuspid stenosis and may result in right to left atrial shunting and cyanosis if the foramen ovale is patent or if there is an associated interatrial septal defect. If stenosis is severe a large 'A' wave may be evident in the jugular venous pulse. The cardiac impulse is inconspicuous.

Auscultation

A low left sternal border diastolic murmur is the most common auscultatory feature of tricuspid stenosis. In the author's experience this murmur is mid-diastolic and without presystolic accentuation (Fig. 16.6). The murmur of tricuspid stenosis is usually subtle and is easily missed, especially if there are associated anomalies. There may be no diastolic murmur at all, even with severe stenosis, if there is an interatrial communication with right to left shunting. The right atrium then decompresses through the interatrial communication, keeping tricuspid flow low and the gradient small. Such decompression is especially likely to occur if there is severe right ventricular outflow obstruction; after relief of the obstruction a prominent diastolic murmur of tricuspid stenosis may appear

for the first time. The murmur of tricuspid stenosis may show considerable respiratory variation, increasing in intensity with inspiration and fading or even disappearing with expiration (Fig. 16.7). Patients with tricuspid stenosis may occasionally demonstrate an opening snap of the tricuspid valve (Fig. 16.8) but it is usually difficult to be sure the snap is not of mitral origin.

EBSTEIN'S ANOMALY OF THE TRICUSPID VALVE

The anomaly

The essence of Ebstein's anomaly of the tricuspid valve is distal displacement of the origin of the septal and inferior leaflets from the tricuspid annulus to a position within the right ventricle. The origin of the anterior leaflet is normal and at the annulus, but the leaflet itself is often large and 'sail-like' and may be perforated. In many patients with Ebstein's anomaly the distal attachments of the tricuspid leaflets are abnormal as well, and in some cases, including the original patient reported by Ebstein, the combination of abnormal proximal and distal attachments results in a fibrous or fibromuscular membrane which partially or completely partitions the right ventricle (Schiebler et al, 1968; Zuberbuhler et al, 1979). The distal displacement of the tricuspid leaflets results in 'physiologic atrialization' of a portion of the right ventricle, with atrial pressure recordable in this area. There may be 'anatomic atrialization' as well, with thinning of the right ventricular free wall between the annulus and the origin of the displaced leaflets.

Clinical course

There is a wide spectrum of clinical presentation and course in patients with Ebstein's anomaly. Intense cyanosis and signs of right heart failure are common in the neonate with this entity and are related to a combination of right heart dysfunction and elevated pulmonary vascular resistance. (The cyanosis is due to right to left atrial shunting through the foramen ovale.) Hypoxemia and congestive heart failure may progress inexorably to death in early infancy, or improvement may follow the fall in pulmonary vascular resistance

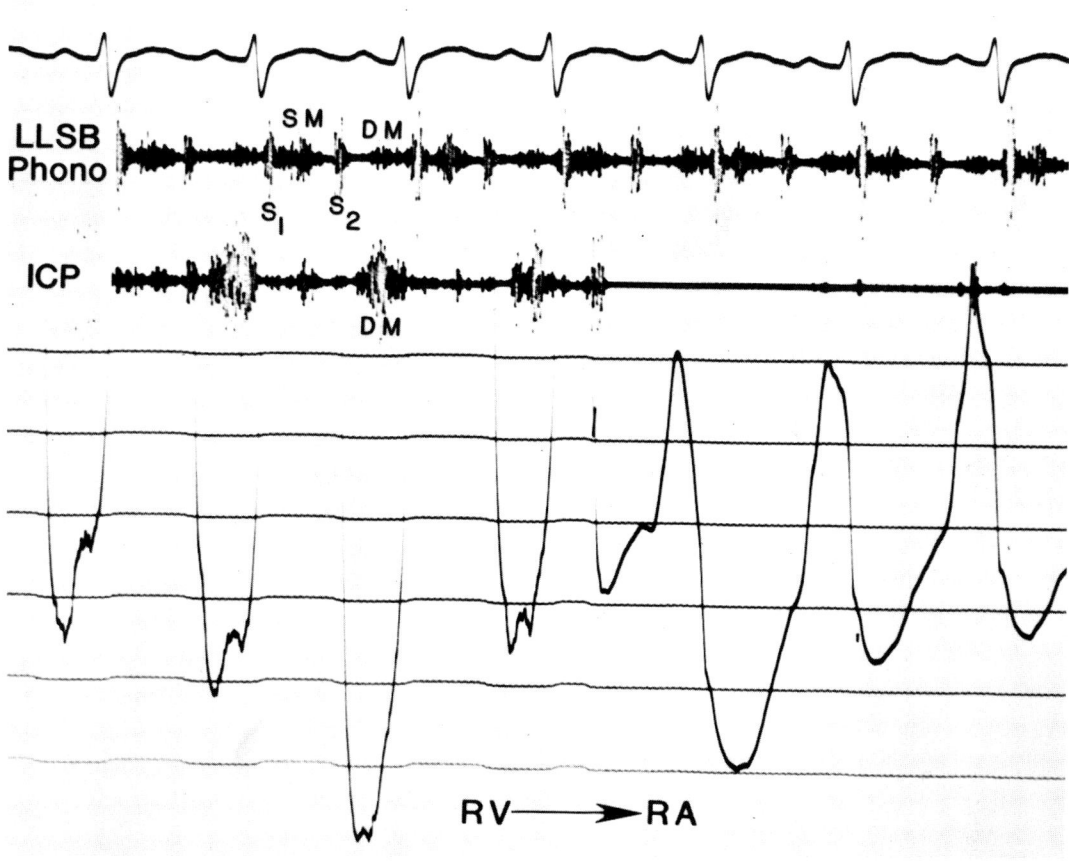

Fig. 16.6 Infant with a ventricular septal defect, severe pulmonary hypertension, a hypoplastic right ventricle and tricuspid stenosis. A mid diastolic murmur (DM) is evident in the low left sternal border phonocardiogram. Its tricuspid valve origin is indicated by its presence in the right ventricle and absence in the right atrium. Both pressure and sound (ICP) were recorded using a micromanometer tipped catheter.

which normally occurs during the first few days of life. Other individuals with Ebstein's anomaly have no difficulty in infancy and the onset of symptoms may be delayed for several years. Eventually, almost all with Ebstein's anomaly experience either congestive heart failure or cyanosis, or develop serious and sometimes life threatening arrhythmias. The latter are sometimes related to the Wolff–Parkinson–White syndrome.

Physical findings

General

The jugular venous pulse is usually normal even in patients with right atrial pressure high enough to produce right to left shunting through an interatrial septal defect or patent foramen ovale, since the 'A' or 'V' waves expected with vigorous atrial systole or tricuspid regurgitation, respectively, are damped by the large volume of blood in the capacious right atrium. A mid or low left sternal border impulse is rarely prominent, even with considerable tricuspid regurgitation, since right ventricular pressure is normal or low. In addition, the functional portion of the right ventricle is confined to the infundibulum and to a lateral crescent of trabeculated ventricle in individuals with marked tricuspid valve displacement (Fig. 16.9).

Auscultation

Heart sounds. In Ebstein's anomaly the auscultatory findings are often so distinctive as to permit

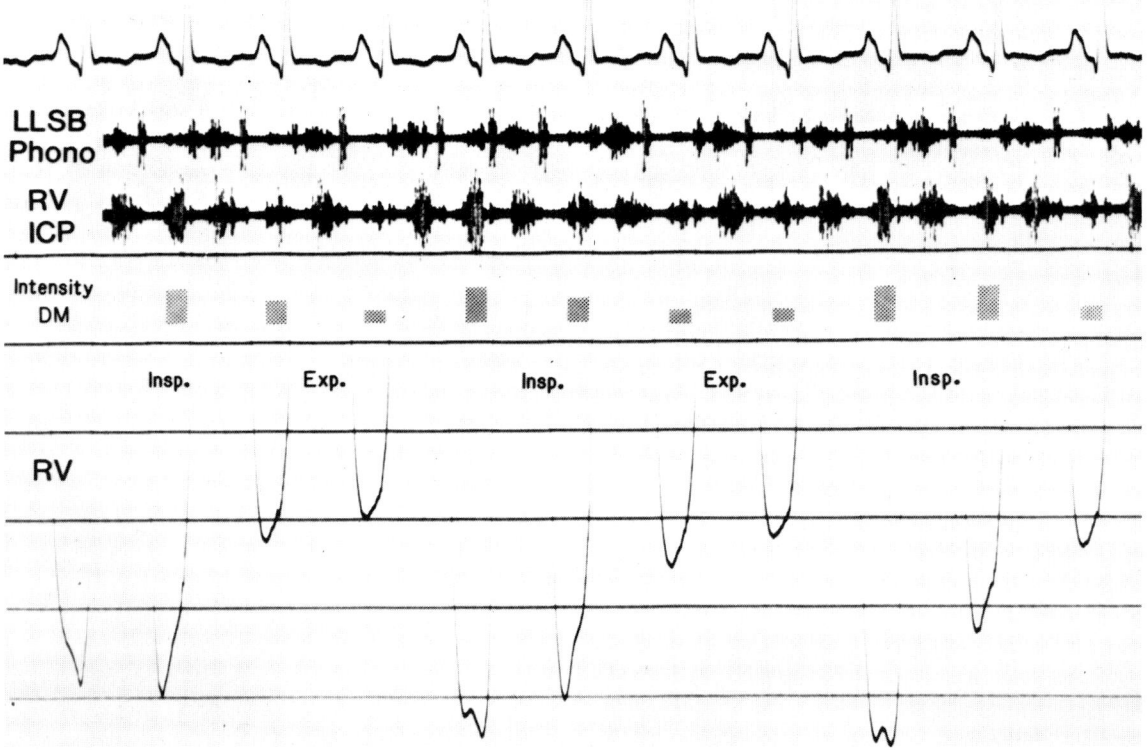

Fig. 16.7 Same infant as Figure 16.6. There is inspiratory augmentation of the diastolic murmur, both in the external phonocardiogram and in the right ventricular sound recording (RV ICP).

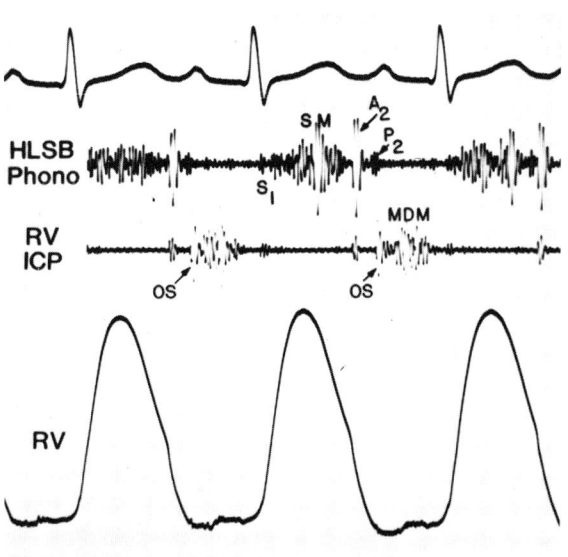

Fig. 16.8 Infant with both valvar pulmonic stenosis and congenital tricupid stenosis. The mid diastolic murmur (MDM) of the tricuspid stenosis is introduced by an opening snap (OS) in the right ventricular sound recording (RV ICP).

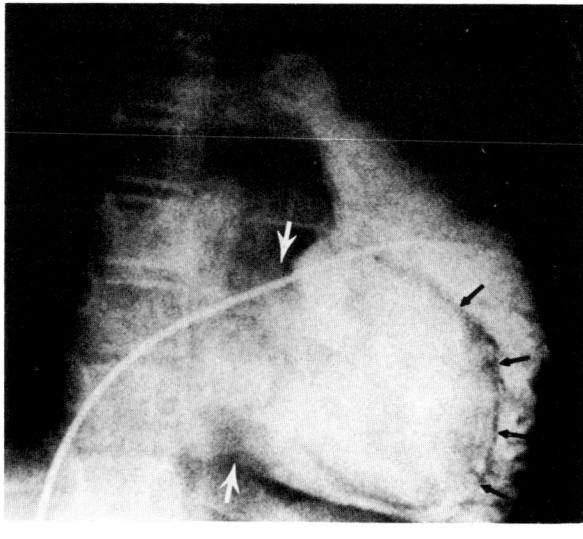

Fig. 16.9 Cineangiogram of a child with Ebstein's anomaly of the tricuspid valve. The tricuspid annulus (white arrows) is normally positioned. The distal attachment of the anterior leaflet is linear (black arrows). The densely opacified right ventricle to the right of the black arrows is the trabecular portion. The inlet portion to the left is 'physiologically atrialized'.

a firm clinical diagnosis. The first sound is usually widely split. The second (tricuspid) component is characteristically loud and quite delayed and has been termed a 'sail sound' (Fontana & Wooley, 1972). The coincidence of tricuspid valve closure and this early systolic sound can be demonstrated echocardiographically. The echocardiogram also documents the large anterior leaflet excursion, which is probably related to the loudness and delay of the sound (Fig. 16.10) (Crews et al, 1972). The second heart sound is usually widely but variably split and a third and fourth sound are common. If split first and second heart sounds and a third and fourth sound are all present phonocardiography may be necessary to sort out the plethora of audible events in the cardiac cycle. The very abundance of sounds in some patients with Ebstein's anomaly may be enough to suggest the diagnosis.

Murmurs. Tricuspid regurgitation is common in Ebstein's anomaly. The resulting systolic murmur may be maximal in the usual location at the lower left sternal border or may be displaced toward the apex. The murmur is often short, ending well before the second heart sound, and is commonly of medium pitch and 'scratchy' quality (Fig. 16.10). These unusual characteristics are probably related to low right ventricular pressure and consequent low velocity of the regurgitant stream. A short low left sternal border mid diastolic murmur is common and is due either to anatomic tricuspid stenosis (Fig. 16.11) or to the increased tricuspid diastolic flow which is a consequence of tricuspid regurgitation.

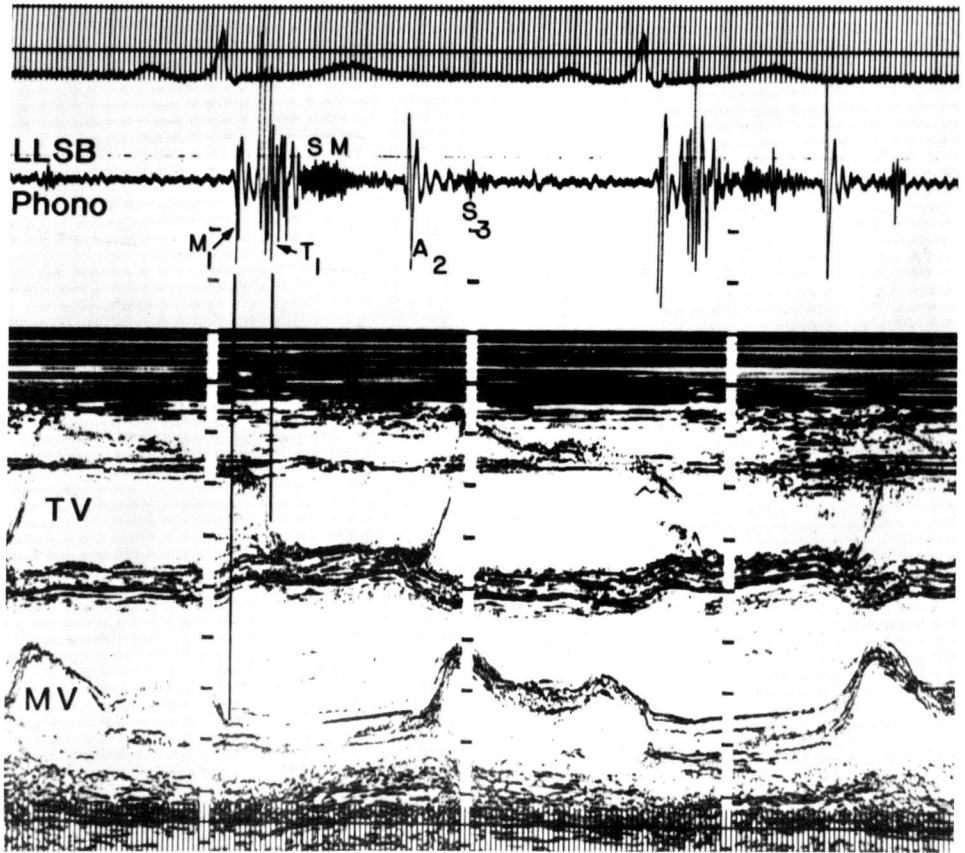

Fig. 16.10 Adolescent with Ebstein's anomaly of the tricuspid valve. In the echocardiogram the mitral valve closure corresponds temporally with the first component of the first heart sound (M_1). Tricuspid closure is delayed and coincides with the second and louder component (T_1). There is a prominent third sound (S_3) and a short systolic murmur (SM).

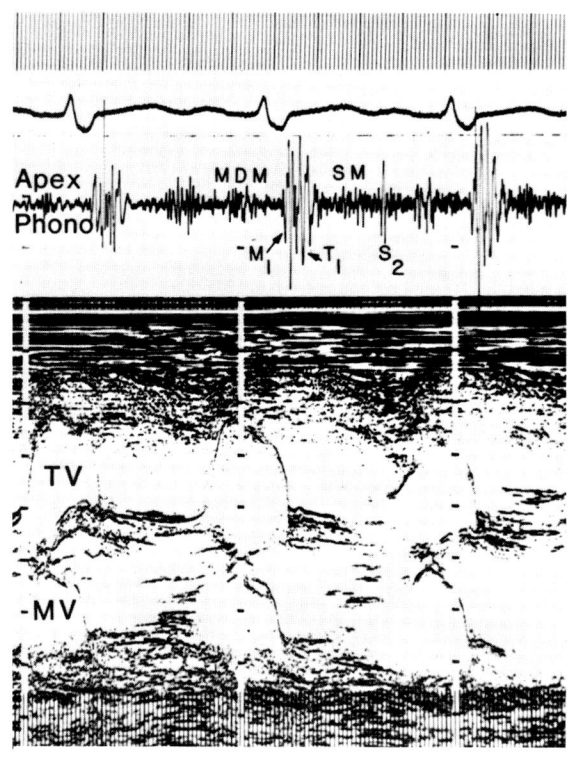

The neonate

As in so many varieties of congenital heart disease, physical findings in the neonate may be quite different from those in the older child. If tricuspid regurgitation is present the systolic murmur is more likely to be high pitched and long, since high right ventricular pressure is usual in the newborn. Gallop sounds and a split first heart sound are less common in this age group than in older children and adults. The second heart sound may be single or split. The clinical picture of Ebstein's anomaly may be dominated by intense cyanosis and in some neonates with this entity the resemblance to pulmonary atresia with intact ventricular septum can be striking, especially if the second heart sound is single and diminished and there is a murmur of tricuspid regurgitation. In such patients differentiation is possible only at cardiac catheterization.

Fig. 16.11 (*left*) Ebstein's anomaly. There is slight asynchrony of mitral and tricuspid closure in the echocardiogram and narrow splitting of the first sound (M_1–T_1) in the phonocardiogram. The mid diastolic murmur (MDM) is due to organic tricuspid stenosis, since the accompanying tricuspid regurgitation was very mild.

REFERENCES

Antia A U, Osunkoya B O 1969 Congenital tricuspid incompetence. British Heart Journal 31 : 664

Becker A E, Becker M J, Edwards J E 1971 Pathologic spectrum of dysplasia of the tricuspid valve: features in common with Ebstein's malformation. Archives of Pathology 91 : 167

Crews T L, Pridie R B, Benham R, Leatham A 1972 Auscultatory and phonocardiographic findings in Ebstein's anomaly: correlation of first heart sound with ultrasonic records of tricuspid valve movement. American Heart Journal 34 : 681

Fontana M E, Wooley C F 1972 Sail sound in Ebstein's anomaly of the tricuspid valve. Circulation 46 : 115

Freymann R, Kallfelz H C 1975 Transient tricuspid incompetence in a newborn. European Journal of Cardiology 2 : 467

Kanjuh V I, Stevenson J E, Amplatz K, Edwards J E 1964 Congenitally unguarded tricuspid orifice with coexistent pulmonary atresia. Circulation 30 : 911

Rivero-Carvallo J M 1946 New diagnostic sign of tricuspid insufficiency. Archivas del Instituto de Cardiologia de Mexico 16 : 531

Schiebler G L, Gravenstein J S, Van Mierop L H S 1968 Ebstein's anomaly of the tricuspid valve: translation of original description with comments. American Journal of Cardiology 22 : 867

Zuberbuhler J R, Allwork S P, Anderson R H 1979 The spectrum of Ebstein's anomaly of the tricuspid valve. Journal of Thoracic and Cardiovascular Surgery 77 : 202

Zuberbuhler J R, Anderson R H 1979 Morphologic variations in pulmonary atresia with intact ventricular septum. British Heart Journal 41 : 281

17

Valvar atresia

TRICUSPID ATRESIA

The anomaly

When the tricuspid valve is atretic systemic venous blood must exit the right atrium through a patent foramen ovale or an interatrial septal defect. It then enters the left atrium and crosses the mitral valve into the left ventricle. A variable amount of left ventricular blood re-enters the right heart via an interventricular septal defect (outlet foramen) (Fig. 17.1). (The only exception to this general rule is when pulmonary atresia accompanies tricuspid atresia. Here, the right ventricle is absent or merely a slit-like cavity and hemodynamically this entity closely resembles pulmonary atresia with intact ventricular septum.) Anatomically, tricuspid atresia is not simply absence of the tricuspid valve leaflets. A dimple in the floor of the right atrium is the only vestige of tricuspid valve in most cases, and relates to the left ventricle rather than the right (Rosenquist et al, 1970). (A needle inserted into this dimple exits into the left ventricle.) The hypoplastic 'right ventricle' of tricuspid atresia differs in no important way from the 'outlet chamber' of right ventricular type commonly present in univentricular hearts. In fact, tricuspid atresia can be considered a variety of univentricular heart in which the right-sided atrioventricular valve did not fully develop (Anderson et al, 1977).

Clinical course and physical findings

General

There are several anatomic variables which determine both the clinical course and the physical findings in a patient with tricuspid atresia. These include the size of the interatrial communication, presence or absence of obstruction between the left ventricle and the artery supported by the 'right ventricle', and ventriculoarterial connection. In our experience the interatrial opening is rarely obstructive, but when it is, vigorous contractions of the hypertrophied right atrium produce large 'A' waves in the jugular venous pulse and palpable presystolic pulsations of the liver (Fig. 17.2) (Lenox & Zuberbuhler, 1970).

Obstruction between the left ventricle and the anterior great artery may be at a restrictive

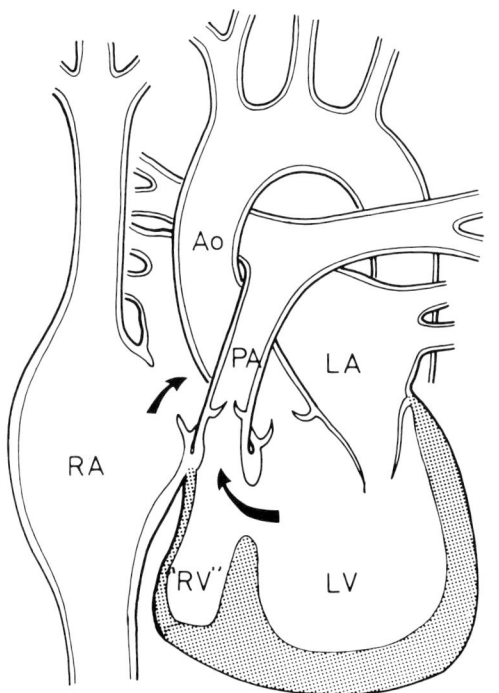

Fig. 17.1 Diagram of tricuspid atresia. There is a right to left shunt at atrial level and a left to right shunt at ventricular level (arrows).

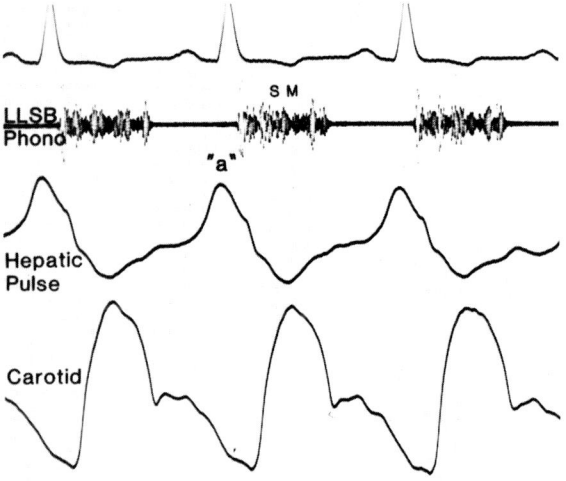

Fig. 17.2 Tricuspid atresia and restrictive interatrial communication. There is a large presystolic 'A' wave in the pulse tracing recorded below the right costal margin.

ventricular septal defect or, more commonly, within the 'right ventricular' cavity (infundibular pulmonic stenosis) or at the pulmonic valve. If obstruction is severe, pulmonary blood flow is small and arterial desaturation and cyanosis will be marked. If there is no obstruction pulmonary blood flow is torrential and congestive heart failure results. If there is moderate pulmonic stenosis, cyanosis is mild and congestive heart failure absent. In summary, if there is severe pulmonic stenosis presentation is in early infancy with intense cyanosis. If there is no pulmonic stenosis, presentation is also early but is with congestive heart failure. With an 'ideal' degree of pulmonic stenosis, cyanosis and physical limitation may be mild for years. Such individuals have been known to survive for several decades.

Since there is complete mixing of systemic and pulmonary venous returns by the time they reach the left ventricle, ventriculo-arterial discordance does not directly influence arterial oxygen saturation. However, there is a strong positive correlation between pulmonic stenosis and normal ventriculo-arterial connection and a strong negative correlation between pulmonic stenosis and ventriculo-arterial discordance. Thus, children with ventriculo-arterial discordance usually present with congestive heart failure, those with ventriculo-arterial concordance more often present with cyanosis. In an occasional individual with ventriculo-arterial discordance, a restrictive ventricular septal defect constitutes subaortic stenosis. One such reported child had episodes of chest pain, sweating and ST segment depression highly suggestive of myocardial ischemia (Neches et al, 1973).

Infants and children with tricuspid atresia usually have no major noncardiac anomalies. Cyanosis is variable and, as dicussed above, is related to the degree of pulmonic stenosis. Peripheral pulses and blood pressure are normal unless there is coarctation of the aorta, which sometimes occurs when ventriculo-arterial discordance accompanies tricuspid atresia (Rudolph et al, 1972). As mentioned above, the jugular venous pulse is abnormal and there may be a presystolic hepatic pulse if the interatrial opening is restrictive (Fig. 17.2). The left parasternal area is quiet in individuals with tricuspid atresia but the apical impulse may be quite active, especially if there is little or no pulmonic stenosis.

Auscultation

The second heart sound is soft and single at the high left sternal border if there is severe pulmonic stenosis, but may be audibly split if pulmonic stenosis is mild. If there is ventriculo-arterial discordance the second heart sound is usually loud and single at the base, representing aortic valve closure. A third heart sound is common if there is increased pulmonary blood flow. Most individuals with tricuspid atresia have a systolic murmur which is loudest at the mid or low left sternal border. It may be either pansystolic and plateau or crescendo-decrescendo (Fig. 17.3), and originates either at the site of right ventricular outflow tract obstruction or at a restrictive ventricular septal defect. The shape, quality and location of the murmur do not reliably distinguish the two sites of obstruction. This distinction is made with assurance only by entering the right ventricle at the time of cardiac catheterization. As in tetralogy of Fallot, there tends to be an inverse relationship between the loudness of the murmur and the severity of the pulmonic stenosis.

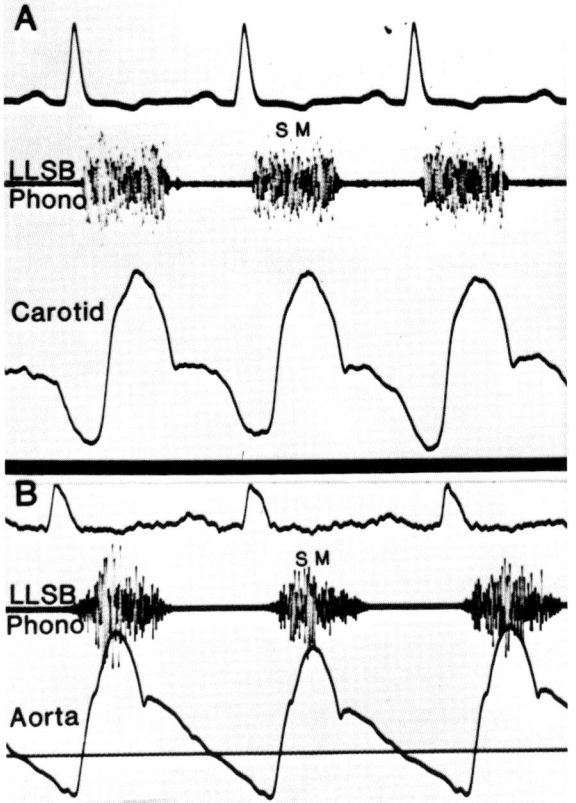

Fig. 17.3 Phonocardiograms from two children with tricuspid atresia. Both have pulmonic stenosis, but in A the murmur is holosystolic and plateau, while in B it is crescendo-decrescendo.

PULMONARY ATRESIA WITH INTACT VENTRICULAR SEPTUM

The clinical course and physical findings associated with complete right ventricular outflow tract obstruction are influenced by the presence or absence of a ventricular septal defect. Pulmonary atresia with a ventricular septal defect is dealt with in Chapter 18, pulmonary atresia with intact ventricular septum is considered here.

The anomaly

The only constant morphologic feature of pulmonary atresia with intact ventricular septum is absence of a patent pulmonary orifice, although certain other right heart structures are usually abnormal as well. Right ventricular cavity size constitutes a wide spectrum, ranging from diminutive to large. The tricuspid annular dimension is also variable and tends to be proportional to the right ventricular cavity size. Structural abnormalities of the tricuspid leaflets are very common (Zuberbuhler & Anderson, 1979) and the tricuspid valve may be regurgitant or may be stenotic out of proportion to hypoplasia of the right ventricle. (Tricuspid stenosis is of no functional significance unless pulmonary valvotomy or outflow tract reconstruction is successful.)

Clinical course

Hemodynamically, this entity has two inevitable consequences. There is obligatory right to left shunting at atrial level, usually via a patent foramen ovale, and left to right shunting must occur at great artery level, almost always through a patent ductus arteriosus (Fig. 17.4). Obstruction to right to left atrial flow is uncommon but left to right shunting at great artery level is less stable, since there is a strong tendency for the ductus arteriosus to close in the neonatal period. Since the ductus is

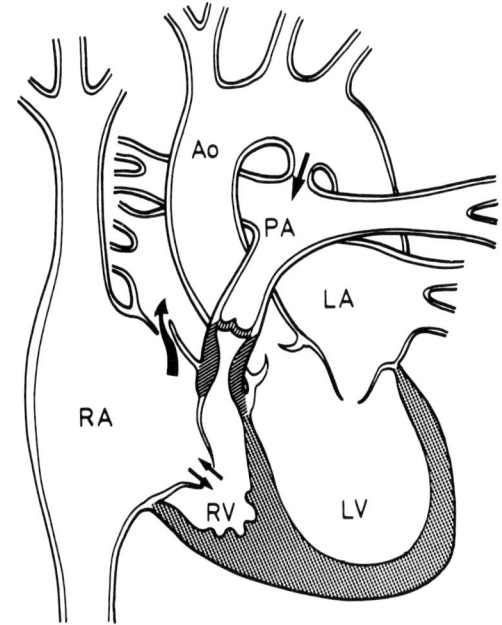

Fig. 17.4 Diagram of pulmonary atresia with intact ventricular septum. There is right to left shunting through the foramen ovale and left to right shunting through the patent ductus arteriosus (arrows).

the sole source of pulmonary blood flow, severe hypoxemia results as the ductus narrows and intense cyanosis dominates the clinical picture. Tachypnea, also on the basis of hypoxemia, is common but congestive heart failure is unusual. Death usually occurs within the first few days or weeks of life unless a stable source of pulmonary blood flow is established surgically.

Physical findings

General

Infants with pulmonary atresia and an intact ventricular septum usually have no other important non-cardiac anomalies and the general examination is unremarkable. Blood pressure and arterial pulses are normal unless the infant is in extremis. Although one might expect the jugular venous pulse to show large 'A' waves from a vigorously contracting right atrium or 'V' waves from tricuspid regurgitation, these findings are unusual since the jugular venous pulse is so hard to see in an infant. The precordium is usually quiet, although a vigorous low left sternal border systolic impulse may be present if there is major tricuspid regurgitation (Schrire et al, 1961).

Auscultation

The second heart sound is always single and is almost always soft at the high left sternal border. The first heart sound is of normal intensity and neither a third or fourth heart sound is part of the auscultatory picture. There is no early systolic ejection sound in this variety of pulmonary atresia, being common only if there is an associated ventricular septal defect. A blowing pansystolic murmur of tricuspid regurgitation may be present at the low left sternal border and is the best single clinical marker of a relatively normal right ventricular cavity size. If the tricuspid regurgitation is of large volume, the short medium pitched mid diastolic murmur of relative tricuspid stenosis may be present at the low left sternal border. Organic tricuspid stenosis out of proportion to the ventricular cavity size occurs but is not detectable clinically, since there is little or no forward flow across the tricuspid valve. Following successful pulmonary valvulotomy, however, a diastolic murmur of tricuspid stenosis may become evident (Fig. 17.5). A patent ductus arteriosus may give rise to a continuous murmur at the high left sternal border. This murmur is almost always soft and high pitched and is so subtle that it is easily obscured by breath sounds or the noise of an oxygen line or an incubator. It is usually missed unless specifically searched for. Some infants with pulmonary atresia have no murmur at all.

Summary

In summary, infants with pulmonary atresia and intact ventricular septum become intensely cyanotic in the newborn period. In such a setting either the systolic murmur of tricuspid regurgitation or the continuous murmur of a patent ductus arteriosus should suggest the diagnosis, especially if the second heart sound is soft and single at the high left sternal border and if there is no ejection sound. It must be noted that critical valvar pulmonic stenosis may be clinically indistinguishable from pulmonary atresia.

MITRAL ATRESIA

The anomaly and its clinical course

When the mitral valve is atretic, other cardiac anomalies are always present. Although very complex malformations are often found, all cases of mitral atresia have certain features in common. By definition, left atrial blood cannot enter the left ventricle directly. It passes instead to the right atrium, usually via an interatrial communication but occasionally by way of a left atrial connection to the coronary sinus or to a systemic vein. Then, the combined systemic and pulmonary venous returns cross the tricuspid valve into the right ventricle. Right ventricular blood is distributed, in a variety of ways, to both pulmonary artery and aorta. The right ventricle may support both great arteries, there being no left ventricular chamber. In other cases the right ventricle supports only one great artery, usually the pulmonary artery. If there is a ventricular septal defect, a left ventricular chamber will be present and supports the other great artery (Fig. 17.6). The left ventricular

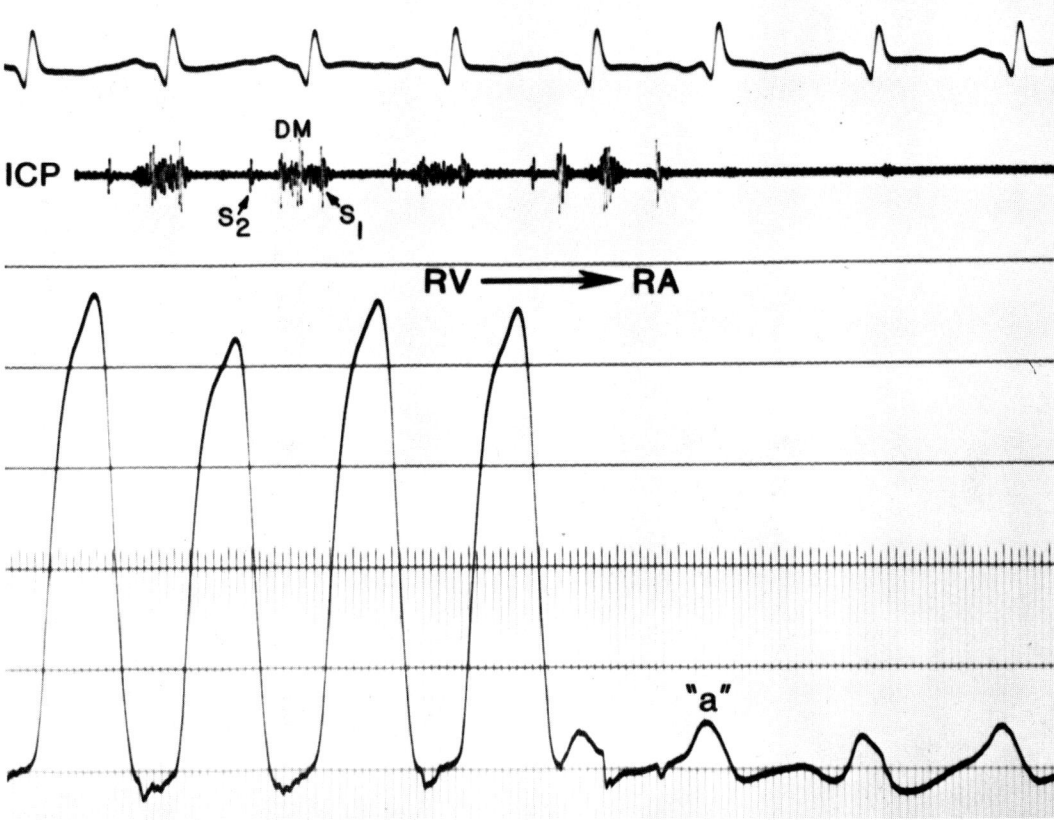

Fig. 17.5 Child with pulmonary atresia who had successful valvotomy in early infancy. A prominent diastolic murmur of tricuspid stenosis is present in the right ventricular inlet but not in the right atrium. Both sound (ICP) and pressure were recorded using a micromanometer tipped catheter.

chamber is usually hypoplastic. If there is no ventricular septal defect, the aortic valve is atretic and the aorta fills only by way of a patent ductus arteriosus.

The clinical spectrum of mitral atresia is wide and is largely determined by the size of the interatrial communication and the morphology of ventricular outlet. Exit from the left atrium is most commonly via an opening in the interatrial septum which has been created by herniation of the flap of the foramen ovale through the foramen into the right atrium (Eliot et al, 1965). This opening is usually restrictive (Fig. 17.7), leading to elevation of left atrial and pulmonary venous pressure and thus to tachypnea, which is often a prominent clinical sign in this entity. Ventriculo-arterial connections do not, per se, influence the clinical picture of mitral atresia. Associated pulmonic or aortic stenosis does. Pulmonic stenosis reduces pulmonary blood flow, and, if stenosis is severe, cyanosis will be intense. If there is no pulmonary stenosis, pulmonary blood flow will be large and cyanosis slight or even inapparent. The clinical picture is then dominated by congestive heart failure. If arterial unsaturation is not obvious such an infant may clinically seem to have a simple left to right shunt at ventricular level. Aortic stenosis tends to reduce systemic flow and to increase output into the pulmonic circuit, contributing to congestive failure.

Individuals with mitral atresia usually become symptomatic in early infancy, but in an occasional patient the combination of a sizable interatrial defect, moderate pulmonic stenosis and unobstructed outflow to the aorta permits late onset of symptoms and relatively prolonged survival.

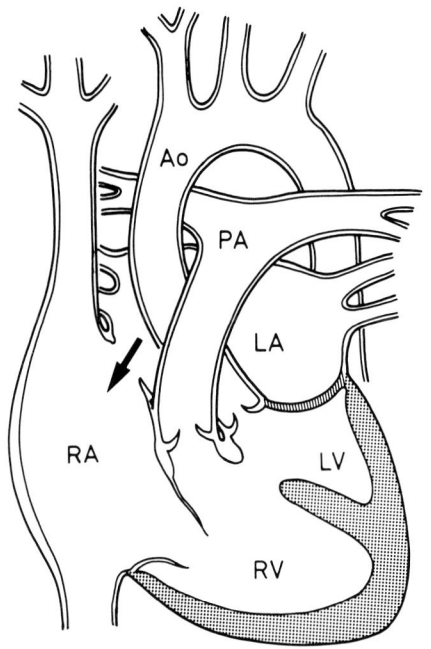

Fig. 17.6 Diagram of mitral atresia. In the variety of mitral atresia pictured here there is an interventricular septal defect, a small left ventricle and ventriculo-arterial concordance. The arrow indicates left to right shunting through an interatrial communication.

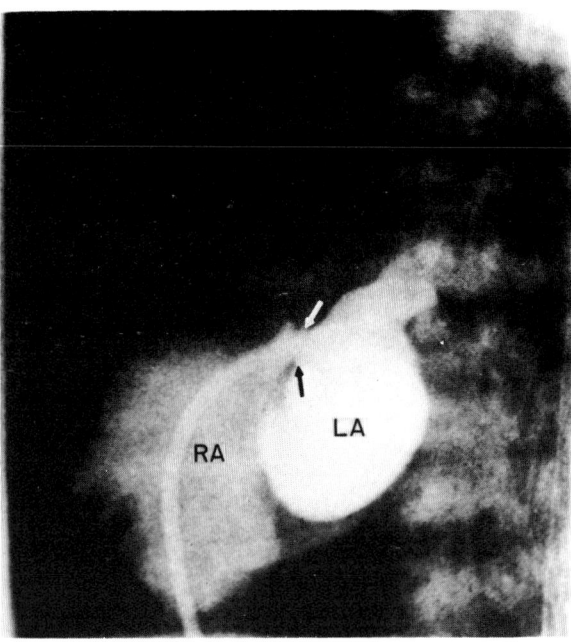

Fig. 17.7 Selective left atrial cineangiogram in an infant with mitral atresia. The interatrial communication (arrows) is quite small and restrictive.

Physical findings

General

As mentioned above, cyanosis is variable in patients with mitral atresia and in general is inversely proportional to pulmonary blood flow. Arterial pulses are decreased or absent if there is associated aortic stenosis or atresia or if there is torrential pulmonary blood flow. Coarctation of the aorta, which may be associated with mitral atresia, causes decreased or absent pulses in the lower extremities (Watson et al, 1960). The jugular venous pulse is usually normal. There is usually a prominent left parasternal lift, since the right ventricle is both pressure and volume overloaded. The apical impulse is quiet or absent.

Auscultation

In infancy, the second heart sound is usually loud and single at the high left sternal border. It may be split, especially if there is mild pulmonic stenosis. In older children the second heart sound is commonly split. The first heart sound is of normal intensity, in spite of the lack of a mitral component. When the interatrial communication is restrictive a continuous 'humming' or 'roaring' murmur may be present, usually over the lower sternum (Ross et al, 1963; Zuberbuhler et al, 1975) (Fig. 17.8). The murmur usually has a diastolic accentuation and may be audible only in diastole. In some patients the murmur is augmented during straining (Zuberbuhler et al, 1975), but in others it is louder during inspiration and decreases with a Valsalva maneuver (Ross et al, 1963). A loud mid or high left sternal border systolic murmur suggests associated pulmonic stenosis. In infants without pulmonic stenosis a soft systolic murmur is usually present at the mid and high left sternal border and often across the back. It is generated by increased flow across the pulmonic valve and through the pulmonary arteries. A short, medium pitched mid-diastolic murmur of relative tricuspid stenosis is common in such patients and results from the obligatory passage of combined systemic and pulmonary venous returns across the tricuspid valve. The systolic murmur of organic tricuspid regurgitation may appear in individuals who survive childhood.

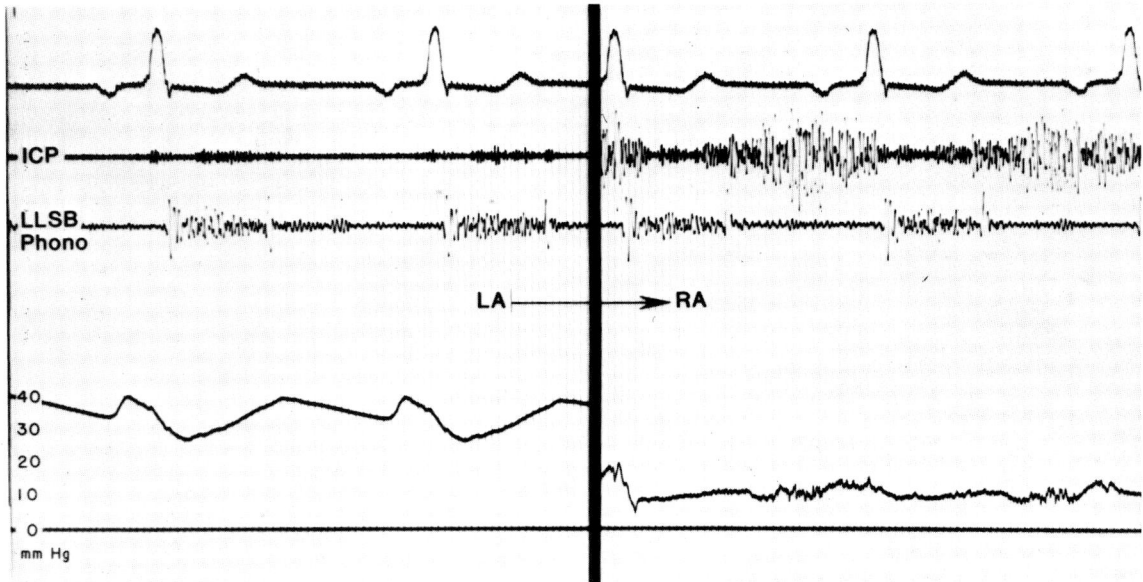

Fig. 17.8 Child with mitral atresia and a restrictive interatrial defect. A loud continuous murmur with diastolic accentuation was recorded in the right but not the left atrium (ICP).

Summary

In summary, in an infant the clinical finding which most strongly suggests the possibility of mitral atresia is tachypnea out of proportion to the severity of congestive heart failure or intensity of cyanosis. In the presence of cyanosis, either a continuous murmur or 'hum' along the right sternal border or a split second heart sound should also suggest the possibility of mitral atresia.

AORTIC ATRESIA

The anomaly

When the aortic valve is atretic, other left heart structures are characteristically very abnormal as well (Fig. 17.9). The ascending aorta is hypoplastic (Fig. 17.10), the left ventricular cavity absent or a mere slit and the mitral valve atretic or very small (Noonan & Nadas, 1958). Aortic atresia is a lethal anomaly and in our institution is one of the most common cardiac causes of death during the first week of life. With aortic atresia, pulmonary venous return leaves the left atrium only via a patent foramen ovale. Systemic and pulmonary venous returns then mix in the right atrium and enter the right ventricle and subsequently the pulmonary artery. The sole ingress to the aorta is via a patent ductus arteriosus. Life is completely dependent on patency of both the foramen ovale and the ductus.

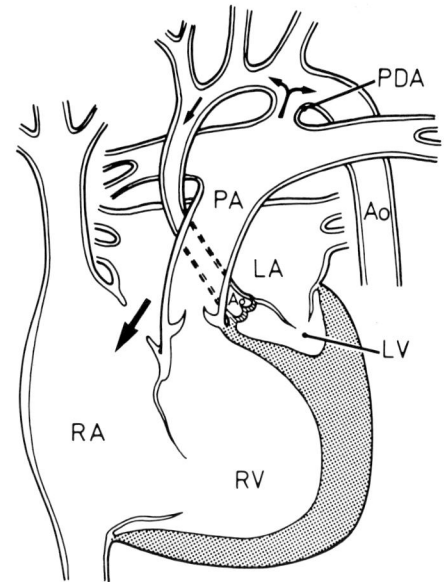

Fig. 17.9 Diagram of aortic atresia. A large arrow indicates flow from left to right atrium. The small branched arrow shows flow from the pulmonary artery to the aorta through the patent ductus arteriosus (PDA). Both the left ventricle (LV) and the ascending aorta are diminutive.

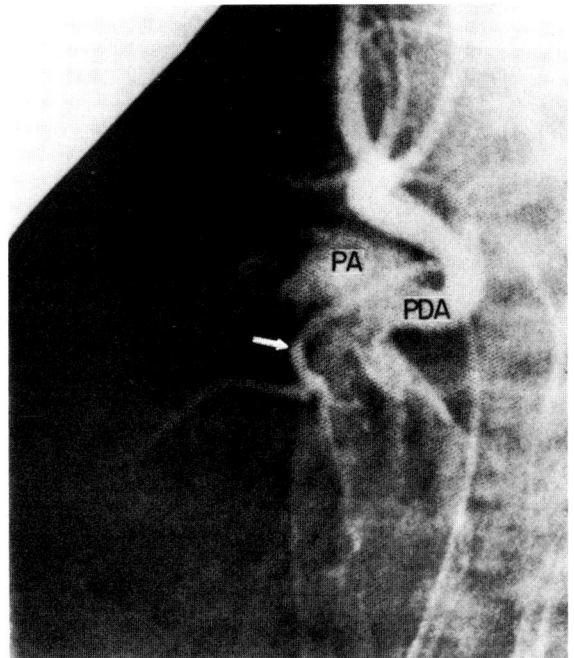

Fig. 17.10 Cineangiogram of aortic atresia. A patent ductus arteriosus is the sole source of systemic blood flow. The ascending aorta (arrow) is very hypoplastic.

Cyanosis is present but is rarely as intense as in an infant with transposition of the great arteries or pulmonary atresia. Instead, the neonate's color is more ashen gray than deep blue. Mottling and poor capillary filling add to the picture of shock.

Although arterial pulses may remain normal for a few hours to a day or two after birth, they soon become weak and disappear as the ductus arteriosus contracts and becomes more restrictive. (In an occasional newborn, leg pulses are stronger than arm pulses, probably because of hypoplasia of the aortic isthmus.) In contrast to the decreased arterial pulse the left parasternal area is usually strikingly active (Fig. 17.11). The labors of the right ventricle are futile, however, serving only to pump more blood to the already overloaded pulmonary circuit. In spite of intense vasoconstriction systemic arterial pressure is low. The jugular venous pulse is, as usual, hard to visualize in the neonate and is not useful.

Clinical course

While an infant with aortic atresia may appear normal at birth, symptoms quickly appear and survival is rarely for more than a few days. Because of the morphology of its flap, the foramen ovale restricts left to right atrial flow and as a consequence left atrial pressure is high. The ductus arteriosus tends to contract and become restrictive shortly after birth and the hemodynamic consequences of ductal closure are even more disastrous. Systemic blood flow falls and congestive heart failure and shock appear.

Physical findings

General

Tachypnea is a prominent early sign in infants with aortic atresia and is reflexly induced by the high pressure in the left atrium and pulmonary veins. The liver enlarges as the picture of florid congestive heart failure emerges. The neonate becomes weak and flaccid and is obviously very ill.

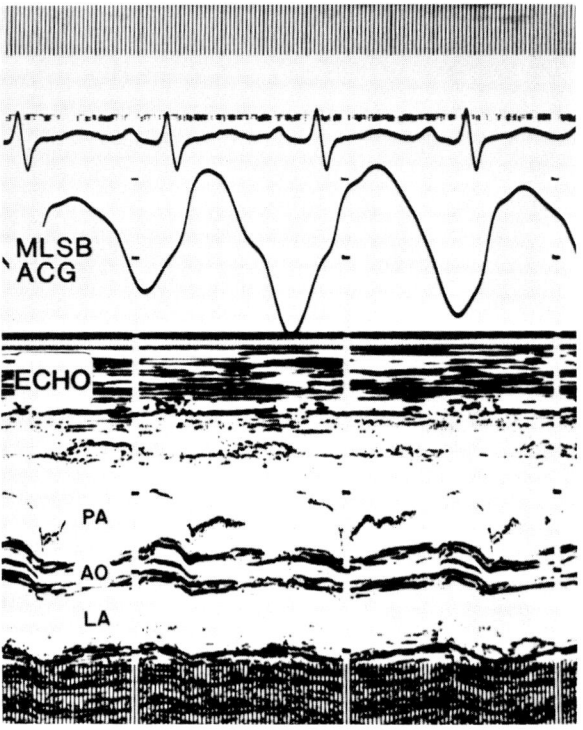

Fig. 17.11 Newborn with aortic atresia. There is a very prominent right ventricular lift in the left sternal border pulse tracing (MLSB ACG). The pulmonary artery (PA) is large and the aorta (AO) very small on the echocardiogram.

Auscultation

The second heart sound is loud and single at the high left sternal border and is generated by forceful closure of the pulmonic valve by the high pulmonary artery pressure. The atretic aortic valve is silent. A gallop is usual. The first heart sound is single and is often loud at the low left sternal border, being generated by tricuspid closure. If a murmur is present, it is soft and heard at the mid and high left sternal border and sometimes over the back. It is generated by rapid flow across the pulmonic valve and through the pulmonary arterial tree.

Differential diagnosis

The differential diagnosis includes critical aortic stenosis, interrupted aortic arch, aortic coarctation involving both subclavian arteries (origin of the left subclavian at the coarctation plus retroesophageal right subclavian artery), severe myocardial disease, and any condition which causes profound peripheral vascular collapse. The presence of a high right sternal border systolic ejection murmur and/or an aortic early systolic ejection sound suggests stenosis rather than atresia of the aortic valve. With coarctation of the aorta carotid pulses are normal or increased, the second heart sound may be split, and the right ventricular impulse is usually less prominent than with aortic atresia. Echocardiography is often useful in the differential diagnosis (Meyer & Kaplan, 1973). If an aortic valve is visualized and the ascending aorta is of normal size, a diagnosis of aortic atresia is untenable. Cardiac catheterization may be necessary to establish a diagnosis of aortic atresia.

Summary

In summary, the physical findings of aortic atresia are usually sufficiently distinctive to permit a clinical diagnosis. They include tachypnea, poor arterial pulses, and signs of rapidly developing congestive heart failure and shock. The diagnosis is especially likely in a newborn baby with very weak pulses and a hyperactive left parasternal impulse.

REFERENCES

Anderson R H, Wilkinson J L, Gerlis L M, Smith A, Becker A E 1977 Atresia of the right atrioventricular orifice. British Heart Journal 39: 414

Eliot R S, Shone J D, Kanjuh V I, Ruttenberg H D, Carey L S, Edwards J E 1965 Mitral atresia. American Heart Journal 70: 6

Lenox C C, Zuberbuhler J R 1970 Balloon septostomy in tricuspid atresia after infancy. American Journal of Cardiology 25: 723

Meyer R A, Kaplan S 1973 Noninvasive techniques in pediatric cardiovascular disease. Progress in Cardiovascular Diseases 15: 341

Neches W H, Park S C, Lenox C C, Zuberbuhler J R, Bahnson H T 1973 Tricuspid atresia with transposition of the great arteries and closing ventricular septal defect. Journal of Thoracic and Cardiovascular Surgery 65: 538

Noonan J A, Nadas A S 1958 The hypoplastic left heart syndrome. An analysis of 101 cases. Pediatric Clinics of North America 5: 1029

Rosenquist G C, Levy R J, Rowe R D 1970 Right atrial — left ventricular relationships in tricuspid atresia: position of the presumed site of atretic valve as determined by transillumination. American Heart Journal 80: 493

Ross J, Braunwald E, Mason D T, Braunwald N S, Morrow A G 1963 Interatrial communication and left atrial hypertension: a cause of continuous murmur. Circulation 28: 853

Rudolph A M, Heymann M A, Spitznas U 1972 Hemodynamic considerations in the development of narrowing of the aorta. American Journal of Cardiology 30: 514

Schrire V, Sutin G J, Barnard C N 1971 Organic and functional pulmonary atresia with intact ventricular septum. American Journal of Cardiology 8: 100

Watson D G, Rowe R D, Conen P E, Duckworth J W A 1960 Mitral atresia with normal aortic valve. Pediatrics 25: 450

Zuberbuhler J R, Anderson R J 1979 Morphologic variations in pulmonary atresia with intact ventricular septum. British Heart Journal 41: 281

Zuberbuhler J R, Lenox C C, Park S C, Neches W H 1975 Continuous murmurs in the newborn. Physiologic principles of heart sounds and murmurs. American Heart Association Monograph 46. The American Heart Association, New York, p 209

Tetralogy of Fallot

The anomaly

As described by Fallot, (quoted by Willius & Keys, 1941) the tetralogy consists of a ventricular septal defect, pulmonic stenosis, overriding of the aorta and right ventricular hypertrophy (Fig. 18.1). Of these, the ventricular septal defect and the pulmonic stenosis are of central importance. (Right ventricular hypertrophy is secondary to the right ventricular outflow obstruction and the override of the aorta has little hemodynamic effect.) In this chapter the term tetralogy of Fallot will be restricted to patients with a ventricular septal defect, equal right and left ventricular peak systolic pressure and sufficient pulmonary stenosis to reduce pulmonary artery pressure to normal or subnormal level. The ventricular septal defect is almost always large and unrestrictive, though rarely it may be partially obstructed by the septal leaflet of the tricuspid valve.

Clinical spectrum

The clinical spectrum of tetralogy of Fallot ranges from the severely symptomatic infant to the minimally limited young adult. There is a corresponding spectrum of physical findings, and both spectra can be related to certain variations in pathologic anatomy. Both site and severity of the pulmonic stenosis are variable, but the most common locus of the obstruction is the infundibulum. The pulmonic valve is usually bicuspid (Sherman, 1963) and, uncommonly, obstruction may be solely or predominately at valvar level. In a few patients the obstruction is subinfundibular and consists of an hypertrophied muscle band which traverses the right ventricular cavity. Although such patients may have 'tetralogy' hemodynamics, anatomically they are quite different from the usual tetralogy; the ventricular septal defect is usually small, the infundibulum is not hypoplastic and there is no aortic override.

The most important anatomic variable in tetralogy of Fallot is the severity of the pulmonic stenosis. It determines the relative resistance to outflow from the two ventricles and, hence, the direction and magnitude of blood flow across the ventricular septal defect. If pulmonic stenosis is relatively mild, a left to right shunt will predominate and the patient will not be cyanotic. If the pulmonic stenosis is very severe, a large right to left shunt will occur and there will be marked arterial unsaturation and intense cyanosis. There

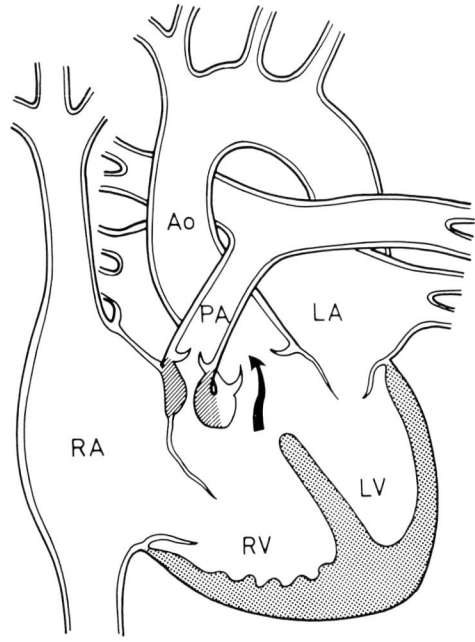

Fig. 18.1 Diagram of tetralogy of Fallot.

is a spectrum of severity between these extremes. Both growth retardation and exercise intolerance are related to the degree of arterial unsaturation and therefore to the severity of the pulmonic stenosis.

Although there is a tendency for the right ventricular outflow tract obstruction to become more severe with the passage of time, the natural history of the pulmonic stenosis is highly variable. Severe stenosis and intense cyanosis may be present at birth, or stenosis may be relatively mild and the onset of cyanosis delayed for months or years. Some patients, in fact, exhibit no clinical or hemodynamic evidence of pulmonic stenosis in early infancy, their clinical picture being that of a large interventricular septal defect. Such patients may even go into congestive failure, but pulmonic stenosis eventually develops and a typical tetralogy of Fallot emerges. Still other young patients are pink, active and without symptoms much of the time, but they experience 'spells', characterized by intense cyanosis, tachypnea and respiratory distress, and sometimes by loss of consciousness. Such spells are more common after awakening from sleep, and are thought to be caused by a transient increase in severity of infundibular pulmonic stenosis, presumably because of increased contraction of infundibular muscle. Evidence for this concept includes softening or disappearance of the systolic murmur during the spell (Fig. 18.2), more severe infundibular pulmonic stenosis demonstrated on cineangiograms just at the onset of a spell (Fig. 18.3), and clinical response to propranolol, a pharmacologic agent which decreases myocardial contractility. A spell may be aborted or ameliorated by squatting, or the squatting equivalent of bringing the knees up to the chest while lying or being held. (Squatting increases systemic resistance and thus pulmonary blood flow, since the balance between pulmonary and systemic flow is determined by relative pulmonary and systemic resistances.) Even in the absence of spells, children who are cyanotic and limited often learn that their symptoms are relieved by squatting, and they assume this posture, especially after exertion.

Congestive heart failure does not occur in uncomplicated tetralogy of Fallot. There may be a history of congestive heart failure in infancy, however, if pulmonic stenosis was mild or non-

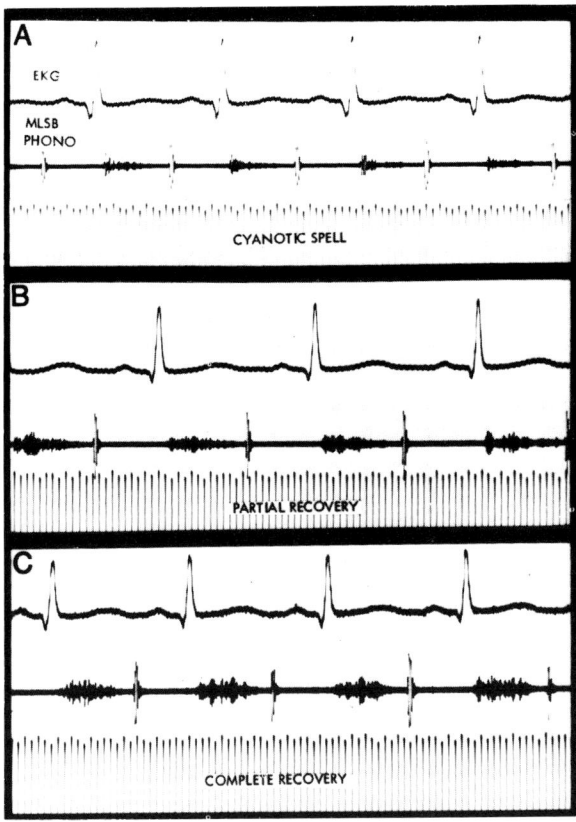

Fig. 18.2 Child with tetralogy of Fallot. Mid left sternal border phonocardiogram taken during the course of a hypercyanotic spell. A. The systolic murmur is very soft and short during the spell. B. & C. It becomes progressively louder and longer with partial and complete recovery. (From Zuberbuhler et al, 1975 by permission of the American Heart Association, Inc.)

existent and the left to right shunt large, or if there was pulmonic regurgitation due to an absent pulmonic valve (Ruttenberg et al, 1964). Failure may also occur in the rare patient with increased pulmonary blood flow from large systemic-pulmonary collateral arteries (Zuberbuhler et al, 1974). If the septal leaflet of the tricuspid valve partially obstructs the ventricular defect, as it may rarely do, right ventricular pressure can rise far above left ventricular and congestive heart failure may develop. Infectious endocarditis can precipitate failure at any age.

Physical findings

General

The large ventricular septal defect of tetralogy of

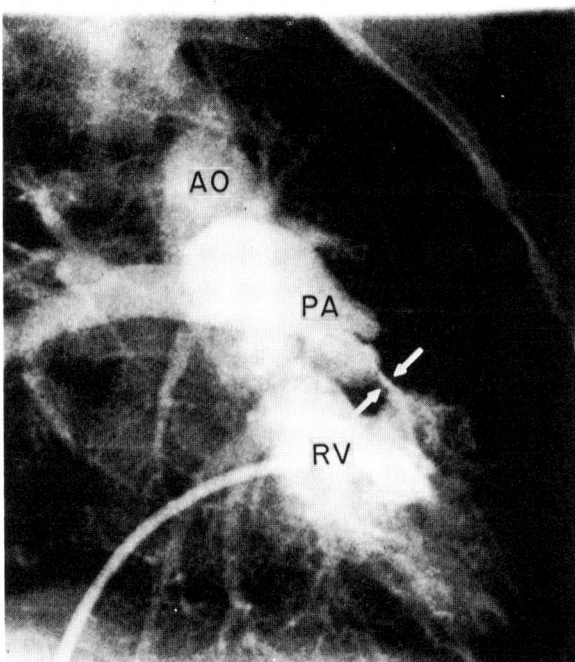

Fig. 18.3 Same patient as 18.2. Cineangiogram frame showing severe infundibular stenosis (arrows).

Fallot permits free flow of blood from the right ventricle to the aorta during systole. This ensures an adequate cardiac output and normal arterial pulses and blood pressure, even in the presence of low pulmonary blood flow and low left ventricular output. Since the large ventricular septal defect prevents right ventricular pressure from rising above left ventricular, no matter how severe the pulmonic stenosis, right ventricular hypertrophy does not become extreme. Right ventricular diastolic pressure remains relatively normal and the right atrium does not become sufficiently hypertrophied to produce the large jugular venous 'A' waves that may occur with very severe 'isolated' pulmonic stenosis. In spite of high right ventricular systolic pressure, tricuspid regurgitation is very rare in unoperated tetralogy of Fallot, and large jugular venous 'V' waves are not present. In the author's experience, precordial motion is usually normal in tetralogy. The absence of a prominent left parasternal impulse is related both to the lack of right ventricular volume overload and to the location of the obstruction within the right ventricle, the infundibular stenosis precluding high pressure in the outflow portion of the ventricle. The work of the left ventricle is not increased in tetralogy of Fallot and the apical impulse is quiet.

Auscultation

Heart sounds. The first heart sound is normal in tetralogy of Fallot. Although the second heart sound is sometimes audibly split in 'pink' tetralogy (Fig. 18.4), it is almost always single to auscultation if cyanosis is present, since pulmonic valve closure is inaudible if pulmonic stenosis is sufficiently severe to cause right to left shunting. Pulmonary vascular disease in a patient with tetralogy of Fallot may result in a split second heart sound, even in the presence of cyanosis. This constitutes a rare exception to the general rule (Fig. 18.5). The second sound is usually loud as well as single at the high left sternal border, since the aortic component is well heard there. Third and fourth heart sounds are not part of the auscultatory spectrum of tetralogy of Fallot. An early systolic ejection sound may be present, originating either at the pulmonic valve or in the dilated ascending aorta. Pulmonic ejection sounds are quite rare in children with tetralogy of Fallot, but are somewhat more common in unoperated young adults — a highly selected group of patients with relatively mild disease (Martin et al, 1973). Aortic ejection sounds are more common in patients with severe tetralogy, a group with a high incidence of large ascending aorta.

Murmurs. A systolic murmur is present in all patients with tetralogy of Fallot save those with complete or nearly complete obstruction between the right ventricle and the pulmonary artery. The murmur originates at the site of obstruction and, since infundibular stenosis is most common, is usually loudest in the third intercostal space at the left sternal border. The murmur may be maximal in the fourth left intercostal space if the obstruction is subinfundibular. In some patients the murmur is clearly crescendo-decrescendo (Fig. 18.4). In others it is plateau and pansystolic, at least with regard to left ventricular mechanical systole, extending from the first heart sound to the aortic closure sound. (The murmur is not pansystolic with regard to right ventricular mechanical systole, but this cannot be judged at the bedside since

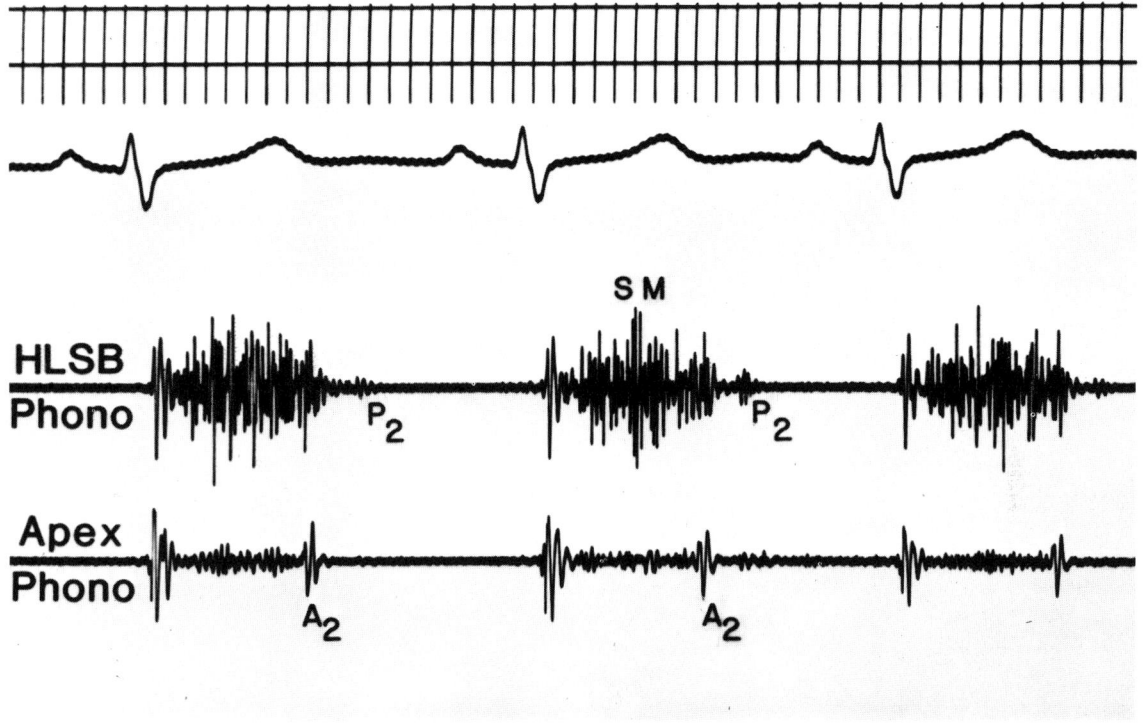

Fig. 18.4 Child with 'pink' tetralogy. The second heart sound is split in the high left sternal border phonocardiogram and the crescendo-decrescendo murmur ends with the aortic component (A_2).

pulmonic closure, the auscultatory marker for the end of right ventricular systole, is inaudible.) The plateau type murmur is identical to the systolic murmur of a small or medium sized ventricular septal defect.

Although the ventricular septal defect itself is silent (Fig. 18.6), its presence modifies the auscultatory features of pulmonic stenosis. With 'isolated' pulmonic stenosis the entire cardiac output traverses the right ventricular outflow tract, and the murmur tends to become louder and longer and to peak later with more severe obstruction (Vogelpoel & Schrire, 1955). If a ventricular septal defect is present the entire right ventricular output need not enter the pulmonary artery, and with increasing obstruction more of the right ventricular stroke volume goes to the aorta. Although the right ventricle-pulmonary artery gradient remains large, the volume of flow becomes so reduced that the murmur softens. The obstruction may become complete in late systole and the murmur is then short as well as soft. In the course of a hypercyanotic spell the murmur may disappear entirely as the right ventricular outflow tract becomes nearly atretic. The soft, short, high-pitched, early systolic murmur of tetralogy of Fallot with very severe infundibular pulmonic stenosis is very like that of a tiny 'closing' ventricular septal defect, and if cyanosis is not present, the diagnosis of tetralogy may be missed. The possibility that such a murmur really represents tetralogy of Fallot is heightened if normal splitting of the second heart sound cannot be heard.

Diastolic murmurs are uncommon in unoperated tetralogy of Fallot, but when present indicate either aortic or pulmonic regurgitation. In a recently reported series of 295 patients with tetralogy of Fallot, a murmur of aortic regurgitation was heard in less than 1 percent of unoperated children and a murmur of pulmonic regurgitation in 3 percent. All of the latter had an absent pulmonic valve (Zuberbuhler et al, 1975).

A continuous murmur is quite unusual in the unoperated child with tetralogy of Fallot. A patent ductus arteriosus, one cause of a continuous murmur, is present in a few very young patients,

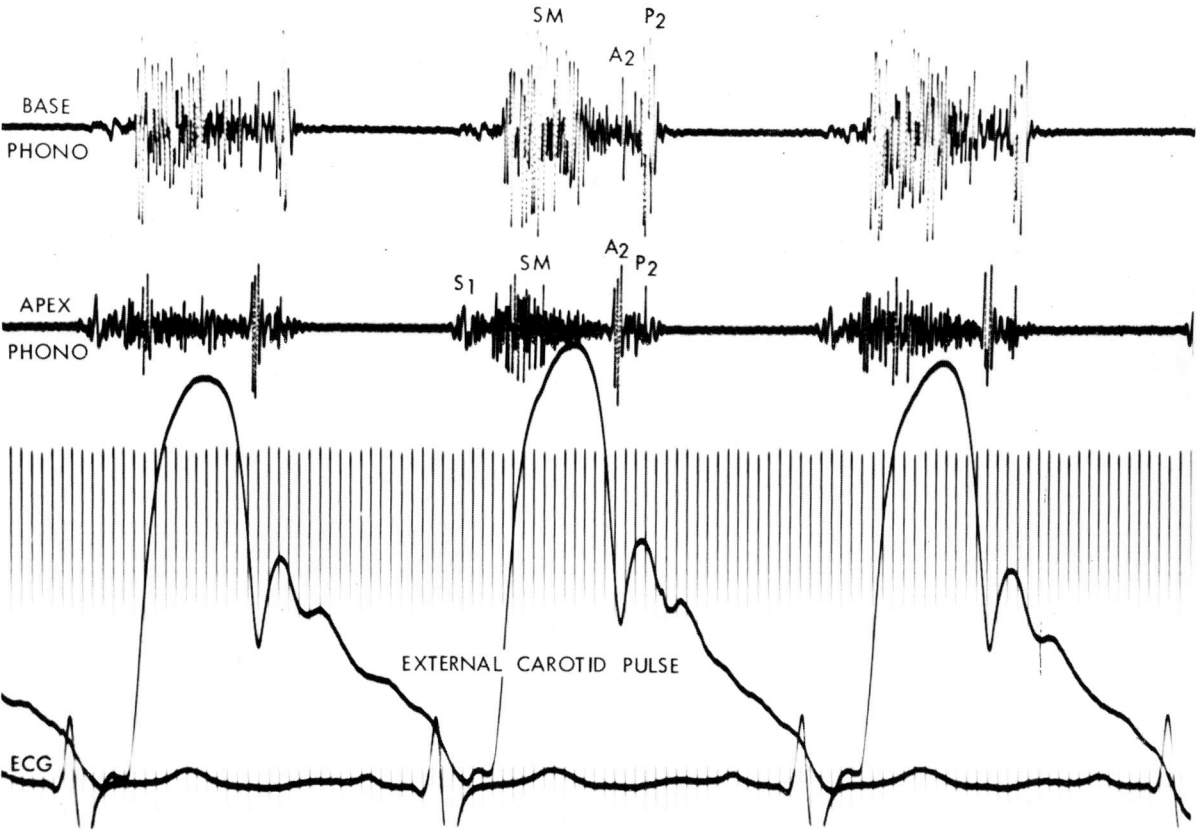

Fig. 18.5 Young adult with tetralogy of Fallot and pulmonary hypertension secondary to aortico-pulmonary artery (Pott's) anastomosis. The pulmonic closure sound (P_2) is loud at the base and prominent even at the apex. (From Zuberbuhler et al, 1975, by permission of the American Heart Association, Inc.)

but is distinctly uncommon beyond early infancy. Systemic-pulmonary collateral arteries, another source of continuous murmurs, are rare in tetralogy unless there is pulmonary atresia. However, if both a continuous murmur and a separate mid left sternal border systolic murmur can be identified, tetralogy of Fallot should be suspected, in spite of a clinical picture otherwise suggestive of pulmonary atresia.

To summarize, the patient with relatively mild pulmonic stenosis is not cyanotic, may have a split second sound and has a loud, harsh, often pansystolic murmur which may resemble that of a ventricular septal defect. With more severe stenosis, cyanosis is evident, the pulmonic closure sound is inaudible and the systolic murmur tends to be crescendo-decrescendo. Severe cyanosis, a single second heart sound, a soft short systolic murmur and, commonly, an aortic ejection sound characterize the patient with tetralogy of Fallot and very severe obstruction.

Postoperative findings

Physical findings are altered by operation. If a palliative systemic-pulmonary artery shunt has been constructed, a continuous murmur is expected. Regardless of the type of shunt the murmur is usually well heard over the anterior and posterior thorax and is louder on the ipsilateral side. The murmur may not be continuous if the systemic-pulmonary communication is either very large or very small. A descending aorta to left pulmonary artery shunt (Potts) or ascending aorta to right pulmonary artery shunt (Waterston) may be so large as to equalize aortic and pulmonary artery

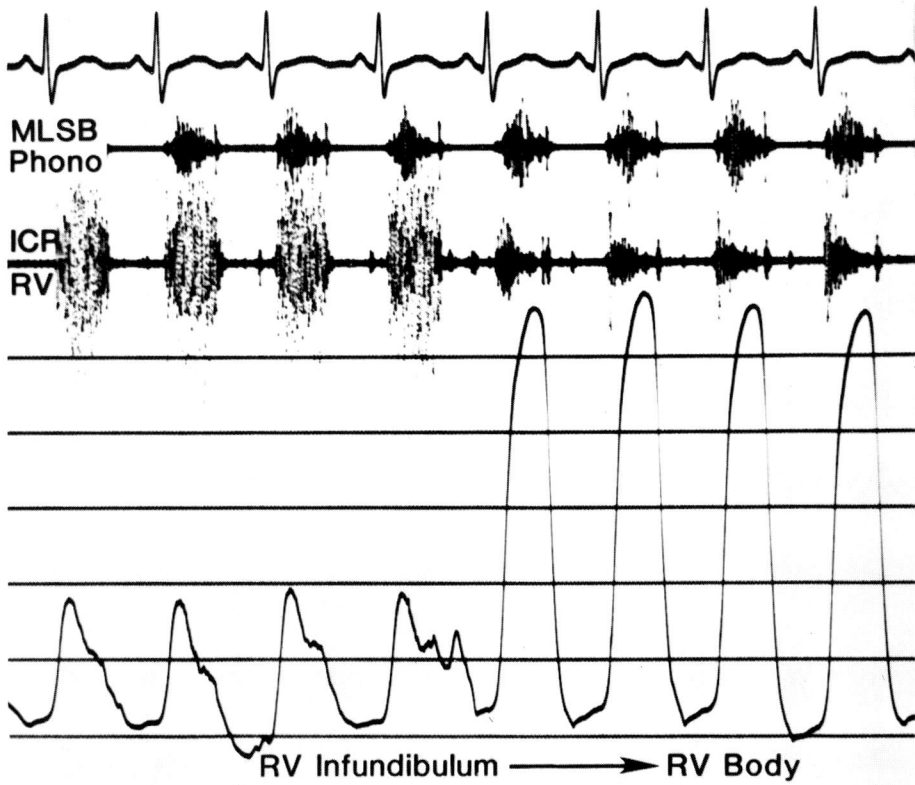

Fig. 18.6 Child with tetralogy of Fallot. The murmur is much louder in the infundibulum, indicating origin at the site of obstruction rather than at the ventricular septal defect.

diastolic pressures and then may generate only a systolic murmur. A subclavian to pulmonary artery shunt (Blalock-Taussig) is rarely too large, but if the shunt is very small, the murmur may be soft and heard only in systole.

Although cyanosis disappears after successful repair of tetralogy, the cardiac physical examination is rarely normal. A left sternal border systolic murmur is usually heard and may represent residual pulmonic stenosis or a residual ventricular septal defect. A diastolic murmur of pulmonic regurgitation is quite common, being present in 50 percent of operated patients (Zuberbuhler et al, 1975). (At operation, the valve may have been excised or a patch placed across the annulus to relieve right ventricular outflow tract obstruction; in either case there is pulmonic regurgitation.) No pulmonic closure sound is audible but the murmur of pulmonic regurgitation begins well after the aortic closure sound (Fig. 3.10). Aortic regurgitation is much less common, but may result from trauma to the aortic valve during patching of the ventricular septal defect. If the anterior wall of the right ventricle has been thinned excessively during resection of the infundibular pulmonic stenosis, the area may become aneurysmal and move paradoxically during ventricular systole. The resultant prolonged systolic outward movement is usually most marked in the third intercostal space to the left of the sternum (Fig. 18.7). The same lift occurs if the right ventricular outflow tract has been enlarged with a pericardial or synthetic patch.

TETRALOGY WITH PULMONARY ATRESIA

The physical findings of tetralogy with pulmonary atresia differ in some respects from those of tetralogy with pulmonary stenosis. As with 'ordinary' tetralogy, the degree of cyanosis depends

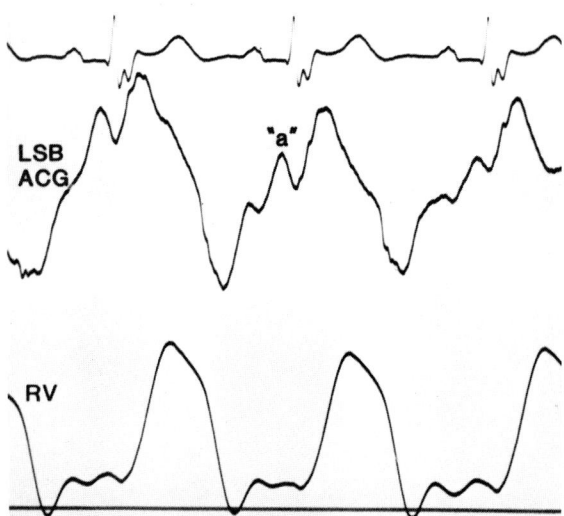

Fig. 18.7 Patient with a right ventricular outflow tract aneurysm following repair of tetralogy of Fallot. The pulse tracing recorded in the third intercostal space at the left sternal border (LSB ACG) shows prominent presystolic and systolic impulses.

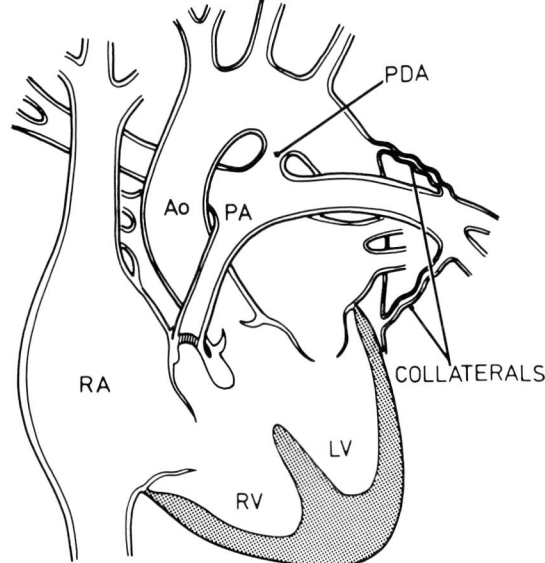

Fig. 18.8 Diagram of tetralogy of Fallot with pulmonary atresia. Pulmonary blood flow may be via a patent ductus arteriosus or systemic-pulmonary collateral arteries.

upon the magnitude of pulmonary blood flow. But with pulmonary atresia, flow depends on the size of a patent ductus arteriosus or of collateral arteries (Fig. 18.8). Since a patent ductus arteriosus has a strong tendency to close, patients without systemic-pulmonary collateral arteries are usually quite cyanotic and clinically unstable. When large collateral arteries are present, cyanosis may be quite mild.

The first heart sound is normal. The second heart sound is single and usually loud at the high left sternal border. It is generated by aortic valve closure. An early systolic ejection sound is usually audible in older children with tetralogy and pulmonary atresia and originates in the dilated ascending aorta. It may be absent in the infant, particularly if pulmonary blood flow is via a patent ductus arteriosus (Zuberbuhler et al, 1975).

With pulmonary atresia, the ventricular septal defect and right ventricular outflow tract are both 'silent', and the soft systolic murmur that is sometimes heard is probably generated at the aortic valve — since both right and left ventricular outputs are via the aorta. A continuous murmur is common in tetralogy with pulmonary atresia, originating either in a patent ductus arteriosus or in a systemic-pulmonary collateral artery. If the ductus is tiny or the collaterals small and inadequate, there may be no murmur at all. Cyanosis is then intense.

REFERENCES

Martin C E, Reddy P S, Leon D F, & Shaver J A 1973 Genesis, frequency, and diagnosic significance of ejection sound in adults with tetralogy of Fallot. British Heart Journal 35:402

Ruttenberg H D, Carey L S, Adams P, & Edwards J E 1964 Absence of the pulmonary valve in the tetralogy of Fallot. American Journal of Roentgenology 91:500

Sherman F E 1963 An atlas of congenital heart disease. Lea & Febiger, Philadelphia, p 192

Vogelpoel L, Schrire V 1955 The role of auscultation in the differentiation of Fallot's tetralogy from severe pulmonary stenosis with intact ventricular septum and right-to-left interatrial shunt. Circulation 11:714

Willius F A, Keys T E 1941 Cardiac classics. Mosby, St. Louis

Zuberbuhler J R, Lenox C C, Neches W H, Park S C, Shaver J A 1975 Auscultatory spectrum of tetralogy of Fallot. Physiologic principles of heart sounds and murmurs. American Heart Association Monograph 46. American Heart Association, New York: p 187

Zuberbuhler J R, Dankner E, Zoltun R, Burkholder J, Bahnson H T 1974 Tissue adhesive closure of aortic-pulmonary communications. American Heart Journal 88:41

19

Transposition of the great arteries

COMPLETE TRANSPOSITION

The anomaly

Transposition of the great arteries may be defined either in terms of the spatial relationship of the aorta and pulmonary artery or in terms of their connection to the ventricles. As a relationship, 'transposition' describes an aorta which is anterior to the pulmonary artery (de la Cruz et al, 1976). As a connection, 'transposition' is synonymous with 'ventriculo-arterial discordance', the right ventricle connecting to the aorta and the left ventricle to the pulmonary artery (Van Praagh, 1971). It is in the latter sense that the term will be used here, since abnormal connection, not position, determines abnormal hemodynamics.

Clinical course

Before birth, there seems to be no adverse effect from ventriculo-arterial discordance and at birth infants with this anomaly tend to be large and well developed. Following birth, two parallel and more or less separate circulations exist, with systemic venous blood being returned to the body via the right heart and pulmonary venous blood returning to the lungs via the left heart (Fig. 19.1). The inevitable consequence of this arrangement is arterial oxygen unsaturation. If there were no mixing of blood between the two circuits, life could not be sustained for more than a few minutes following birth. In fact, the early clinical course of the infant with transposition is largely determined by the amount of mixing which can take place through various communications between the two circuits. If the only communications are a patent foramen ovale and a patent ductus arteriosus, the newborn will become intensely cyanotic as the ductus closes. If there is a large communication at atrial, ventricular, or great artery level there is usually better mixing and therefore less cyanosis.

The size of an interventricular or great artery communication and the presence or absence of pulmonic stenosis are other important determinants of clinical course. If there is a large ventricular septal defect or patent ductus arteriosus, pulmonary artery pressure remains high from birth. Pulmonary blood flow increases markedly as pulmonary vascular resistance falls, and signs of congestive heart failure usually appear during the first month or two of life. Severe pulmonic stenosis, on the other hand, reduces pulmonary blood flow

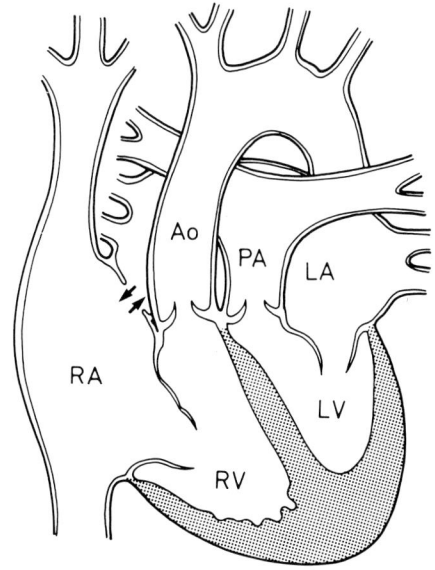

Fig. 19.1 Diagram of complete transposition of the great arteries. The arrows indicate bidirectional shunting through an interatrial communication.

and eliminates the major cause of congestive heart failure. Although congestive failure is unlikely in an infant with transposition and pulmonic stenosis, cyanosis may be intense, especially if the stenosis is severe.

Physical findings

Ventriculo-arterial discordance

The most striking physical finding directly attributable to ventriculo-arterial discordance is cyanosis. There may be little else on physical examination which points to congenital heart disease in general or to transposition of the great arteries in particular. Although right ventricular pressure is always high the left parasternal impulse may or may not be prominent in patients with transposition (Fig. 19.2). Pulses are normal and the jugular venous pulse is usually unremarkable. Ventriculo-arterial discordance does not, per se, result in any auscultatory abnormalities but the anterior 'relationship' of the aorta which is so common does have auscultatory consequences. The aortic closure sound tends to be loud and the

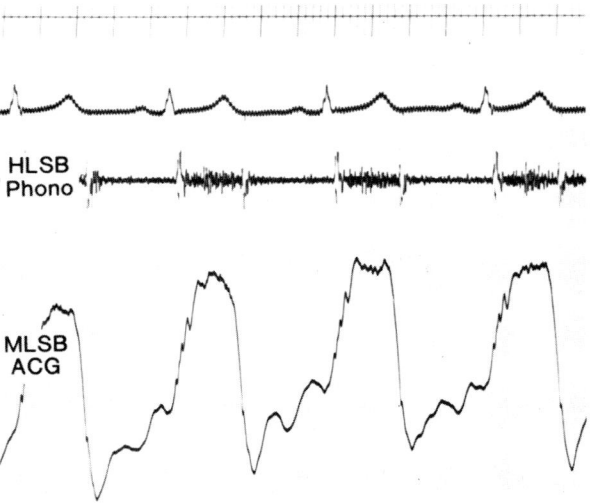

Fig. 19.2 Prominent left sternal border lift (MLSB ACG) in a child with transposition of the great arteries.

pulmonic closure sound soft or inaudible, since the pulmonary artery is posterior to the aorta and relatively far from the anterior chest wall (Fig. 19.3). The second sound is thus commonly both

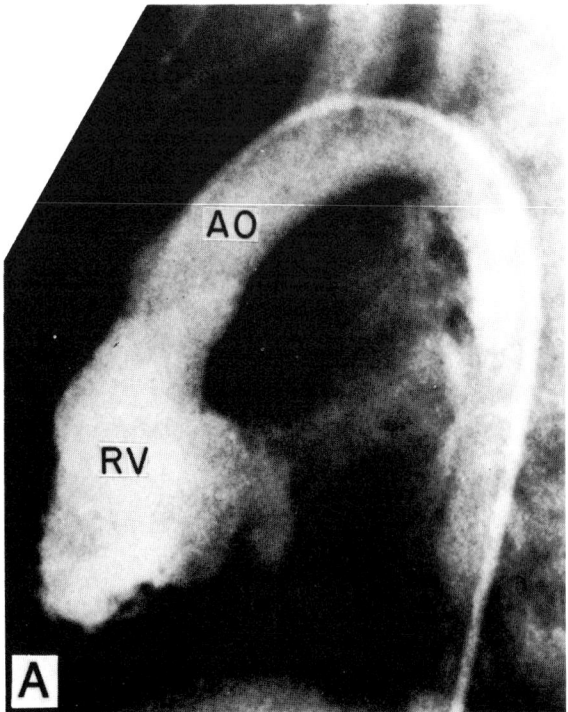
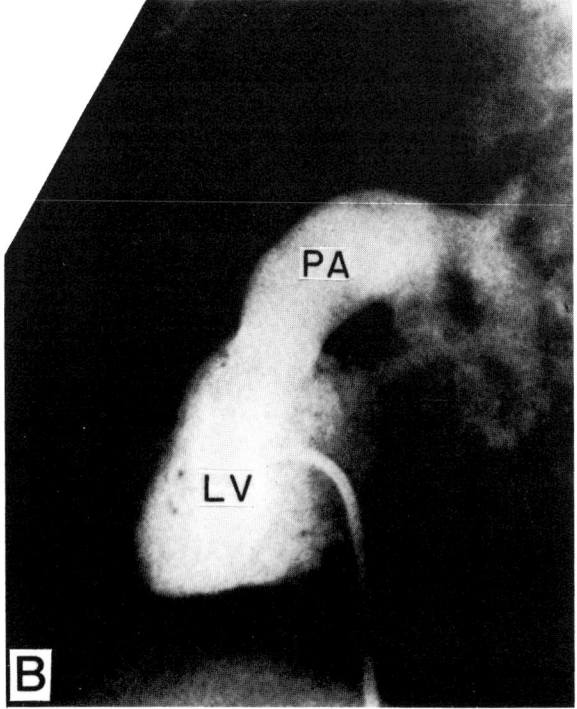

Fig. 19.3 Lateral right (A) and left (B) ventriculogram frames showing the posterior position of the pulmonary artery in a child with complete transposition of the great arteries.

loud and single at the high left sternal border in infants with complete transposition of the great arteries. In such infants there is often no murmur, or only a soft one, presumably generated by rapid flow across the aortic or pulmonic valve or through the pulmonary arterial tree. It is rare to have a diastolic murmur of relative tricuspid or mitral stenosis if there is no ventricular septal defect or patent ductus arteriosus (Moss et al, 1977).

Ventricular septal defect

In an infant with transposition a ventricular septal defect may influence physical findings in several ways. If the defect is large, mixing between the two circulations may be good and cyanosis mild or even inapparent. Instead, signs of congestive heart failure appear early in infancy, usually between two and six weeks of age. The auscultatory findings depend upon the size of the ventricular defect. If it is very small, the systolic murmur is rather high pitched and maximal at the mid or low left sternal border. If the defect is larger but still restrictive, the murmur is loud, harsh and pansystolic and there is often a mid diastolic apical rumble. If the defect is large and unrestrictive, the mid or low left sternal border systolic murmur is soft or absent but there is often a soft systolic ejection murmur at the base and across the back, generated by rapid flow across the pulmonic valve and through the pulmonary arteries. In such patients, too, an apical mid diastolic rumble is common. The second sound is more commonly audibly split in the presence of a large ventricular septal defect, because of higher pressure in the pulmonary artery and also because of a higher incidence of a side by side relationship of the great arteries (Fig. 19.4).

Patent ductus arteriosus

The physical findings associated with a patent ductus arteriosus are also dependent upon the size of the communication. A small ductus generates a continuous murmur at the left base. Pulses may be normal or somewhat increased. If there is a large ductus the murmur may be only systolic or even absent and pulses are strikingly increased. Also, a mid diastolic murmur of relative tricuspid stenosis

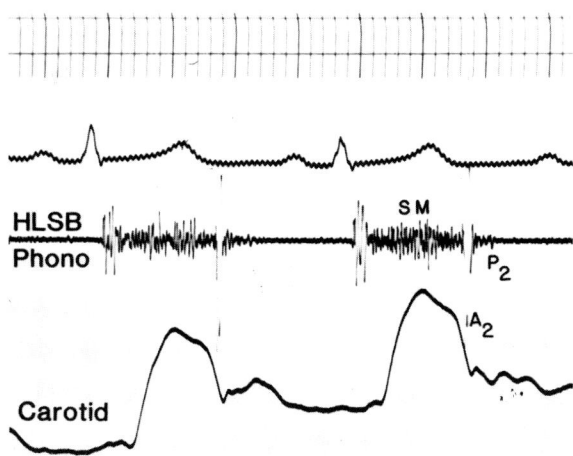

Fig. 19.4 Split second heart sound (A_2 & P_2) in a child with transposition, a ventricular septal defect and mild pulmonic stenosis.

may be audible at the low left sternal border, especially if the ventricular septum is intact (Fig. 19.5). (Since a balance must be maintained between right to left and left to right shunting in transposition, the flow through the ductus to the pulmonary circuit must be matched by a similar volume of blood exiting from the pulmonary circuit. If there is no ventricular septal defect, then flow out of the pulmonary circuit must be at atrial level and there will then be increased diastolic flow across the tricuspid valve.) Cyanosis may be slight but congestive heart failure is common in infants with transposition and a large patent ductus arteriosus.

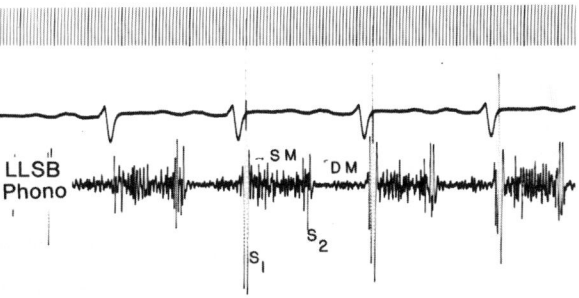

Fig. 19.5 Infant with transposition of the great arteries and a large patent ductus arteriosus. The low left sternal border phonocardiogram shows a mid diastolic murmur of relative tricuspid stenosis.

Pulmonic stenosis

The severity of pulmonic stenosis is difficult to assess on clinical grounds. Since the pulmonic closure sound is often soft or absent in complete transposition of the great arteries, the lack of an audible pulmonic closure sound in an infant with transposition is not reliable evidence of severe pulmonic stenosis, and a very useful gauge of severity is lost. A systolic murmur usually accompanies pulmonic stenosis whether or not transposition is present, but the murmur itself is a poor guide to the severity of the obstruction in the infant with transposition. With 'isolated' pulmonic stenosis without transposition, a short systolic murmur implies mild obstruction. With transposition, even severe pulmonic stenosis may generate only a short systolic murmur which ends well before the end of the left ventricular systole. There may be no murmur, even with very significant left ventricular outflow tract obstruction. This apparent lack of correlation between the characteristics of the systolic murmur and the severity of pulmonic stenosis is unexplained.

Pulmonary hypertension

Pulmonary hypertension is frequent in patients with transposition of the great arteries, especially if there is a large communication at ventricular or great artery level, but it is very difficult to recognize or quantitate pulmonary hypertension clinically. The association of a loud and single or closely split second heart sound with a right ventricular lift is usually good evidence of pulmonary hypertension if there is ventriculo-arterial concordance. These findings are common in complete transposition however, whether or not pressure is high in the pulmonary artery. Neither can cyanosis be used as evidence of advanced pulmonary vascular disease and 'reversed' shunt, since it too is a consequence of ventriculo-arterial discordance per se. When there is high pulmonary vascular resistance in a patient with transposition and a patent ductus, reversal of flow through the ductus causes an increase in arterial oxygen saturation in the lower half of the body. The feet are then less cyanotic than the hands or lips. Such differential cyanosis is a very rare finding, however.

Summary

To summarize, the clinical picture of an infant with transposition of the great arteries and inadequate mixing is dominated by intense cyanosis. There is commonly no murmur, or an unimpressive one, and the second heart sound tends to be loud and single. None of these findings are specific for transposition of the great arteries or even of congenital heart disease. A high index of suspicion in any cyanotic newborn is the best assurance of early definitive diagnosis, which can be made only at cardiac catheterization. The clinical picture of an infant with an associated interventricular or great artery communication is quite different. Cyanosis is less striking than in an infant with less mixing and may be so mild that transposition is not suspected until cardiac catheterization is carried out. The clinical picture of such an infant is often dominated by congestive heart failure. A patent ductus arteriosus may be suggested by a continuous murmur and/or bounding pulses and a ventricular septal defect by the systolic murmur. Pulmonic stenosis is difficult to assess by physical examination, as is pulmonary hypertension and pulmonary vascular disease. Since pulmonary vascular disease tends to develop early, has disastrous consequences, and is currently impossible to reliably assess clinically, serial cardiac catheterizations are still necessary in infants whose open heart repair has not yet been accomplished.

Postoperative findings

As of this writing the Mustard operation is the most commonly used technique of repair. It consists of inserting an interatrial baffle to redirect systemic and pulmonary venous returns. Hemodynamic abnormalities are common following operation and may be residual or iatrogenic. The most common abnormalities include obstruction to systemic or pulmonary venous return, tricuspid regurgitation and residual septal defect. The most common site of obstruction to systemic venous return is just below the junction between the superior vena cava and the systemic venous atrium and is related to placement of the baffle suture line in that area. If there is adequate run off through the azygos venous system there may be nothing to suggest superior vena cava obstruction on physical examination. More commonly, the jugular veins are distended (Fig. 19.6). A prominent 'A' wave is rare, since there is usually little contracting right atrium above the site of obstruction. Since a continuous pressure gradient can exist between the superior vena cava and the right atrium, a continuous murmur should theoretically be possible but has never been noted by the author. (Figure 19.7 shows a continuous murmur recorded in the right atrium of a patient with superior vena cava obstruction. The murmur was inaudible externally.) Severe inferior vena cava obstruction is much less common, but may cause nonpulsatile hepatic enlargement. Obstruction to systemic venous return may result in a prominent cutaneous venous pattern over the thorax (Fig. 19.6).

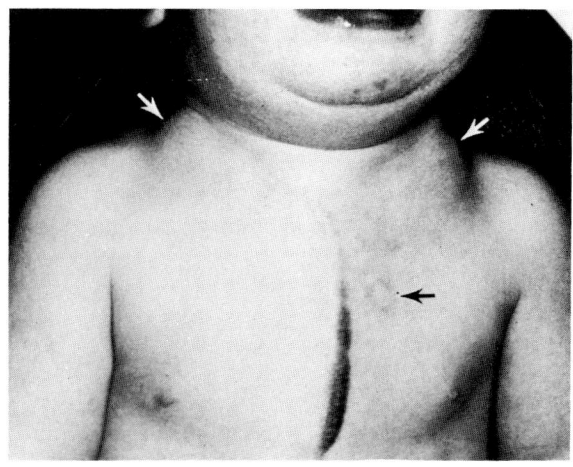

Fig. 19.6 Distended jugular veins (white arrows) in a child with superior vena caval obstruction following Mustard operation for transposition of the great arteries. Cutaneous veins are visible (black arrow).

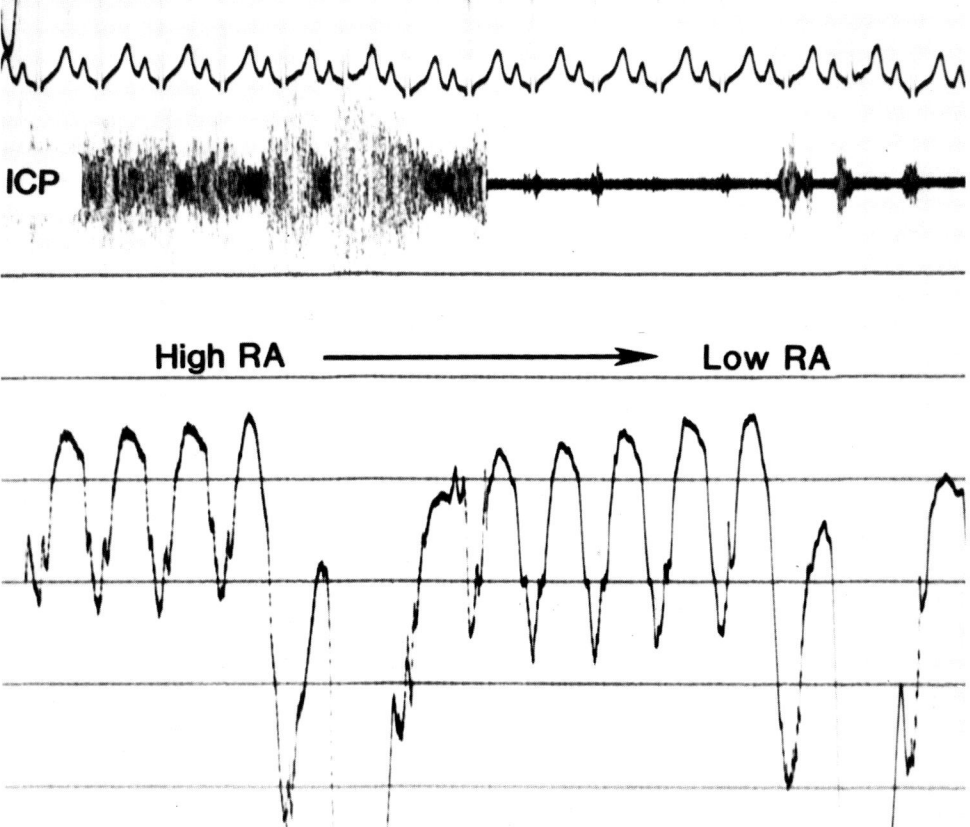

Fig. 19.7 Same patient as Figure 19.6. The intracardiac sound recording (ICP) shows a loud continuous murmur in the high systemic venous atrium near the entrance of the severely obstructed superior vena cava.

Postoperative obstruction to pulmonary venous return occurs, not in the pulmonary veins themselves, but within the pulmonary venous atrium. The usual etiology is redundancy of the baffle. In a recent report, a continuous murmur was described in each of three cases with severe pulmonary venous obstruction (Park et al, 1976). The murmur was shown to originate at the site of obstruction (Fig. 19.8) and disappeared following surgical relief of the narrowing.

Postoperative tricuspid regurgitation may be due to surgical trauma to the tricuspid valve apparatus or may be a consequence of continuing high right ventricular pressure. There is usually a soft high pitched pansystolic murmur at the low left sternal border and the murmur is clinically indistinguishable from that of a small residual ventricular septal defect, unless the regurgitation is severe. The murmur of tricuspid regurgitation does not accentuate with inspiration, since inspiration increases return to the anatomic left rather than the anatomic right ventricle after Mustard's operation. Similarly, tricuspid regurgitation does not cause large 'V' waves in the jugular venous pulse or a pulsatile liver since the tricuspid valve now communicates with the pulmonary rather than the systemic venous atrium.

Paradoxic splitting of the second heart sound may result from right bundle branch block in patients with transposition of the great arteries (Fig. 19.9) (Zuberbuhler et al, 1967). Continuing cyanosis following Mustard's operation is most commonly due to a residual interatrial defect at the baffle margin.

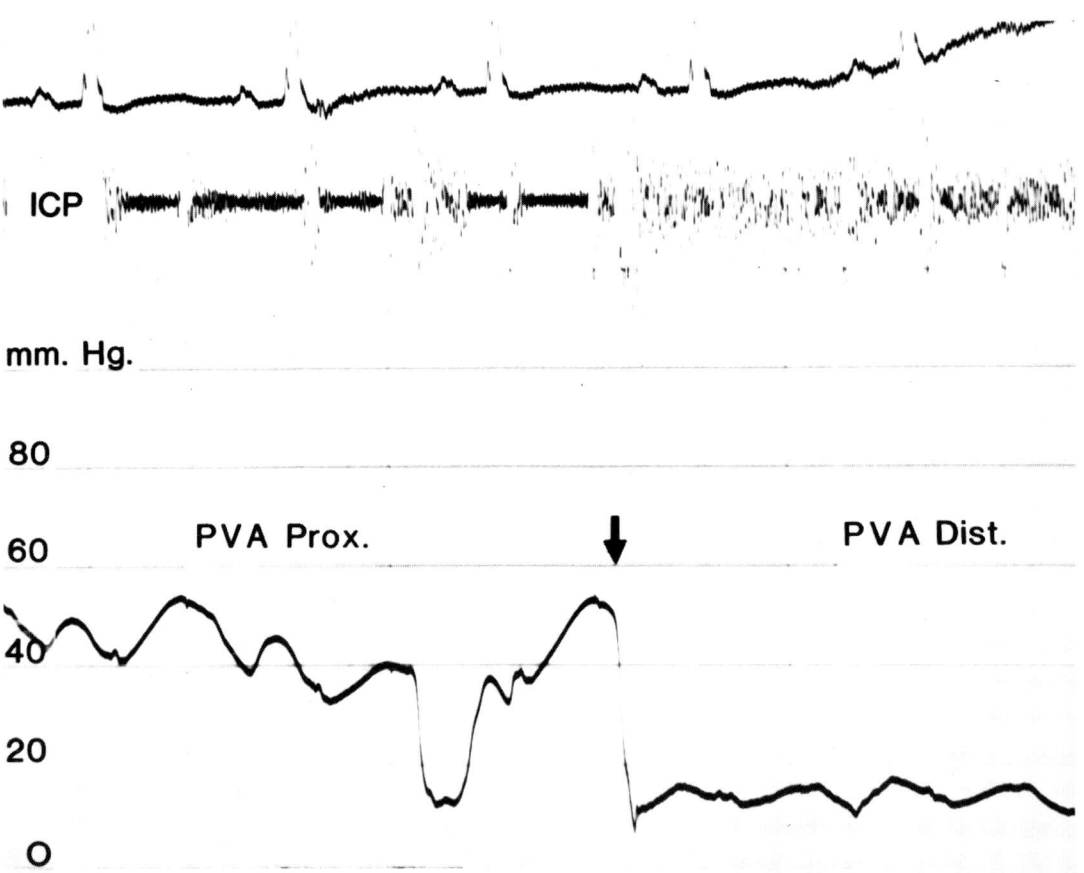

Fig. 19.8 Intracardiac pressure and sound (ICP) recordings in a child with pulmonary venous obstruction following Mustard operation for transposition of the great arteries. A loud continuous murmur is recorded in the pulmonary venous atrium (PVA) distal to the obstruction (arrow).

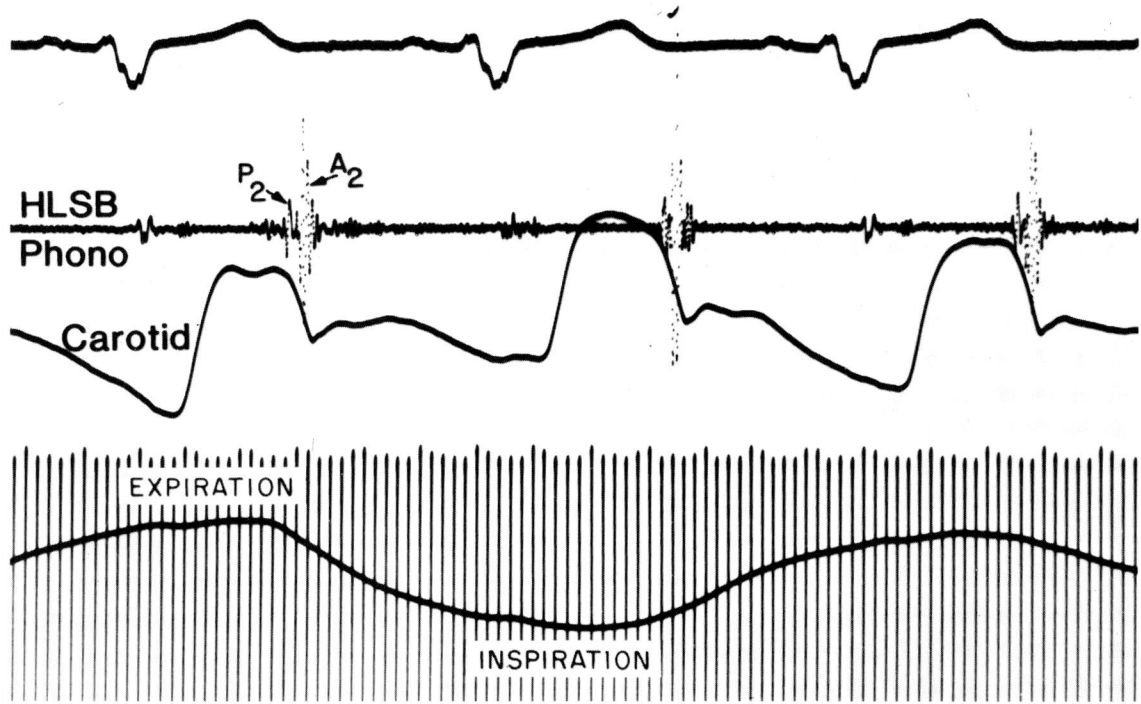

Fig. 19.9 Child with transposition of the great arteries following Mustard operation. There is right bundle branch block and paradoxic splitting of the second sound at the high left sternal border.

CORRECTED TRANSPOSITION

The anomaly

The essence of congenital corrected transposition of the great arteries is discordance of both atrioventricular and ventriculoarterial connections. In other words, the right atrium connects to the morphologic left ventricle and the left atrium to the morphologic right ventricle; the morphologic left ventricle connects to the pulmonary artery and the morphologic right ventricle to the aorta (Fig. 19.10). Rokitansky, in the original description of the anomaly, first used the term 'corrected', since the abnormal connections did not, per se, alter the *course* of blood flow (quoted by Schiebler et al, 1961). Systemic venous return proceeds to the pulmonary artery while pulmonary venous return eventually enters the aorta, although the ventricle in each circuit is not the appropriate one. Since the atrioventricular valves 'go with' the ventricles, the mitral valve is right sided as is the anatomic left ventricle, and the tricuspid valve leads from the left atrium to the left sided but

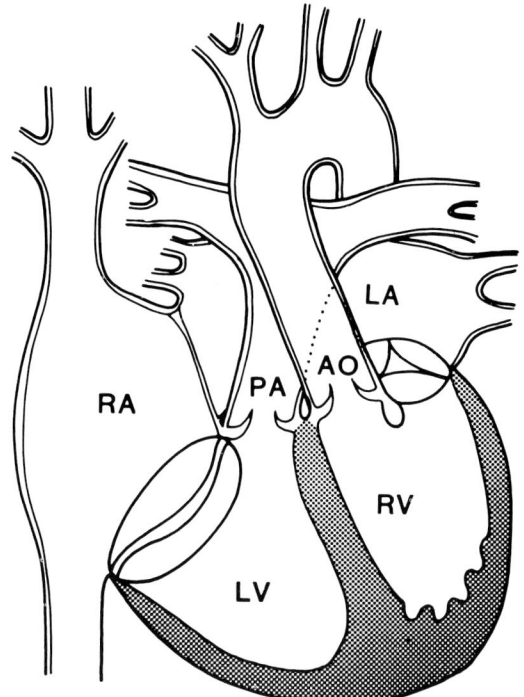

Fig. 19.10 Diagram of corrected transposition of the great arteries.

anatomic right ventricle. The aorta is to the left of the pulmonary artery and is usually, but not always, somewhat more anterior. The aortic valve approximates the position of the pulmonic valve in the normal individual.

Associated anomalies

Associated anomalies are usually present and include ventricular septal defect, pulmonic stenosis, left atrioventricular valve abnormality, and atrioventricular block. A ventricular septal defect is the most common of these and is found in about 75 percent of cases of corrected transposition. The defect is usually large (Allwork et al, 1976). Pulmonic stenosis is also common and is usually subvalvar. The most common morphologic abnormality of the left atrioventricular valve is a distal displacement of the origin of the septal and inferior leaflets (Ebstein's anomaly) (Jaffe, 1976). Atrioventricular block may be first, second or third degree and may be present at birth or appear later. The block occurs because the ventricular septum immediately below the atrioventricular node is entirely fibrous in corrected transposition, preventing passage of an electrical impulse. There is usually another more anteriorly placed atrioventricular node, however, which does connect to the ventricular myocardium, but via a longer and more tortuous conduction pathway. This elongated bundle seems to be subject to fibrosis, explaining the late onset of atrioventricular block in some patients with corrected transposition (Anderson et al, 1974).

Nomenclature

The nomenclature of this anomaly remains in some dispute. The term 'congenitally corrected transposition' has been criticized because 'corrected' seems to imply normality, and in most cases significant associated anomalies preclude a normal circulation. The term 'corrected' also may be confused with surgically 'correcting' complete transposition. 'Atrioventricular discordance plus ventriculoarterial discordance' is an accurate and descriptive term but is ponderous. The term 'l-transposition of the great arteries' refers to the supposed embryologic origin of corrected transposition from an l-loop, while 'd-transposition' describes the more common 'complete' transposition (Van Praagh et al, 1964). Unfortunately, 'd' and 'l' terms seem to assign prime importance to the positional relationship of the great arteries and position does not always reflect the atrioventricular and ventriculo-arterial connections. For instance, in complete, or 'd' transposition, the aorta is sometimes to the left of the pulmonary artery rather than to the right.

In summary, 'congenitally corrected transposition', or more briefly, 'corrected transposition', is the most widely used term, seems less confusing than most and will be used subsequently in this section, with the caveat that 'corrected' does not imply 'normal'.

Clinical course

Rarely, corrected transposition is 'isolated' and without important other cardiac anomalies. Long survival has been reported (Lieberson et al, 1969), although failure of the systemic (anatomic right) ventricle may occur prematurely even though no structural abnormalities are present (Nagle et al, 1971). The clinical course of most cases of corrected transposition is determined by the associated anomalies. The most common anomaly, a ventricular septal defect, can result in poor growth and develpment or in frank congestive heart failure during infancy.

If an 'ideal' degree of pulmonic stenosis accompanies the ventricular defect, symptoms may not appear for many years and cyanosis may be mild or absent. If more severe pulmonic stenosis accompanies a ventricular septal defect, there is a strong clinical resemblance to tetralogy of Fallot, and cyanosis may appear early in life and dominate the clinical picture. If there is severe left atrioventricular valve regurgitation, congestive heart failure results and may appear in early infancy. The atrioventricular block of corrected transposition is usually 'suprahisian' and a stable pacemaker controls the ventricle. Even with a stable pacemaker, however, the slow rate may be poorly tolerated if there is an associated hemodynamically important anomaly such as a large ventricular septal defect. In an occasional patient with congenital block, the natural pacemaker is unstable and Stokes-Adams attacks may occur.

Physical findings

Positional

Since the abnormal connections which constitute corrected transposition do not, per se, produce hemodynamic abnormalities, any abnormal physical findings are related either to certain inherent positional abnormalities or to associated anomalies. The positional deviations which may cause abnormal physical findings include an abnormal orientation of the interventricular septum (Caufield et al, 1967), the anterior and leftward position of the aortic root, and dextrocardia. The interventricular septum has an unusual anteroposterior orientation in corrected transposition, with the ventricles being side by side. (Normally the septum runs obliquely, so that the right ventricle is both to the right and anterior to the left ventricle.) The left sided ventricle thus underlies the left sternal border as well as the 'apex' (Fig. 19.11). Hemodynamic abnormalities which increase the vigor of contraction of this left sided systemic ventricle (e.g. left atrioventricular valve regurgitation) may thus produce a left parasternal lift which mimics overload of the right sided ventricle and suggests pulmonary hypertension. The abnormal anterior and leftward position of the aorta may heighten

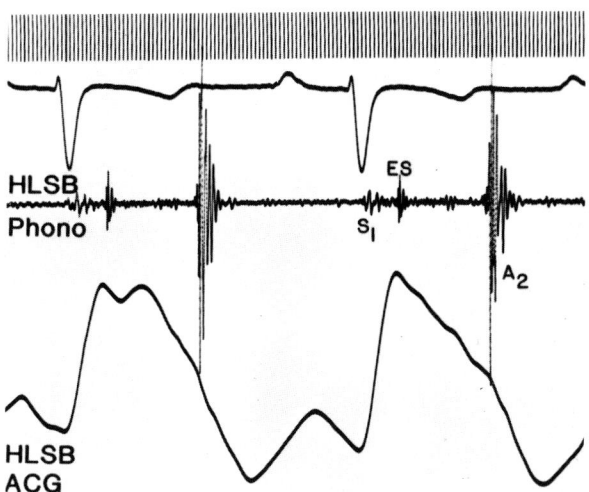

Fig. 19.12 Child with corrected transposition of the great arteries. The high left sternal border phonocardiogram shows a very loud and single second heart sound (A_2) and an ejection sound (ES). A pulse tracing recorded in the same area (HLSB ACG) shows a prominent systolic outward movement. Both the pulse and the loud second sound are due to the anterior position of the aorta.

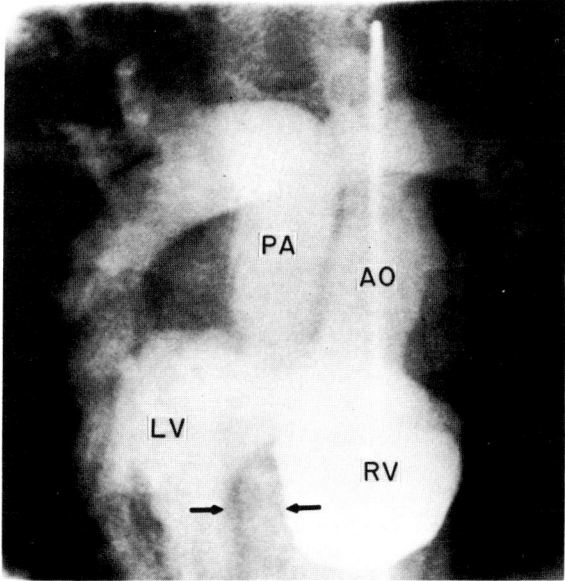

Fig. 19.11 Cineangiogram frame showing the anteroposterior position of the interventricular septum (arrows) in a child with corrected transposition.

the impression of pulmonary hypertension by producing a palpable systolic impulse in the second or third left intercostal space (Fig. 19.12). The pulmonic closure sound is usually inaudible and the loud single second sound is indistinguishable from the loud pulmonic closure sound of pulmonary hypertension. Audible splitting of the second heart sound at the high right sternal border has been described as a characteristic finding in corrected transposition (Gasul et al, 1959). This has been a very uncommon finding in the author's experience, probably because the posterior position of the pulmonic valve causes the pulmonic component to be very soft. The presence of dextrocardia is evidenced by the location of the apical impulse and the heart sounds over the right hemithorax.

Associated anomalies

Abnormal physical findings may be due to associated cardiac anomalies. The findings of an associated ventricular septal defect do not differ appreciably from those of an isolated ventricular septal defect. Since the defect is usually large in corrected transposition, secondary pulmonary hypertension is common and may result in pulmonary vascular disease. Pulmonic regurgitation eventually develops in some patients with secondary pulmonary hypertension. Its presence is signaled by a decrescendo diastolic murmur (Fig. 3.23). (As mentioned above the loud aortic closure sound at the high left sternal border may falsely suggest secondary pulmonary hypertension. Aortic regurgitation, if present, is difficult to clinically distinguish from hypertensive pulmonic regurgitation.)

The murmur of associated pulmonic stenosis is typically maximal at the mid sternal level, either to the right or left of the sternum or directly over it. The murmur closely resembles that heard in tetralogy of Fallot, its loudness and duration tending to vary inversely with the severity of the obstruction. If the ventricular septum is intact and obstruction severe, the murmur of pulmonic stenosis may be long and extend through the aortic component of the second heart sound (Fig. 19.13).

The murmur of left atrioventricular valve regurgitation may be apical and closely resemble ordinary mitral regurgitation, but the unusual orientation of the septum may make the murmur as loud or louder at the low left sternal border. If the regurgitation is severe there may be a mid diastolic murmur of relative stenosis of the left atrioventricular valve (anatomic tricuspid valve). In the author's experience, this murmur is less low pitched than the usual diastolic murmur accompanying severe mitral regurgitation and more closely resembles the medium pitched diastolic murmur of relative tricuspid stenosis. This suggests that the differing pitch of the murmurs of tricuspid and mitral stenosis is related to different anatomy of the two valves, rather than to their relative position within the thorax.

The physical findings accompanying an associated atrioventricular block are the same as in an individual without corrected transposition. (Chap. 24). The first heart sound may be soft if there is

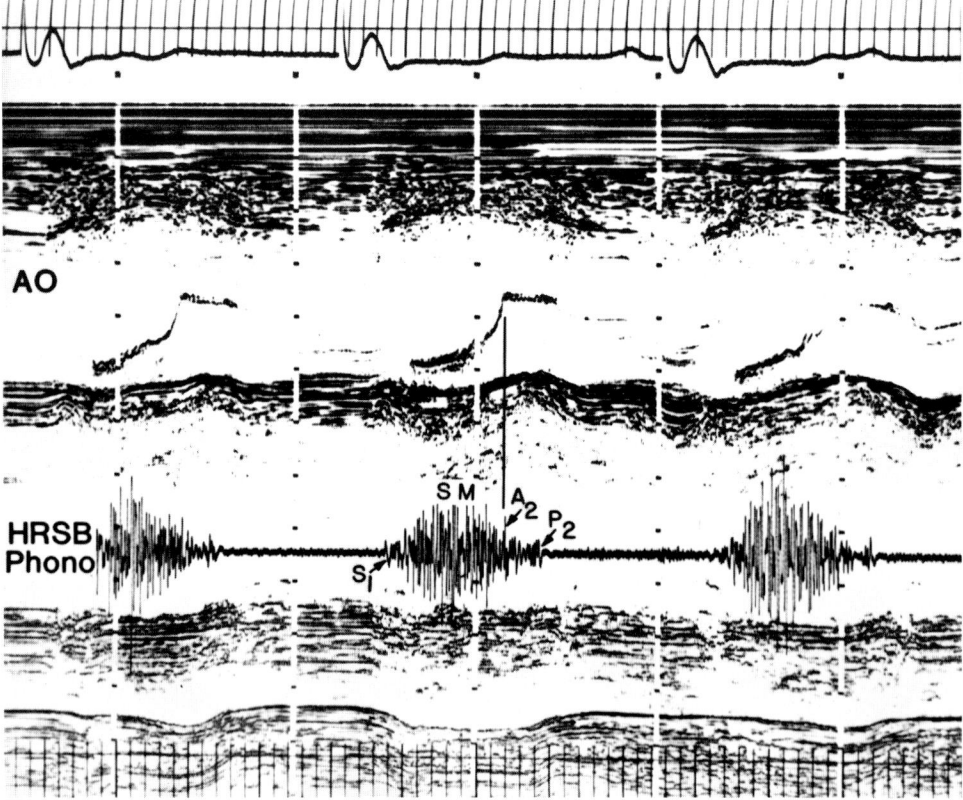

Fig. 19.13 Child with corrected transposition and pulmonic stenosis. The systolic murmur is crescendo-decrescendo and extends beyond aortic closure, as timed by the aortic valve echo (AO). (Note the anterior position of the aortic valve).

first degree block and of variable intensity with third degree block, changing with the apparent PR interval. An intermittant protodiastolic sound and intermittant cannon waves in the jugular venous pulse are other findings in third degree block.

Summary

In summary, the physical findings which suggest corrected transposition are a slow pulse (with other physical trappings of third degree atrioventricular block), unexplained 'mitral' regurgitation (especially if the associated diastolic murmur is medium pitched) and signs suggesting secondary pulmonary hypertension (loud single second heart sound, left sternal border lift) when pulmonary hypertension seems unlikely to be present.

REFERENCES

Allwork S P, Bentall H H, Becker A E, Cameron H, Gerlis L M, Wilkinson J L, Anderson R H 1976 Congenitally corrected transposition of the great arteries: morphologic study of 32 cases. American Journal of Cardiology 38:910

Anderson R H, Becker A E, Arnold R, Wilkinson J L 1974 The conducting tissue in congenitally corrected transposition. Circulation 50:911

Caulfield W H Jr, Bostock B, Perloff J K, 1967 Corrected transposition of the great vessels with isolated pulmonic stenosis. American Journal of Cardiology 19:285

de la Cruz M V, Berrazueta J R, Arteaga M, Attie F, Soni J 1976 Rules for diagnosis of arteioventricular discordances and spatial indentification of ventricles. British Heart Journal 38:341

Gasul B M, Graettinger J S, Bucheleres G 1959 Corrected transposition of the great vessels. Journal of Pediatrics 55:180

Jaffe R B 1976 Systemic atrioventricular valve regurgitation in corrected transposition of the great vessels. American Journal of Cardiology 37:395

Lieberson A D, Schumacher R R, Childress R H, Genovese P D 1969 Corrected transposition of the great vessels in a 73-year-old man. Circulation 39:96

Moss A I, Adams F H, Emmanoulides G C 1977 Heart disease in infants, children and adolescents. Williams & Wilkins, Baltimore, p 310

Nagle J P, Cheitlin M D, McCarty R J 1971 Corrected transposition of the great vessels without associated anomalies: report of a case with congestive failure at age 45. Chest 60:367

Park S C, Weiss F H, Siewers R D, Neches W H, Zuberbuhler J R, Lenox C C 1976 Continuous murmur following Mustard operation for transposition of the great arteries: a sign of pulmonary venous obstruction. Circulation 54:684

Schiebler G L, Edwards J E, Burchell H B, DuSchane J W, Ongley P A, Wood E H 1961 Congenital corrected transposition of the great vessels: a study of 33 cases. Pediatrics 27:851

Van Praagh R 1971 Transposition of the great arteries. American Journal of Cardiology 28:739

Van Praagh R, Van Praagh S, Vlad P, Keith J D 1964 Anatomic types of congenital dextrocardia: diagnostic and embryologic implications. American Journal of Cardiology 13:510

Zuberbuhler J R, Bauersfeld S R, Pontius R G 1967 Paradoxic splitting of the second sound with transposition of the great vessels. American Heart Journal 74:816

Arterial anomalies

SYSTEMIC ARTERIOVENOUS FISTULA

Clinical course

Systemic arteriovenous fistulae are rare. They may be intracranial (Silverman et al, 1955; Cunliffe, 1974) intrahepatic (Martin et al, 1965), cervical, thoracic (Atwood et al, 1975) or in an extremity. The clinical course of an individual with an arteriovenous fistula is determined by the magnitude of blood flow through it. A small fistula is well tolerated but congestive heart failure may occur if the fistula is large. Failure is occasionally evident at birth if flow through the fistula is especially great.

Physical findings

General

Any large systemic arteriovenous fistula increases the output of both right and left ventricles, and both left sternal border and apical pulsations may be prominent. Since a large fistula constitutes a low resistance exit from the aorta, diastolic pressure in the aorta is low and pulse pressure wide. Peripheral arterial pulses therefore tend to be increased, even in the face of congestive heart failure.

Physical findings are influenced not only by the size of a fistula but also by its location. If the fistula is intracranial and very large, carotid pulses may be full and pulses elsewhere weak or even absent (Rowe & Mehrizi, 1968). Neck veins are often prominent and pulsatile with an intracranial fistula. The jugular venous distension is due both to the large venous return from the fistula and to elevated right atrial pressure. Jugular venous distension is so uncommonly seen in infants with other cardiovascular anomalies that its presence should suggest the possibility of an intracranial fistula. Hepatic pulsations may occur with an intrahepatic arteriovenous fistula and thoracic wall or cervical pulsations may accompany fistulae in those areas. A thrill or pulsatile mass may signal the presence of an arteriovenous fistula in an extremity, and hypertrophy of the involved extremity is common. Heart rate reflexly decreases with sudden compression of a peripheral arteriovenous fistula (Fig. 20.1) (Branham, 1890). Although a systemic arteriovenous fistula does not, per se, produce arterial unsaturation, cyanosis can occur if torrential systemic venous return from a large fistula raises right atrial pressure sufficiently to cause right to left shunting through a patent foramen ovale (Walker et al, 1969).

Auscultation

The second heart sound is usually physiologically split in a patient with a systemic arteriovenous fistula. The pulmonic closure sound is accentuated if there is secondary pulmonary hypertension. A third heart sound is common.

The rapid flow and abrupt pressure drop across an arteriovenous fistula usually produces a continuous murmur. When timed by heart sounds, this continuous murmur may seem to have a late systolic or even diastolic accentuation, but this is due to the delay in pulse transmission to the periphery (Fig. 20.2). The continuous murmur of an arteriovenous fistula may be missed unless specifically searched for, since most fistulae are in regions that are not routinely auscultated, such as the head, liver, or extremities. These areas should

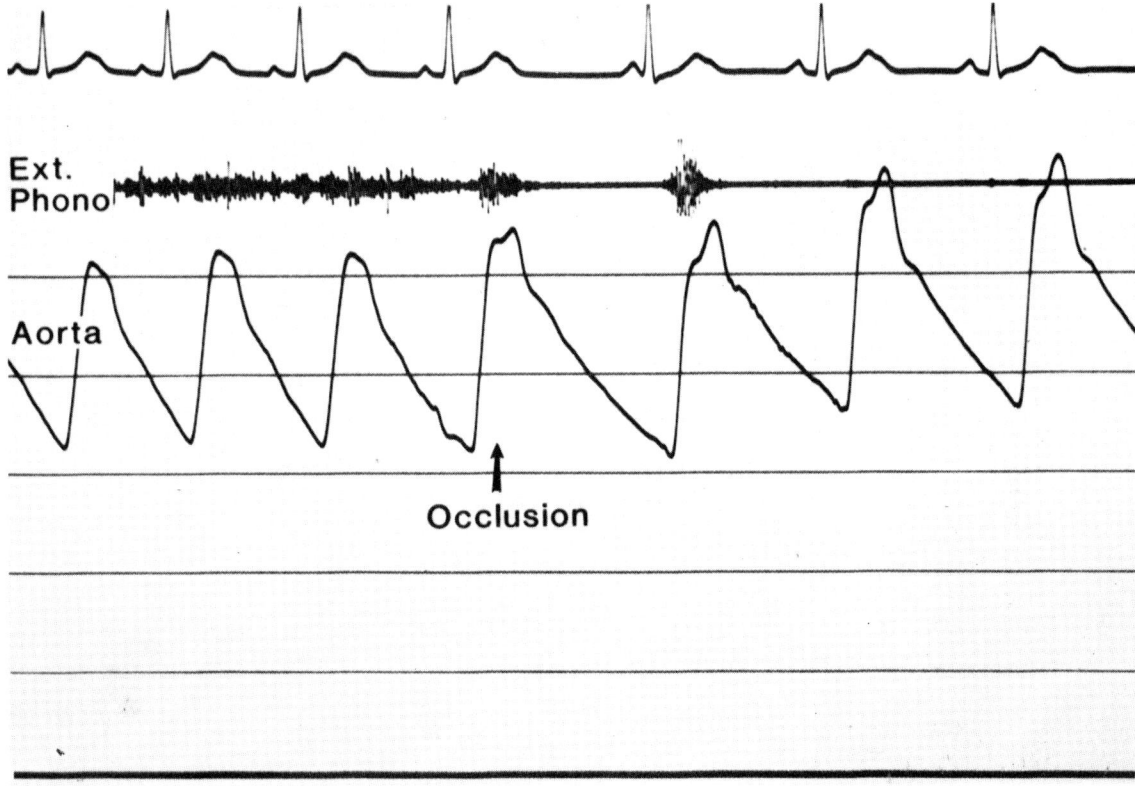

Fig. 20.1 Child with cervical arteriovenous fistula. The continuous murmur disappears and there is slowing of the heart rate and increase in aortic pressure with intra-arterial balloon occlusion of the fistula.

be carefully listened to in any infant with unexplained congestive heart failure, especially if pulses are more prominent than expected in the setting of congestive heart failure. It must be emphasized that not all intracranial fistulae produce an audible murmur, and that not all bruits heard over the head emanate from a fistula. Indeed, most do not since a faint continuous murmur can be heard over the head of many normal children. The co-existence of a head bruit and congestive heart failure is highly suggestive, however, especially if pulses are full and neck pulsations are visible (Cunliffe, 1974). With any large systemic arteriovenous fistula a soft systolic murmur may be generated by rapid flow across the aortic and/or pulmonic valves and be audible at the base.

Differential diagnosis

The differential diagnosis of a systemic arteriovenous fistula is usually that of a continuous murmur or of abnormally increased pulses. Localization of a continuous murmur to the head, neck, abdomen, extremities, or to a thoracic region away from the usual 'ductal' area should point to the correct diagnosis. (An arteriovenous fistula in the left cervical area may generate a continuous murmur which is well heard at the high left sternal border. The correct diagnosis is obvious, however, if it is recognized that the murmur is louder above than below the left clavicle.) Strong carotid pulses associated with weak pulses elsewhere suggest a large intracranial fistula but can also occur with a coarctation of the aorta if the coarctation involves the left subclavian artery and is associated with distal origin of the right subclavian artery. Although prominent jugular venous pulsations also occur with tricuspid atresia and a restrictive interatrial septal defect or with severe tricuspid regurgitation, the combination of prominent arterial *and* jugular venous neck pulsations in a neonate is almost pathognomonic of a large

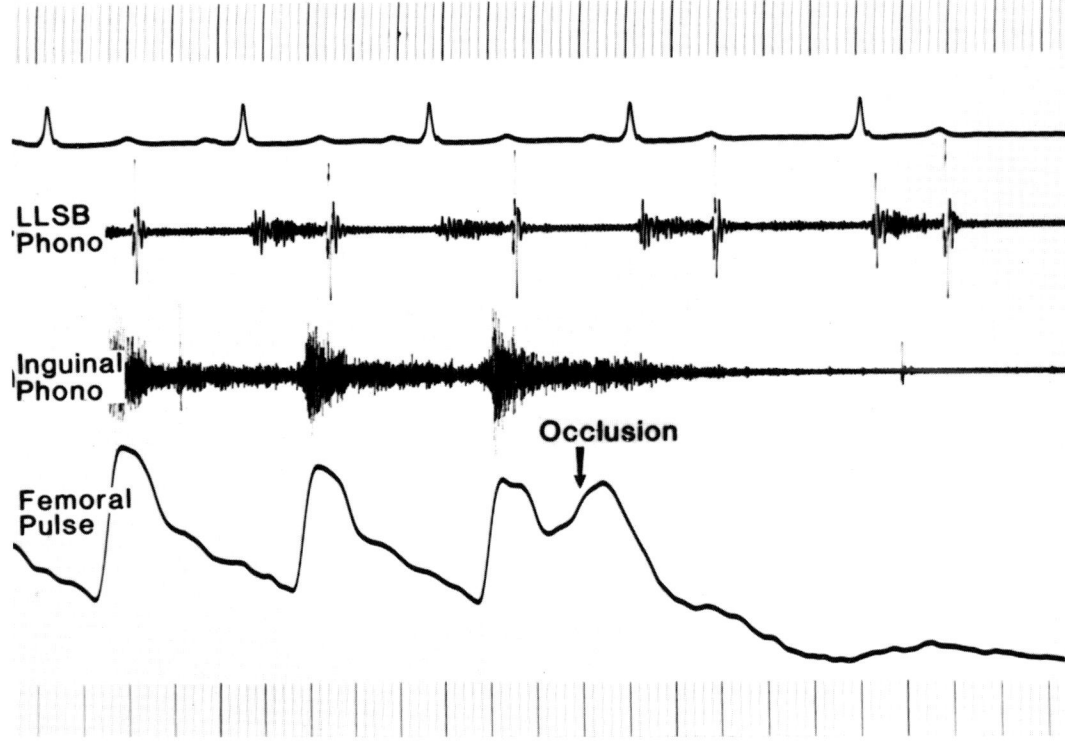

Fig. 20.2 Child with femoral arteriovenous fistula and a small ventricular septal defect. The apparent late systolic peaking of the inguinal murmur is due to normal delay in transmission of the pulse to the periphery. The murmur disappears with local pressure.

intracranial arteriovenous fistula. Congestive heart failure which occurs in utero and which is, therefore, evident at the time of birth as fetal hydrops is quite rare and suggests the possibility of an arteriovenous fistula. (Other causes of such failure include congenital tricuspid regurgitation, absent pulmonic valve and in utero arrhythmia or myocarditis.)

A systolic or continuous murmur is occasionally heard along the sternal borders or over the breasts in late pregnancy (mammary souffle of pregnancy) (Tabatznik et al, 1960). It results from increased arterial blood supply to the breast and may superficially simulate a patent ductus arteriosus or an arteriovenous fistula in the thoracic wall. The murmur may be accentuated with light stethoscope pressure and obliterated with firm pressure with the stethoscope or with digital compression. It also tends to become softer or disappear with standing and spontaneously disappears shortly after termination of pregnancy or the cessation of lactation.

PULMONARY ARTERIOVENOUS FISTULA

The anomaly

Congenital pulmonary arteriovenous fistulae are quite rare, and may be isolated (Moyer et el, 1962) or part of the Rendu-Osler-Weber Syndrome (hereditary hemorrhagic telangiectasia) (Hodgson et al, 1959). In the latter entity telangiectases, nosebleeds, gastrointestinal hemorrhage and a positive family history point to the correct diagnosis.

Clinical course and physical findings

General

The most common clinical manifestation of a pulmonary arteriovenous fistula is cyanosis. Although pulmonary arterial blood which traverses the fistula bypasses the pulmonary capillary bed, the resulting arterial unsaturation may not result in cyanosis if flow through the fistula is small or if there is anemia (especially common with telangiectasia). Dyspnea and easy fatigue are usually absent or mild, even with a large fistula which causes considerable arterial unsaturation and obvious cyanosis. Complications include rupture of the fistula, brain abscess and the hemorrhagic or thrombotic sequellae of polycythemia.

Auscultation

The cardiac examination is normal. A murmur may or may not be audible over the chest wall overlying the fistula. If present it may be either systolic or continuous and is characteristically louder with inspiration (Moyer et al, 1962). The murmur becomes softer and disappears with expiration or with the strain phase of a Valsalva maneuver. These changes in intensity are doubtless due to the alteration in systemic venous return and right ventricular stroke volume which accompany changes in intrathoracic pressure.

PULMONARY-LEFT ATRIAL FISTULA

A pulmonary arteriovenous fistula may take the form of a direct pulmonary artery to left atrial communication. In one cyanotic 14-year-old boy, a large channel connected the right pulmonary artery and the left atrium. (Bauersfeld et al, 1964). The cardiac examination was completely normal and no murmur was heard over the lung fields. When the fistula was transiently occluded with a balloon catheter, arterial saturation rose from 65 percent to 95 percent and cyanosis disappeared. The fistula was successfully treated by surgical ligation.

CORONARY ARTERY FISTULA

Coronary artery fistulae usually drain to a cardiac chamber (Sakakibara et al, 1966) but rarely may enter the pulmonary artery (Gobel et al, 1970) or the coronary sinus (Vlodaver et al, 1973). By far the most common sites of drainage are the right ventricle and the right atrium. Flow through a coronary artery fistula is usually small and symptoms are unusual. Flow may occasionally be large,

however, and cause congestive heart failure. This is quite rare in infancy (Verani & Lauer, 1975). Angina like chest pain has been described, even with small fistulae (Gobel et al, 1970), and infectious endocarditis may occur. In most cases, however, organic heart disease is first suspected when a continuous murmur is heard incidentally in an asymptomatic individual. If the run-off through the fistula is small, arterial pulses, blood pressure, jugular venous pulse, precordial motion and heart sounds will be normal. In the occasional patient with a large fistula arterial pulses are full and pulse pressure wide.

Auscultation

The most characteristic auscultatory feature of a coronary artery fistula is a continuous murmur, and the location of the murmur often suggests the drainage site of the fistula (Sakakibara et al, 1966). If the fistula is to the right ventricle, the continuous murmur is usually maximal at the mid or low left sternal border. (Exceptions do occur, and in an unusual case of coronary to right ventricle fistula seen in our institution the continuous murmur was maximal at the mid right sternal border and had both systolic and diastolic accentuations (Figs. 20.3

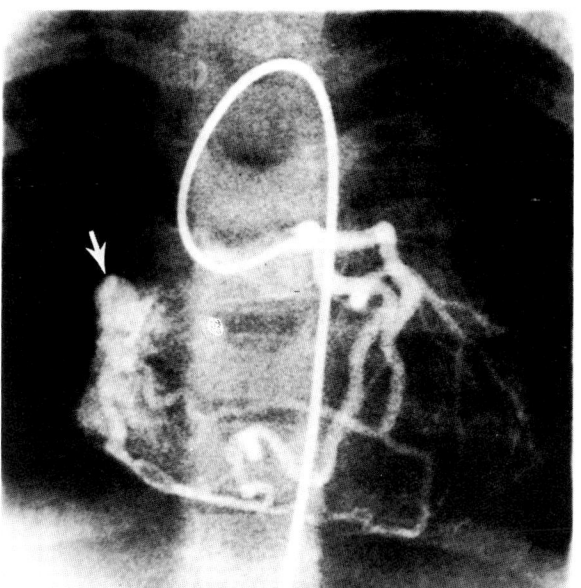

Fig. 20.3 Cineangiogram frame from a child with a coronary-cardiac fistula. The fistula (arrow) drains to the right ventricle.

and 20.4). The direction of the jet entering the right ventricle varied with the phase of the cardiac cycle and the intracardiac murmur varied strikingly in intensity and shape with slight differences in catheter position.) If the fistula enters the right atrium the murmur is usually better heard along the right sternal border. If the fistula is to the pulmonary artery the murmur is maximal at the high left sternal border and is indistinguishable from the continuous murmur of a patent ductus arteriosus. Rarely, a coronary artery to pulmonary artery fistula is associated with pulmonary atresia and a ventricular septal defect and is the sole source of pulmonary blood flow (Krongrad et al, 1972). Here, also, the fistula is clinically indistinguishable from a patent ductus arteriosus. In most cases of coronary-cardiac fistula, however, the continuous murmur is not maximal in the usual 'ductal' location at the high left sternal border. A continuous murmur in an 'atypical' location should always suggest the possibility of a coronary artery fistula, especially if the patient is without symptoms and is acyanotic. If a coronary artery fistula enters the left ventricle, a diastolic murmur may be the only auscultatory finding (Eguchi et al, 1970).

ANOMALOUS ORIGIN OF A CORONARY ARTERY

Clinical course

Several anomalies involving the origin of one or more coronary arteries have been described. Most consist of an unusual number of coronary ostia in the aortic root, either a single orifice or three or more. Rarely, one of the coronary arteries — or

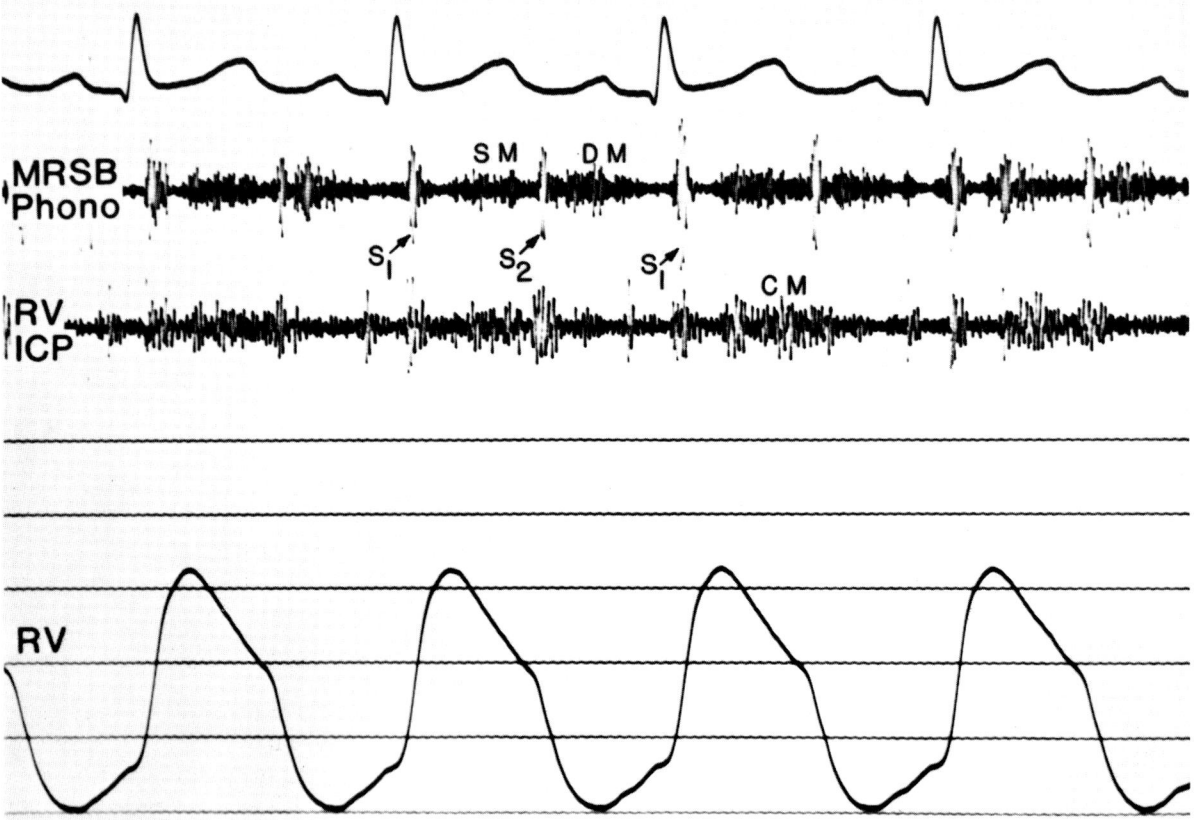

Fig. 20.4 Same child as Figure 20.3. The mid right sternal border phonocardiogram (MRSB Phono) shows a to and fro murmur with systolic (SM) and diastolic (DM) components. The right ventricular phonocardiogram (RV ICP) demonstrates a continuous murmur which is louder in systole.

even both of them — may arise from the pulmonary artery. The left coronary artery is more commonly involved than the right and will be discussed first. The anomaly poses no problem in utero, since high pulmonary artery pressure ensures adequate myocardial perfusion. With the normal fall in pulmonary vascular resistance and pulmonary artery pressure after birth forward flow through the left coronary artery ceases. If there are intercoronary collateral arteries there will be retrograde flow from right coronary artery through these collaterals to the left coronary artery and eventually into the pulmonary artery. The adequacy of these collaterals largely determines the clinical course. (Liebman et al, 1963; Talner et al, 1965). If they are sparse the left ventricular myocardium suffers the consequences of poor perfusion and may show decreased contractility, infarction, endocardial fibroelastosis, or papillary muscle dysfunction leading to mitral regurgitation.

An infant with an anomalous left coronary artery usually seems normal at birth and for a variable period thereafter, but signs of congestive heart failure usually appear within the first few months. The infant may experience episodes of irritability, sweating, dyspnea, and pallor which are thought to be due to myocardial ischemia and to be the equivalent of angina. These episodes are often brought on by feeding but may occur at rest. Most infants with an anomalous left coronary artery and poor intercoronary collaterals die during the first year of life but spontaneous clinical improvement occasionally occurs (Liebman et al, 1963). If the intercoronary anastomoses are large, left ventricular function may be normal and congenital heart disease unsuspected during infancy and childhood. Mitral regurgitation, congestive heart failure, angina, or sudden death eventually occur in most individuals with this anomaly. Even with large intercoronary anastomoses the volume of blood shunted from aorta to pulmonary artery through the anomalous coronary artery is trivial; poor myocardial perfusion is the important hemodynamic abnormality.

Physical findings

In the symptomatic infant with anomalous origin of a coronary artery the usual physical signs of congestive heart failure are present, including tachypenea, dyspnea and hepatomegaly. Since the aortic run-off is small, pulses are normal, or decreased if congestive heart failure is severe. The jugular venous pulse is difficult to see and is not helpful. The apical impulse may be active, especially if there is important mitral regurgitation. There may be a prominent left sternal border systolic impulse if left ventricular dysfunction has resulted in pulmonary hypertension. There is usually a gallop, but heart sounds are otherwise normal.

Patients with anomalous origin of the left coronary artery may have an apical systolic murmur of mitral regurgitation (Noren et al, 1964). Diastolic and continuous murmurs have been reported and have been postulated to originate in the normally arising but dilated right coronary artery or in intercoronary collaterals (Liebman et al, 1963). Each of two older children with this anomaly seen in our institution had a peculiar mid left sternal border murmur which was soft and high pitched and which varied strikingly from beat to beat, being sometimes continuous, sometimes only diastolic and sometimes disappearing altogether. (In the second case the unusual characteristics of the murmur first raised the suspicion of an anomalous coronary artery.) In each case the murmur disappeared after the left coronary artery was surgically implanted in the aortic root.

Differential diagnosis

In infancy the important differential diagnoses include primary myocardial disease and congenital mitral regurgitation. In older children rheumatic mitral regurgitation must be added. Although an electrocardiographic pattern of myocardial infarction suggests the presence of an anomalous left coronary artery, a definitive diagnosis can be made only by aortography or, preferably, selective coronary arteriography. The anomaly is potentially surgically correctable, even in symptomatic infants with abnormal left ventricular function. A high index of suspicion in any infant with unexplained congestive heart failure or mitral regurgitation is important, whether or not there is a 'typical' electrocardiogram.

An anomalous right coronary artery is usually more benign. Although symptoms are rare and survival to age 90 years has been reported (Cronk et al, 1951), sudden death may occur (Wald et al, 1971). Origin of both coronary arteries from the pulmonary artery is exceedingly rare and is not compatible with life beyond early infancy (Colmers & Siderides, 1963).

REFERENCES

Atwood G F, King T D, Graham T P Jr, Canent R V, Ebert P A, Spach M S 1975 Thoracic arteriovenous fistula: venous connection to right iliac vein. American Journal of Diseases of Children 129:233

Bauersfeld S R, Zuberbuhler J R, Ford W B 1964 Right pulmonary artery-left atrial communication. American Heart Journal 67:244

Branham H H 1890 Aneurysmal varix of the femoral artery and vein, following a gunshot wound. International Journal of Surgery 36:250

Colmers R A, Siderides C I 1963 Anomalous origin of both coronary arteries from pulmonary trunk. American Journal of Cardiology 12:263

Cronk E S, Sinclair J G, Rigdon R H 1951 An anomalous coronary artery arising from the pulmonary artery. American Heart Journal 42:906

Cunliffe P N 1974 Cerebral arteriovenous aneurysm presenting with heart failure. British Heart Journal 36:919

Eguchi S, Nitta H, Asano K, Tanaka M, Hoshini K 1970 Congenital fistula of the right coronary artery to the left ventricle. American Heart Journal 80:242

Gobel F L, Anderson C F, Baltaxe H A, Amplatz K, Wang Y 1970 Shunts between the coronary and pulmonary arteries with normal origin of the coronary arteries. American Journal of Cardiology 25:655

Hodgson C H, Burchell H B, Good C A, Clagett O T 1959 Hereditary hemorrhagic telangiectasia and pulmonary arteriovenous fistula. New England Journal of Medicine 26:625

Krongrad E, Ritter D G, Hawe A, Kincaid O W, McGoon D C 1972 Pulmonary atresia or severe stenosis and coronary artery-to-pulmonary artery fistula. Circulation 46:1005

Liebman J, Hallerstein H K, Ankeney J L, Tucker A 1963 The problem of the anomalous left coronary artery arising from the pulmonary artery in older children. New England Journal of Medicine 269:486

Martin L W, Benzing G, Kaplan S 1965 Congenital intrahepatic arteriovenous fistula. Annals of Surgery 161:209

Moyer J H, Glantz G, Brest A N 1962 Pulmonary arteriovenous fistulas. American Journal of Medicine 32:417

Noren G R, Raghib G, Moller J H, Amplatz K, Adams P, Edwards J E 1964 Anomalous origin of the left coronary artery from the pulmonary trunk with special reference to the occurrence of mitral insufficiency. Circulation 30:171

Rowe R D, Mehrizi A 1968 The neonate with congenital heart disease. Saunders, Philadelphia, p 375

Sakakibara S, Yokoyama M, Takao A, Nogi M, Gomi H 1966 Coronary arteriovenous fistula. American Heart Journal 72:307

Silverman B K, Breckx T, Craig J, Nadas A S 1955 Congenital failure in the newborn caused by cerebral A-V fistula. American Journal of Diseases of Children 89:539

Tabatznik B, Randall T W, Hersch C 1960 The mammary souffle of pregnancy and lactation. Circulation 22:1069

Talner N S, Halloran K H, Mahdavy M, Gardner T H, Hipona F 1965 Anomalous origin of the left coronary artery from the pulmonary artery. American Journal of Cardiology 15:689

Verani M S, Lauer R M 1975 Echocardiographic findings in right coronary arterial-right ventricular fistula. American Journal of Cardiology 35:444

Vlodaver Z, Johnson T, Karnegis J N, Edwards J E, Castaneda A R 1973 Clinical pathologic conference. American Heart Journal 85:689

Wald S, Stonecipher K, Baldwin B J, Nutter D O 1971 Anomalous origin of the right coronary artery from the pulmonary artery. American Journal of Cardiology 27:677

Walker W J, Mullins C E, Knovick G 1964 Cyanosis, cardiomegaly and weak pulses: a manifestation of massive congenital systemic arteriovenous fistula. Circulation 29:777

21

Pericardial disease

ACUTE PERICARDITIS

The pericardium is the 'silent partner' of the myocardium and endocardium. Only when it is abnormal in some way does it show evidence of its presence. In childhood, disease processes involving the pericardium are most often inflammatory and include infection, acute rheumatic fever, post pericardiotomy syndrome and collagen vascular disease (especially systemic lupus erythematosis and rheumatoid arthritis). Neoplasms, especially lymphoma, may occasionally involve the pericardium. Other rare causes of pericardial disease include renal failure (uremic pericarditis) and trauma.

In the acute phase of pericarditis there may be substernal chest pain. The pain is often accentuated with inspiration, and a patient can sometimes relieve his discomfort by sitting forward and pressing his chest against a pillow or his folded forearms. Pericardial disease may also evidence its presence by a large intrapericardial fluid collection (pericardial effusion).

Pericardial rub

A pericardial friction rub is the most characteristic physical finding of acute pericarditis. It is produced as 'sticky' visceral and parietal pericardial surfaces pass over each other, and resembles the sound produced by rubbing the stethoscope head against the back of one's hand or by rubbing a tuft of hair between one's thumb and forefinger. It is usually maximal along the left sternal border and at the apex and is best heard with the diaphragm of the stethoscope. A rub may have 1, 2 or 3 components, produced by cardiac motion during ventricular systole, ventricular protodiastole and atrial systole, respectively. A 'rub' heard only in ventricular systole, however, is suspect and must be distinguished from a scratchy systolic murmur. The tendency for a rub to become much louder when the stethoscope head is pressed firmly against the chest wall may be very helpful in differentiating it from such a murmur. Also, a 'rub' which persists unchanged for more than a few days is more likely to be a systolic murmur, since a pericardial rub is characteristically changeable and evanescent.

Inflammatory or neoplastic pericardial disease may result in considerable fluid collection in the pericardial space and, as the accumulating fluid separates the visceral and parietal layers of pericardium, a previously audible pericardial rub may disappear. If a large amount of fluid accumulates, heart sounds may become soft. (It must be noted that the presence of a pericardial rub and/or normal heart sounds by no means rules out a large pericardial effusion.) A very large pericardial effusion may compress the left lower lung and result in bronchial breath sounds at the left base posteriorly (Ewart's sign).

TAMPONADE

A small amount of intrapericardial fluid (or even a large amount of fluid slowly accumulated) has no hemodynamic consequences. When fluid collection is sufficiently rapid and/or massive, intrapericardial pressure rises and there is a corresponding increase in systemic venous pressure. If there is sufficient impairment of cardiac filling and cardiac output, tamponade occurs, manifested by distension of jugular veins, hepatomegaly, and tachycardia. The

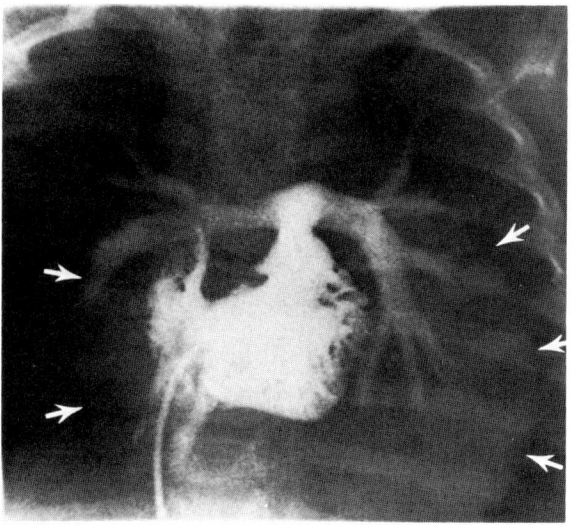

Fig. 21.1 Cineangiogram frame showing a small heart within a large pericardial effusion. Pericardial border indicated by arrows.

precordium is usually quiet and arterial pulses are weak. The first and second heart sounds may or may not be soft, but no gallop is present. In contrast to the peripheral signs of low cardiac output, cineangiography shows a small vigorously contracting heart floating in a sea of pericardial fluid (Fig. 21.1). Echocardiography also demonstrates the striking cardiac motion within the pericardial sac.

Paradoxic pulse

One of the most striking features of tamponade is the respiratory variation in arterial pulse amplitude known, paradoxically, as a 'paradoxical' pulse. This phenomenon is really an exaggeration of the *normal* response to inspiration. During inspiration, intrathoracic pressure falls and there is a resultant increase in systemic venous return. There is also an increase in capacitance of the pulmonary vascular bed, which tends to decrease venous return to the left side of the heart. The net result of the decreased intrathoracic pressure and altered blood flow is a transient inspiratory decrease in blood pressure. This decrease does not normally exceed 10 mm of mercury. With pericardial tamponade there is an exaggerated inspiratory fall in blood pressure which may exceed 20 mm of mercury (Fig. 21.2). The excessive inspiratory fall in blood pressure in patients with tamponade has been postulated to be related to a tightly stretched pericardium and a relatively fixed total intrapericardial space. With tamponade, therefore, intracardiac volume cannot increase with respiration. Since systemic venous return *does* increase with inspiration, there must be a corresponding decrease in pulmonary venous return, blood being transiently stored in the pulmonary vascular bed. With the decrease in pulmonary venous return, left ventricular output is reduced and blood pressure falls. Hence, the paradoxical pulse of tamponade. (Shabetai et al, 1965).

A paradoxic pulse may be appreciated by simply feeling the pulse during quiet respiration and may be quantitated by measuring blood pressure variation during the respiratory cycle. A blood pressure cuff is inflated until no Korotkoff sounds are heard and is then slowly deflated until sounds appear during expiration. The cuff is further deflated until sounds are present throughout the respiratory cycle. The difference between the blood pressure at which sounds first appear during expiration and the pressure at which sounds are heard throughout the cycle is a measure of the degree of 'paradox' and therefore of the degree of restriction of cardiac filling. A respiratory variation of over 20 mm of mercury is highly suggestive of pericardial tamponade (Lange et al, 1966).

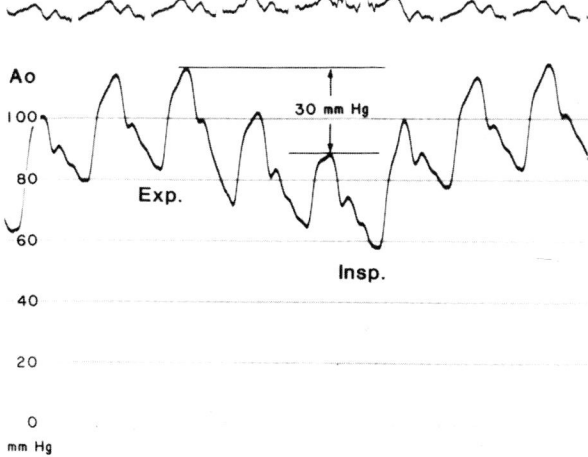

Fig. 21.2 Pulsus paradoxus. Aortic peak systolic pressure is 30 mmHg higher during expiration than during inspiration.

POST PERICARDIOTOMY SYNDROME

The pericardium may become acutely inflamed following surgical procedures which violate the pericardial space. The cause is obscure, but may involve an immune response to trauma. The interval between surgery and pericarditis is highly variable, ranging from a few days to several weeks.

Fever and a pericardial rub are the most common clinical manifestations and the differential diagnosis of fever in the postoperative period should always include the post pericardiotomy syndrome. If there is no sign of a wound infection and if blood cultures are negative a therapeutic trial of aspirin may be useful. Prompt defervescence of fever is consistant with the post pericardiotomy syndrome.

CONSTRICTIVE PERICARDITIS

Pericardial inflammation may lead to a thickening and scarring of the pericardium which results in constriction. At one time, tuberculosis was the infection most likely to lead to constriction, but tuberculous pericarditis is now quite rare and other infectious agents are more common causes. Of five cases of purulent pericarditis seen in our institution within the last 10 years, three have been due to hemophilus influenza and two of these three developed signs of constriction within a month of the onset of infection.

Chronic constrictive pericarditis is likely to have a more subtle onset than pericardial tamponade. Jugular veins are distended and there may be a striking diastolic collapse in the jugular venous pulse known as Friedreick's sign (Wood, 1961). This collapse corresponds to the early diastolic dip seen in right atrial and right ventricular pressure tracings. Kussmaul's sign, an inspiratory increase in filling of the jugular veins, is of more historic than clinical interest, since it is often absent with

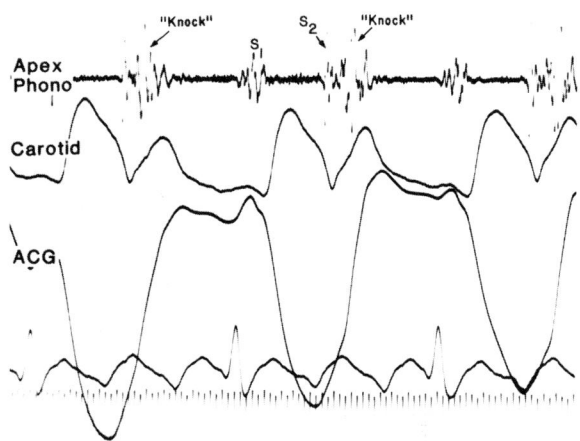

Fig. 21.3 Chronic constrictive pericarditis. There is a very loud protodiastolic sound (pericardial knock) as well as apical systolic retraction on the apexcardiogram (ACG).

constriction and may be present with congestive heart failure (Lange et al, 1966). Peripheral pulses may be decreased with constrictive pericarditis but a paradoxic pulse is rare. There is often hepatomegaly and sometimes ascites and peripheral edema. The precordium is usually quiet with no well-defined apical impulse but in some cases there is a palpable systolic retraction at or near the apex (Fig. 21.3). The second heart sound is often widely split and there may be a very loud protodiastolic sound known as a 'pericardial knock' (Fig. 21.3). A knock usually occurs earlier in diastole than a third heart sound (Mounsey, 1955). There is usually no murmur.

There are many clinical similarities between constrictive pericarditis and chronic restrictive cardiomyopathy. Clinical differentiation may be quite difficult but a murmur of mitral or tricuspid regurgitation, an active apical impulse, or a gallop at the usual time in the cardiac cycle favors cardiomyopathy.

REFERENCES

Lange R L, Botticelli J T, Tsagaris T J, Walker J A, Gani M, Bustamante R A 1966 Diastolic signs in compressive cardiac disorders. Circulation 33:763

Mounsey P 1955 The early diastolic sound of constrictive pericarditis. British Heart Journal 17:143

Shabetai R, Fowler N O, Fenton J C 1965 Restrictive cardiac disease. Pericarditis and the myocardiopathies. American Heart Journal 69:271

Wood P 1961 Chronic constrictive pericarditis. American Journal of Cardiology 7:48

Pulmonary hypertension

'Pulmonary hypertension' and 'pulmonary vascular disease' are not synonymous terms; although all patients with pulmonary vascular disease have pulmonary hypertension, not all patients with pulmonary hypertension have pulmonary vascular disease. The distinction is quite important since presentation, clinical course, and therapy differ, depending on the underlying cause of the elevated pressure. Pulmonary hypertension may result from increased pulmonary blood flow, high pulmonary venous pressure or elevated pulmonary vascular resistance. Although pulmonary arterial systolic pressure may equal aortic systolic pressure with very large pulmonary blood flow and normal pulmonary vascular resistance, equality of diastolic and mean pressures in the pulmonary artery and aorta occurs only with elevated pulmonary vascular resistance.

Etiology

Primary pulmonary hypertension

Pulmonary hypertension may be 'primary' or 'secondary'. In primary pulmonary hypertension, vascular resistance is always high and there is no important associated cardiac anomaly to explain the morphologic changes in the pulmonary arterioles which are responsible for the high resistance. A few patients with supposed primary pulmonary hypertension have high pulmonary vascular resistance on the basis of multiple pulmonary emboli (Fowler et al, 1966), residence at high altitude (Sime et al, 1936), or a more general arteriopathy (Celoria et al, 1960). In most, however, the etiology of the elevated resistance is unknown. At one time primary pulmonary hypertension was thought to be a disease of young women (Wood, 1959) but is now known to occur in infancy and childhood and in both sexes (Thilenius et al, 1965). Effort fatigue, dyspnea, syncope and anginoid chest pain occur and are related to an inability of the right ventricle to increase its output in the face of high vascular resistance (Howarth & Lowe, 1953). Since systemic vascular resistance falls with exertion, systemic pressure also falls if output does not increase, and coronary and cerebral perfusion then may suffer.

Secondary pulmonary hypertension

Secondary pulmonary hypertension may be due to the increased pulmonary blood flow which accompanies a large septal defect or to the elevated pulmonary venous pressure which results from left heart obstruction or left ventricular dysfunction. Although elevation of pulmonary artery pressure may be entirely 'passive' and caused by increased blood flow or by pulmonary venous hypertension, eventually the pulmonary arterioles undergo changes which increase pulmonary vascular resistance. The severity and permanence of this increased resistance vary with different cardiac anomalies and also from individual to individual with the same anomaly. In a patient with an interatrial septal defect, for instance, pulmonary hypertension and pulmonary vascular disease are late phenomena and are uncommon in a child or young adult. At the other end of the spectrum, pulmonary hypertension is an inevitable consequence of a large and unrestrictive ventricular septal defect if there is no associated pulmonic stenosis. Although pulmonary artery pressure is always high in such a patient, pulmonary vascular resistance may or may not be elevated. In most infants with a large ventricular septal defect there is a relatively slow fall in the high levels of pulmonary vascular resistance normally present at birth. Only during the second or third month of life does resistance fall sufficiently to permit a large left to right shunt and only then does congestive heart failure appear (Ch. 5). Pulmonary vascular resistance may then rise secondarily, but usually not until after the first year or two of life. In other infants with a large ventricular defect there is little or no postnatal fall in pulmonary vascular resistance and the fetal pulmonary vascular pattern persists.

The permanence of pulmonary vascular changes depends not only on the severity of the morphologic changes in the arterioles but also on the possibility of reducing pressure or flow in the pulmonary circuit. Excessive pressure and large flow stimulate the development of arteriolar disease and if either or both can be eliminated the progression of disease may be halted or slowed. In some instances the arteriolar changes may actually regress. If neither pressure nor flow can be reduced, pulmonary vascular disease will progress. Thus, surgically relieving mitral stenosis or closing a ventricular septal defect in a patient with large pulmonary blood flow will effect a fall in pulmonary artery pressure and will likely have a favorable affect on the course of pulmonary vascular disease. On the other hand, surgically closing a ventricular septal defect in a patient with equal pulmonary and systemic blood flows will not reduce pulmonary artery pressure and will not favorably affect the course of the vascular disease.

Clinical course

The typical courses of primary and of secondary pulmonary hypertension differ. If a septal defect is present and pulmonary vascular resistance rises sufficiently, right to left shunting and cyanosis occur. Complications of polycythemia and of right to left shunting, such as hemorrhage, thrombosis, or brain abscess are not rare. It is of note that effort syncope and chest pain are less common with secondary pulmonary hypertension than with primary, presumably because right to left shunting through a septal defect permits augmentation of systemic output with exercise. Central cyanosis is uncommon in patients with primary pulmonary hypertension but may occur if there is a patent foramen ovale. Peripheral cyanosis may occur as cardiac output decreases in the late stages of primary pulmonary hypertension but intense cyanosis is not a feature. Sudden death is more common with primary pulmonary hypertension than with the secondary variety but right ventricular failure may be the terminal event in either type.

Physical findings

General

Most children with pulmonary hypertension secondary to a large septal defect show signs of poor growth, especially of slow weight gain, but individuals with primary pulmonary hypertension usually display normal growth and development. As mentioned above, cyanosis will be present if there is a septal defect and if pulmonary vascular resistance exceeds systemic. Arterial pulses and systemic arterial pressure are not affected by pulmonary hypertension, per se. Large 'A' waves may be present in the jugular venous pulse, especially with primary pulmonary hypertension, and are a result of right atrial hypertrophy and vigorous right atrial contractions against elevated right ventricular diastolic pressure. In the clinical

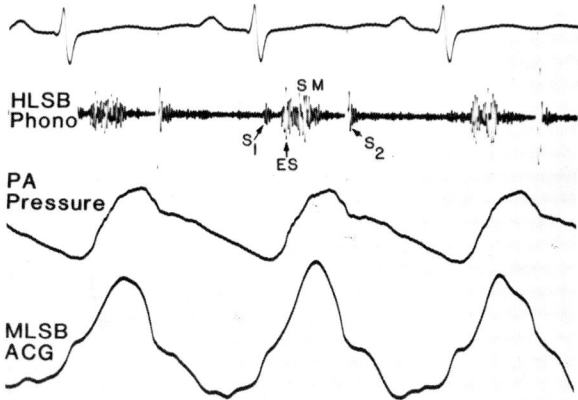

Fig. 22.1 Adolescent with secondary pulmonary hypertension. The high left sternal border phonocardiogram shows a loud and single second heart sound (S2) and a rather delayed pulmonic ejection sound (ES). There is a short systolic murmur. A prominent systolic outward movement is evident in the mid left sternal border pulse tracing (MLSB ACG).

setting of pulmonary hypertension a bifid jugular venous pulse with prominent 'A' and 'V' waves suggests the presence of tricuspid regurgitation. A sustained left parasternal systolic lift is an expected finding in severe pulmonary hypertension (Fig. 22.1) and pulmonary artery pulsations may be palpated at the high left sternal border (Fig. 22.2). Pulmonary valve closure is often palpable in the same area.

Auscultation

Heart sounds. A loud pulmonary valve closure sound is the most characteristic auscultatory finding in pulmonary hypertension (Fig. 22.2). The timing of pulmonary valve closure is influenced both by pulmonary artery pressure and by right ventricular function. High pressure in the pulmonary artery tends to close the pulmonic valve more quickly than usual and as long as right ventricular function is adequate, pulmonary and

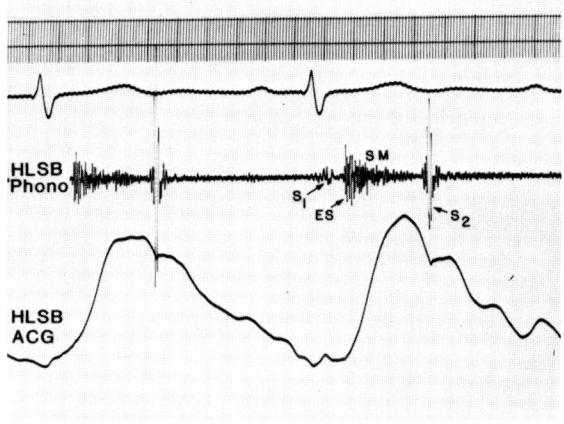

Fig. 22.2 Same patient as Figure 22.1. Transmitted pulmonary artery pulsations are recorded in the high left sternal border pulse tracing (HLSB ACG). The dicrotic notch is coincident with the loud second heart sound.

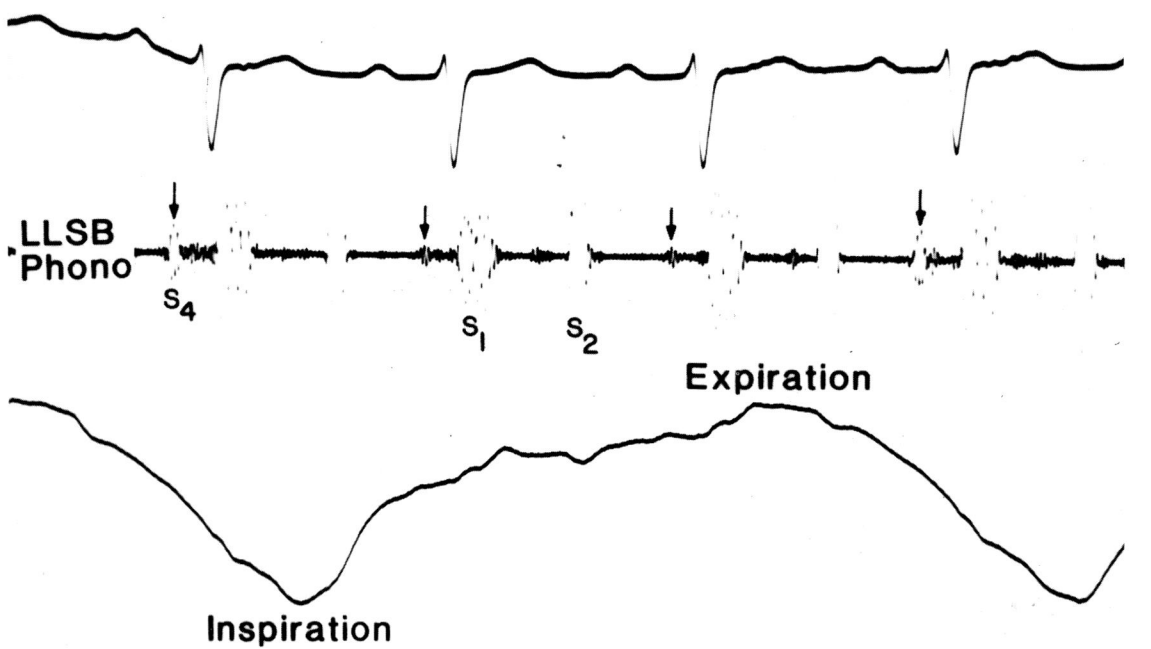

Fig. 22.3 Child with secondary pulmonary hypertension and chronic right ventricular failure. The fourth heart sound (S4, arrows) becomes louder with inspiration.

aortic valves close nearly simultaneously. The second heart sound is then single or very narrowly split. If right ventricular contractility is decreased or if after-load sufficiently increases, ejection is prolonged, pulmonic valve closure is delayed and the second heart sound is widely split (Shaver et al, 1974). (A very loud pulmonic closure sound may obscure a relatively soft preceding aortic closure sound and splitting can be missed. It may be more obvious lower along the left sternal border or at the high right sternal border, where the pulmonic closure sound is less loud.) Splitting may not vary with respiration, since decreased right ventricular function may preclude an inspiratory increase in right ventricular stroke volume. In the clinical setting of pulmonary hypertension a widely and nearly fixed split second heart sound is therefore presumptive evidence of advanced pulmonary vascular disease and of relatively poor right ventricular function. A third heart sound may be present if there is right ventricular failure. A right sided fourth heart sound occasionally occurs and when present is maximal at the low left sternal border. There may be an inspiratory augmentation of this fourth sound (Fig. 22.3). An early systolic ejection sound is another common auscultatory finding in pulmonary hypertension; the sound is high pitched, maximal at the high left sternal border and tends to disappear with inspiration. The sound tends to be later than the ejection sound which accompanies valvar pulmonic stenosis since the pre-ejection period is prolonged in pulmonary hypertension.

Murmurs. The most common and least specific murmur associated with pulmonary hypertension is a soft crescendo-decrescendo systolic murmur at the high left sternal border. The murmur is probably related to dilatation of the main pulmonary artery. With severe long-standing pulmonary hypertension the tricuspid and/or the pulmonic valves may become incompetent. The murmur of tricuspid regurgitation is maximal at the low left sternal border and is usually holosystolic and high pitched. It may, however, have a musical quality and in an occasional patient is harsh and loud. The murmur may increase with inspiration (Rivero-Carvallo, 1946). The murmur of hypertensive pulmonic regurgitation (Fig. 22.4) is usually described as being high pitched, decrescendo and maximal at the high or mid left sternal border (Graham Steelle, quoted by Willius & Keys, 1941). In the author's experience, the murmur is sometimes displaced well laterally from the left sternal border and may be loud, harsh and have an accompanying thrill. Unless carefully timed with an arterial pulse this latter murmur will be assumed to be systolic, since murmurs with these characteristics almost always are systolic.

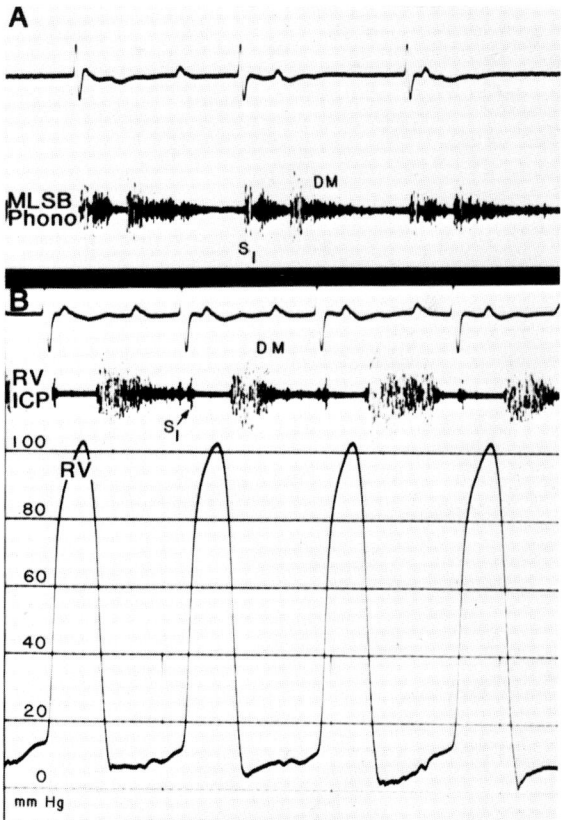

Fig. 22.4 Child with secondary pulmonary hypertension and pulmonic regurgitation. The external phonocardiogram in A shows a decrescendo diastolic murmur which begins with the second heart sound and which is indistinguishable from the murmur of aortic regurgitation. In B the pulmonic origin of the murmur is demonstrated in the phonocardiogram recorded in the right ventricle (RV ICP).

REFERENCES

Celoria G C, Friedell G H, Sommers S C 1960 Raynaud's disease and primary pulmonary hypertension. Circulation 22:1055

Fowler N O, Black-Shaffer B, Scott R C, Gueron M 1966 Idiopathic and thromboembolic pulmonary hypertension. American Journal of Medicine 40:331

Howarth S, Lowe J B 1953 The mechanism of effort syncope in primary pulmonary hypertension and cyanotic congenital heart disease. British Heart Journal 15:47

Rivero-Carvallo J M 1946 New diagnostic sign of tricuspid insufficiency. Archivas del Instituto de Cardiologia de Mexico 16:531

Shaver J A, Nadolny R A, O'Toole J D, Thompson M E, Reddy P S, Leon D F, Curtiss E I 1974 Sound pressure correlates of the second heart sound — an intracardiac sound study. Circulation 49:316

Sime F, Banchero N, Panaloza D, Gamboa R, Cruz J, Marticorena E 1963 Pulmonary hypertension in children born and living at high altitudes. American Journal of Cardiology 11:143

Thilenius O G, Nadas A S, Jockin H 1965 Primary pulmonary vascular obstruction in children. Pediatrics 36;75

Willius F A, Keys T E 1941 Cardiac classics. Mosby, St. Louis p 680

Wood P 1959 Pulmonary hypertension. Modern Concepts of Cardiovascular Disease 28:513

23

Functional murmurs

By definition, 'functional' or 'innocent' murmurs are not caused by structural abnormalities of the cardiovascular system. The terms 'functional' and 'innocent' are usually used interchangeably, but it can be argued that murmurs of high output states such an anemia, fever or thyrotoxicosis are 'functional' since they do not emanate from an abnormal cardiac structure, but are not 'innocent' since they are the result of altered physiology. In this chapter no such distinction will be made.

The importance of differentiating functional from organic murmurs is obvious. Even if the organic murmur arises from a hemodynamically trivial anomaly the risk of infectious endocarditis may be real and require antibiotic prophylaxis in situations likely to produce bacteremia. Fortunately, the differentiation of functional and organic murmurs is usually possible 'at the bedside'.

Basal murmurs

The more common systolic functional murmurs arise in the right or left ventricular outflow tracts and are caused by turbulence resulting from high velocity blood flow. Since velocity reaches a peak early in systole, especially in the left heart, such functional murmurs typically peak in early systole and end well before the second heart sound. Although the functional systolic murmur itself is indistinguishable from the systolic murmur of mild anatomic outflow tract obstruction, the organic murmur can be recognized 'by the company it keeps'. If the murmur is functional the cardiac examination will be otherwise unremarkable. With outflow tract obstruction there is almost always some other finding; another murmur, an abnormal cardiac sound, or abnormal splitting of the second heart sound. Outflow tract murmurs, be they functional or organic, become somewhat louder with the increased cardiac output of exercise, fever or anxiety, but the organic murmur has a greater tendency to become quite loud and to develop an associated thrill.

Pulmonic

A short soft systolic murmur can be heard at the high left sternal border in many normal children, adolescents and young adults. The murmur begins after the first heart sound and is soft and crescendo-decrescendo. It originates at the pulmonic valve and corresponds to the systolic murmur that can be demonstrated by intracardiac phonocardiography in the main pulmonary artery of individuals without right heart disease (Lewis et al, 1959). The functional 'pulmonic' murmur does not differ appreciably in its characteristics from the murmur of mild pulmonic stenosis or of an interatrial septal defect, but clinical differentiation is usually not difficult. The pulmonic stenosis murmur becomes much louder with exercise and often develops an accompanying thrill. In addition, if the pulmonic stenosis is valvar the murmur is almost always accompanied by an early systolic ejection sound. The fixedly split second heart sound and the low left sternal border diastolic murmur of an interatrial septal defect effectively differentiate it from a functional pulmonic murmur.

Aortic

A systolic murmur may be generated at a structurally normal aortic valve, especially if there is anemia, fever, or some other cause of increased cardiac output. This is the only functional murmur that is maximal at the high right sternal border and it must be differentiated from the murmur of a bicuspid aortic valve, with or without mild aortic stenosis. With a bicuspid valve there is virtually always an aortic early systolic ejection sound, usually loudest at the apex and heard best with the patient sitting.

Carotid, cervical and cranial murmurs

In many children a systolic murmur can be heard above the clavicles or over the carotid arteries. The murmur begins well after the first heart sound and is crescendo-decrescendo. It probably arises in the subclavian and carotid arteries and has a wide range of intensity. This murmur is distinguished from the murmur of aortic or pulmonic stenosis by being louder above the clavicles than over the precordium. (A thrill may be present above the clavicles, but never below.) A soft systolic or continuous murmur may be heard over the head of some normal children and is not, in itself, reason to institute a search for an intracranial arteriovenous fistula.

Still's murmur

Another very common functional systolic murmur is that first described by Still (1909). This murmur is maximal at the mid and low left sternal border and out toward the apex. It is recognized by its quality, which is variously described as 'vibratory', 'buzzing', 'groaning', or like a 'twanging string'. It is, in fact, difficult to describe but quite easy to recognize by its characteristic quality. Although Still's murmur may be heard in infants, it is much more common in children over 2 or 3 years of age. It becomes less common after adolescence. The murmur may vary from day to day and typically becomes louder with fever or exertion. The exact origin of this murmur has never been definitely established.

'Physiologic' pulmonary artery stenosis

The murmur of so called 'physiologic' pulmonary artery stenosis (Danilowicz et al, 1972) is heard only in early infancy and is especially common in prematures. It is recognized by its distribution, being nearly equally loud at the base, in the axillae, and across the posterior thorax. This murmur originates in the proximal right and left pulmonary arteries, which are normally somewhat hypoplastic in the newborn and leave the main pulmonary artery at a relatively acute angle. The murmur disappears within the first few months of life unless there are true stenoses in the pulmonary arteries (Ch. 9). The murmur of pulmonary artery stenosis, be it physiologic or organic, must be differentiated from that of increased flow through the pulmonary arteries. With a large left to right shunt, however, there is always other evidence of organic heart disease. The murmur of physiologic pulmonary artery stenosis has nearly the same pitch as breath sounds and can easily be mistaken for them if breathing is not temporarily interrupted during auscultation.

Continuous 'murmurs'

Jugular venous hum

Continuous functional 'murmurs' include the jugular venous hum and the mammary souffle of pregnancy. A jugular venous hum is usually maximal above the clavicles but may radiate well below them. It may be quite loud and is occasionally accompanied by a thrill. It is sometimes much louder on one side than the other. A venous hum must be differentiated from a patent ductus arteriosus or, less commonly, an arteriovenous fistula. Most texts emphasize the importance of head turning and external pressure over the jugular veins to alter the intensity of the hum and confirm the diagnosis, but it is easier simply to listen to the patient in sitting and recumbent positions. The murmur of a patent ductus arteriosus or an arteriovenous fistula is unaltered by position, while a venous hum invariably attenuates or disappears entirely with recumbency. (It should be noted that a venous hum may be induced inadvertently by partially occluding a jugular vein while auscultating the neck.)

Mammary souffle

The mammary souffle of late preganancy and the early postpartum period is heard in the left and/or the right second intercostal spaces. The murmur may be systolic or continuous and can be obliterated with local pressure. Its disappearance after pregnancy and lactation have terminated further help to distinguish it from a patent ductus arteriosus or an arteriovenous fistula.

REFERENCES

Danilowicz D A, Rudolph A M, Hoffman J I E, Heymann M 1972 Physiologic pressure differences between main and branch pulmonary arteries in infants. Circulation 45:410

Lewis D H, Ertugrul A, Deitz G W, Wallace J D, Brown J R Jr, Moghadam A 1959 Intracardiac phonocardiography in the diagnosis of congenital heart disease. Pediatrics 23:837

Still G F 1909 Common disorders and diseases of childhood. Frowde, Hodder & Stoughton, London

Conduction abnormalities

Certain atrioventricular conduction abnormalities have hemodynamic consequences which are reflected in the physical examination. Three will be considered here:

1. Atrioventricular block
2. Bundle branch block
3. Wolff-Parkinson-White syndrome

ATRIOVENTRICULAR BLOCK

Classification

The spectrum of atrioventricular block ranges from delay in propagation of the atrial impulse across the atrioventricular junction (first degree block), to propagation of only some atrial impulses to the ventricles (second degree block), to complete loss of conduction of atrial impulses to the ventricles (third degree block). The most important of these, third degree atrioventricular block, may be congenital or acquired. Congenital block may be 'isolated' or be associated with other congenital cardiac anomalies, especially 'corrected' transposition. In children the most common etiology of the acquired variety is open heart surgery, although occasionally block is related to acute myocarditis, to acute rheumatic fever or to rheumatoid arthritis (Lenox et al, 1978).

Clinical course

First and second degree atrioventricular block are usually benign and produce no symptoms, although high grade second degree block may result in a very slow ventricular rate and be poorly tolerated. The most important determinant of the clinical course and prognosis of third degree block is the stability of the pacemaker controlling the ventricles, the stability being related to the site of block. If the block is above the bundle of His (suprahisian block) the ventricles are driven by a junctional pacemaker, which is generally quite stable. The ventricular rate usually exceeds 40 beats per minute and the slow rate is well tolerated unless there are serious associated cardiac anomalies. If the block is below the bifurcation of the bundle of His (infrahisian block) an idioventricular focus controls the ventricles. Such a focus tends to be quite unstable and Stokes-Adams attacks and/or sudden death are common. In general, most cases of congenital atrioventricular block are suprahisian and have a good prognosis, especially if there is no associated cardiovascular anomaly. Surgically acquired atrioventricular block, on the other hand, is most often infrahisian, carries a grave prognosis and requires insertion of an artificial pacemaker. (Surgical block may be suprahisian and benign but the distinction from infrahisian block usually requires intracardiac electrophysiologic studies.) The ventricular rate in infrahisian block is supposedly slower than in suprahisian block, but this is not necessarily so. Among 36 patients with congenital heart block seen at our institution during the last 10 years, the median heart rate in the group with 'isolated' suprahisian block was 42 beats per minute and was 52 beats per minute in the group with associated congenital cardiac anomalies. In a separate group of patents with surgically-acquired infrahisian block, the median heart rate was 50 beats per minute.

Physical findings

The physical examination may be useful in suggesting the presence of an atrioventricular conduction abnormality. Adequate evaluation of atrioventricular block, however, requires at least a surface electrocardiogram; occasionally, intracardiac electrical recordings are necessary.

Incomplete AV block

First degree atrioventricular block is rarely suspected before an electrocardiogram is done, although, at least in retrospect, the first heart sound is often soft, a consequence of the long PR interval. With second degree atrioventricular block the ventricular rate may be merely slow (2:1 block, 3:1 block, etc.) or may be irregular (3:2 block, 4:3 block, etc.) The differentiation of the irregular rhythm of block from coupled premature beats is difficult without an electrocardiogram.

Complete AV block

Heart sounds. Several physical signs are regularly associated with third degree atrioventricular block. The pulse rate is abnormally slow and, in addition, the intensity of the first heart sound varies from beat to beat, depending upon the length of the apparent PR interval (Fig. 24.1) (Wolferth & Margolies, 1930; Burggraf & Craige, 1974). The most likely cause of this phenomenon is the variable position of the atrioventricular valve leaflets at the onset of ventricular contraction. If the mitral and tricuspid valves are open widely, as they will be if atrial systole has immediately preceded ventricular systole, they will be closed forcefully by ventricular systole and the first heart sound will be loud. If there is a long apparent PR interval and therefore more delay between atrial and ventricular systole, the leaflets will have floated toward the closed position by the time ventricular systole begins. Closure will then be less abrupt and the first heart sound will be soft or even inaudible.

Another consequence of independent atrial and ventricular rates is an intermittent protodiastolic sound, generated when atrial systole and rapid early diastolic filling happen to coincide. The resulting sound is really a summation of third and fourth heart sounds and may occur in certain cases of second degree atrioventricular block (Fig. 24.2) as well as in individuals with complete block.

Cannon waves. Careful inspection of the jugular venous pulse of an individual with third degree block will reveal 'cannon' waves, which occur when atrial and ventricular systole coincide, atrial contraction then being against a closed tricuspid valve (Fig. 24.2). Rather prolonged auscultation of the heart and inspection of the jugular venous pulse may be necessary to demonstrate variability of the first heart sound and cannon waves, respectively, especially if the atrial and ventricular rates are nearly equal or if the atrial rate is nearly an exact multiple of the ventricular rate. Under these circumstances the apparent PR interval may vary only slightly over a considerable period of time.

Murmurs. A basal systolic murmur is common with third degree atrioventricular block and is generated at the aortic and/or pulmonic valves by the compensatory increase in stroke volume. An increased left ventricular stroke volume is also responsible for the prominent apical impulse which is common in complete atrioventricular block.

BUNDLE BRANCH BLOCK

Delay in electrical excitation of one ventricle (bundle branch block) results in a corresponding delay in mechanical events in that ventricle, and closure of the semilunar valve which guards the outflow from the ventricle will occur later than usual. In right bundle branch block the pulmonic valve closure sound is delayed and the second heart

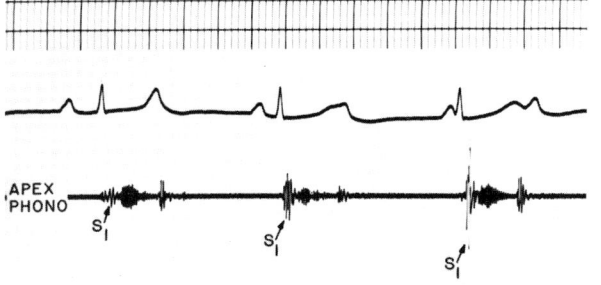

Fig. 24.1 Third degree atrioventricular block. In the three beats shown there is progressive accentuation of the first heart sound (S1) with decreasing apparent PR interval.

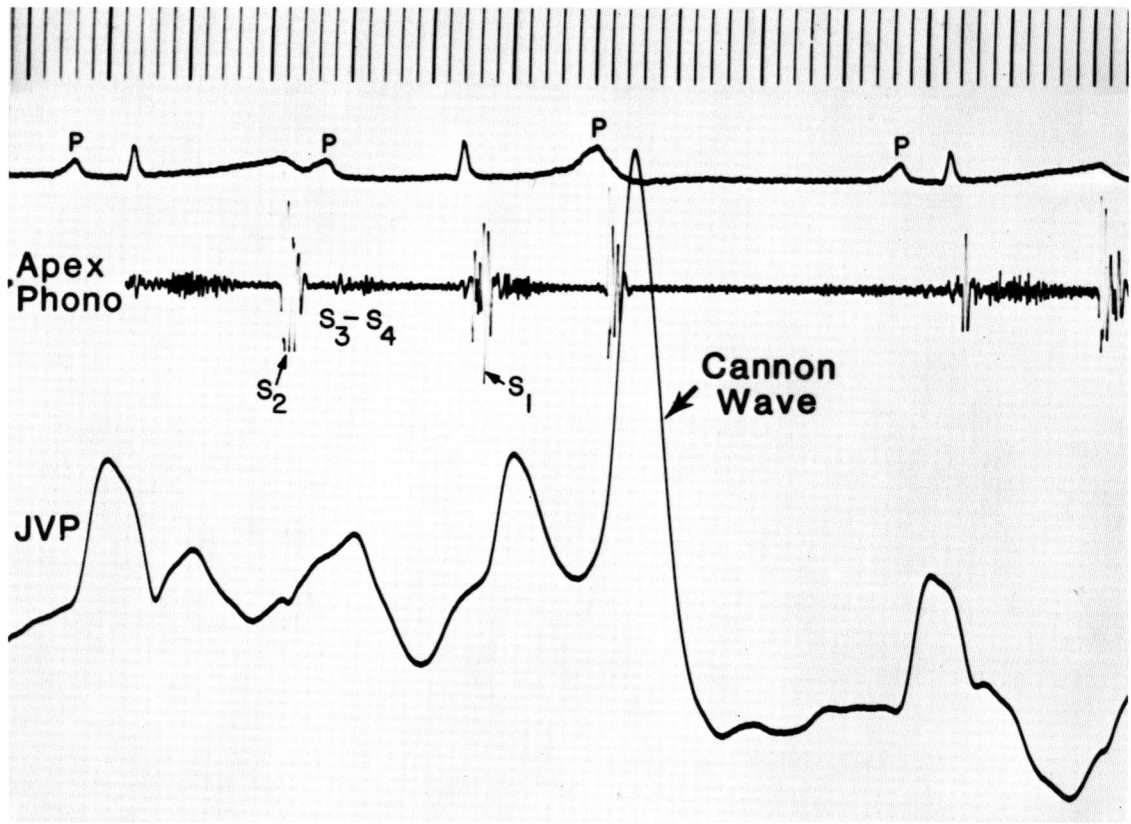

Fig. 24.2 Second degree atrioventricular block with Wenckebach phenomenon. The third P wave falls in late systole; since the tricuspid valve is closed, atrial contraction produces a large 'cannon' wave in the jugular venous pulse. The second atrial systole falls in early diastole and the protodiastolic sound is a combined third and fourth heart sound (S3–S4).

sound is widely split. The first heart sound may also be split with right bundle branch block. In left bundle branch block, aortic valve closure is late and the second heart sound is often paradoxically split (Gray, 1956).

WOLFF-PARKINSON-WHITE SYNDROME

Etiology

The Wolff-Parkinson-White syndrome, also known as the pre-excitation syndrome, is an electrocardiographic diagnosis. The PR interval is short and the initial QRS forces rise or fall slowly (delta waves). In this entity myocardial tissue bridges the atrioventricular sulcus. Conduction is more rapid through the bridge than through the atrioventricular node and the ventricular myocardium adjacent to the bridge is depolarized prematurely, or 'pre-excited', shortening the PR interval and causing the delta waves. The chief clinical importance of the Wolff-Parkinson-White syndrome is in the frequent association of paroxysmal tachycardia.

Physical findings

Electrical pre-excitation may result in early mechanical events in the right or left ventricle, depending upon the distal insertion of the myocardial bridge. In type B Wolff-Parkinson-White syndrome the right ventricle depolarizes early and pulmonic valve closure may precede aortic, resulting in paradoxic splitting of the second heart sound

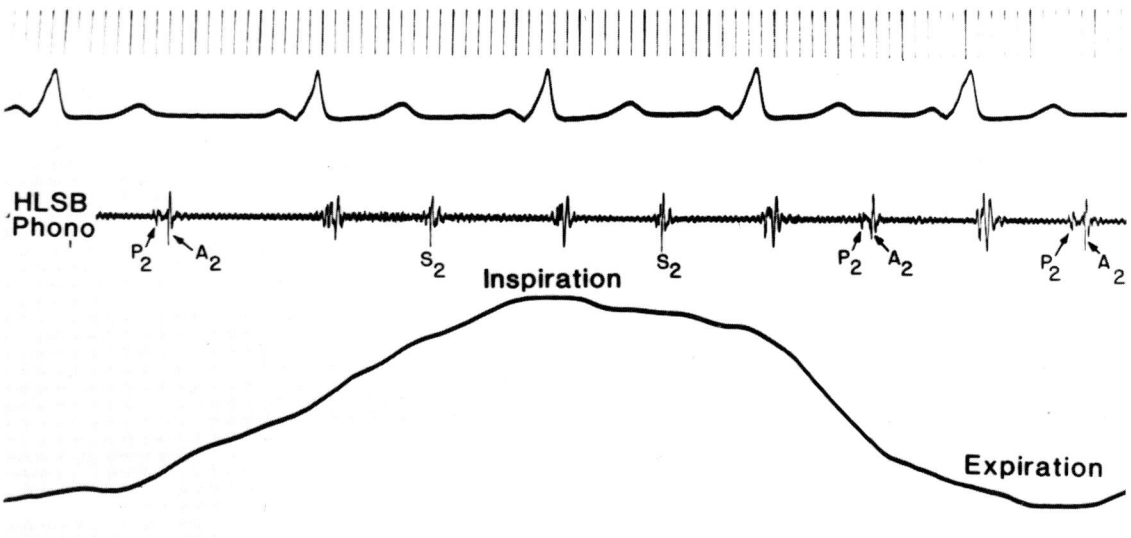

Fig. 24.3 Type B Wolff-Parkinson-White Syndrome. The second heart sound is single during inspiration and splits with expiration (paradoxic splitting).

(Fig. 24.3) (Zuberbuhler & Bauersfeld, 1965). (Paradoxic splitting occurs when pulmonic valve closure precedes aortic; it matters not at all whether the sequence is due to an early pulmonic or to a tardy aortic closure, although the latter is much more common.) Type A Wolff-Parkinson-White syndrome usually results in early depolarization of the left ventricle, although the wide splitting of the second sound which should occur if the aortic closure sound were early has not been noted.

REFERENCES

Burggraf G W, Craige E 1974 The first heart sound in complete heart block. Circulation 50:17

Gray I R 1956 Paradoxic splitting of the second heart sound. British Heart Journal 18:21

Lenox C C, Zuberbuhler J R, Park S C, Neches W H, Mathews R A, Zoltun R A 1978 Arrhythmias and Stokes-Adams attacks in acute rheumatic fever. Pediatrics 61:559

Wolferth C C, Margolies A, 1930 The influence of auricular contraction on the first heart sound and the radial pulse. Archives of Internal Medicine 46:1048

Zuberbuhler J R, Bauersfeld S R 1965 Paradoxic splitting of the second heart sound in the Wolff-Parkinson-White syndrome. American Heart Journal 70:595

Miscellaneous anomalies

COR TRIATRIATUM

The anomaly

Cor triatriatum is a very rare congenital cardiac anomaly in which the left atrium is partitioned by a diaphragm. The proximal portion receives the pulmonary veins; the distal portion includes the left atrial appendage and communicates with the left ventricle through the mitral orifice.

Clinical course

The size of the perforation in the dividing membrane is the most important anatomic variable and largely determines the clinical course. If the orifice is large, the anomaly is a trivial one and is usually diagnosed only at autopsy. There may be only exertional dyspnea if the obstruction is relatively mild but if it is severe tachypnea, dyspnea and pulmonary edema appear in early infancy. The clinical course may be modified by the presence of alternate exits from the proximal chamber, such as a defect in the interatrial septum or an anomalous venous channel leading from the proximal chamber to a systemic vein (Brickman et al, 1970).

Physical findings

General

Abnormal physical findings are largely due to pulmonary venous hypertension and/or secondary pulmonary hypertension. There is usually no cyanosis, unless severe pulmonary venous congestion prevents adequate oxygenation of pulmonary capillary blood. Tachypnea, respiratory distress and, occasionally, the rales of pulmonary edema occur in patients with severe obstruction. In one reported case there was a prolonged febrile course due to repeated intrapulmonary hemorrhages (Brickman et al, 1970).

Arterial and jugular venous pulses are normal. There may be a prominent left parasternal lift if there is pulmonary hypertension. The apical impulse is inconspicuous.

Auscultation

The most consistent auscultatory finding is a loud pulmonic valve closure sound, and on occasion this may be the only abnormal physical finding (Brickman et al, 1970). A variety of murmurs have been reported, including those of pulmonic and tricuspid regurgitation secondary to pulmonary hypertension. Continuous, as well as diastolic murmurs, have been thought to originate at a restrictive perforation in the membrane (Jegier et al, 1963). In one of our cases a high left sternal border continuous murmur was generated in the left superior vena cava, which connected the proximal chamber to the left innominate vein and served as an alternate exit from the proximal chamber. The murmur disappeared following resection of the membrane and ligation of the left superior vena cava (Brickman et al, 1970).

It is not possible to make a firm clinical diagnosis of cor triatraiatum but the entity should be suspected in any patient with unexplained pulmonary venous congestion and/or pulmonary hypertension.

PULMONARY VEIN STENOSIS

The anomaly

Pulmonary vein stenosis is a very rare anomaly and

in our experience the obstruction has most often been at the junction of a pulmonary vein and the left atrium.

Course and physical findings

The hemodynamic consequence of pulmonary vein stenosis is an elevation in pulmonary venous pressure, often with a secondary increase in pulmonary arterial pressure. Only one of our patients with pulmonary vein stenosis had physical findings other than those attributable to pulmonary hypertension. The lone exception was a 2-year-old girl with an ostium primum atrial septal defect, severe pulmonary hypertension and bilateral pulmonary vein stenosis. The vein stenoses were severe and produced a 20 mmHg gradient between the pulmonary arterial wedge pressure and the left atrial pressure. A faint continuous murmur was heard at the mid and low right sternal border and was recorded in the left atrium near the orifice of one of the stenosed pulmonary veins. The murmur disappeared when the micromanometer tipped catheter was withdrawn to the right atrium (Fig. 25.1).

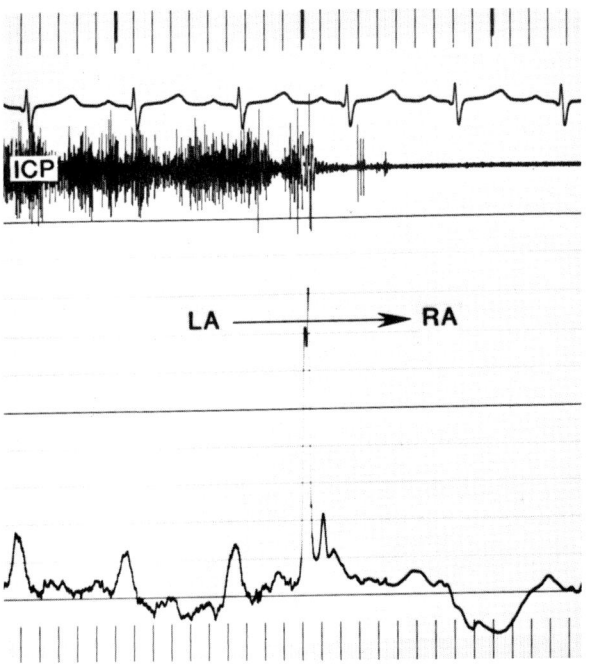

Fig. 25.1 Child with severe bilateral pulmonary vein stenosis. A loud continuous murmur is present in the left but not the right atrium (ICP).

SINUS OF VALSALVA ANEURYSM

The anomaly

A sinus of Valsalva aneurysm is a very uncommon cardiac anomaly. It develops as a finger-like pouch from an area of weakness at the junction of the aortic media and the annulus fibrosis (Edwards & Burchell, 1956). Aneurysms most commonly involve the right coronary or the non-coronary sinus. If the right coronary sinus is involved, the aneurysm may extend into either the right atrium or right ventricle, while non-coronary sinus aneurysms protrude into the right atrium (Sakakibara & Konno, 1962). Unruptured sinus of Valsalva aneurysms are rarely diagnosed pre-mortem, since they usually cause no abnormal signs or symptoms. Occasionally, an unruptured aneurysm distorts the aortic valve and produces aortic regurgitation (London & London, 1961), or interferes with the tricuspid valve and causes tricuspid regurgitation. Unruptured aneurysms also may protrude into the right ventricular outflow tract and cause subpulmonic stenosis (Bulkley et al, 1975).

Clinical course

Aneurysms rarely rupture before adolescence and the diagnosis is rarely made in infancy or childhood (Ainger & Pate, 1963). The actual rupture may be marked by sudden retrosternal chest pain and dyspnea, and patients sometimes describe a sudden 'tearing sensation' or become aware of a 'purring' in the chest. Rupture results in an aortic root runoff, the magnitude of the run-off depending on the size of the tear in the aneurysm. After rupture the clinical course is determined not only by the magnitude of the aortic run-off but also by the rapidity of its development. If a large run-off develops suddenly, congestive heart failure almost invariably ensues. Symptoms may subside after the acute episode, but congestive heart failure usually eventually recurs. A small rupture — or a large one that has developed slowly — may produce no symptoms for many years.

Physical findings

General

The general physical examination is normal, as is

the jugular venous pulse. The magnitude of arterial pulses is quite variable, depending on the size of the rupture. With a large perforation bounding arterial pulses, a capillary pulse, a pistol shot sound over the peripheral arteries and a Duroziez sign may all be present. The apical impulse is active and a left parasternal lift is expected with a large aneurysm, since both right and left ventricles are volume overloaded. The ventricular lift may be especially prominent if large pulmonary blood flow has caused an elevation of right ventricular pressure.

Auscultation

A continuous murmur is the most characteristic physical finding in a patient with a ruptured sinus of Valsalva aneurysm. The location of the murmur is related to the site of rupture. If the rupture is into the right atrium, the continuous murmur may be louder to the right or left of the sternum. If the aneurysm ruptures into the right ventricular inflow area, the continuous murmur is loudest at the mid or low left sternal border, while rupture into the right ventricular outflow tract produces a continuous murmur which is maximal at the high left sternal border (Perloff, 1978). The continuous murmur may be louder in systole or diastole but usually does not peak around the second heart sound, as does the typical murmur of a patent ductus arteriosus. Murmurs which occur before perforation are those of valve distortion or outflow tract obstruction caused by the aneurysm itself. Heart sounds are unremarkable.

Differential diagnosis

The differential diagnosis of a ruptured sinus of Valsalva aneurysm is that of a continuous murmur and peripheral signs of an aortic run-off. A diagnosis of a ruptured aneurysm must be considered when a continuous murmur appears suddenly, with or without chest pain or congestive heart failure. (It must be noted that even with an apparently new continuous murmur, a patent ductus arteriosus is still more likely than a ruptured sinus of Valsalva aneurysm. The author has examined several older children, cared for by competent pediatricians, who were referred because of the apparently sudden appearance of a continuous murmur but who were found at cardiac catheterization to have a typical patent ductus arteriosus.) Other diagnoses which must be considered in the differential are a ventricular septal defect with aortic regurgitation and a coronary-cardiac fistula.

TRUNCUS ARTERIOSUS

The anomaly

The terms truncus arteriosus, persistent truncus arteriosus and truncus arteriosus communis are synonymous. All refer to the presumed embryologic origin of this entity, i.e. lack of septation and division of the truncus arteriosus into aorta and pulmonary artery. Consonant with this concept is the definition of truncus arteriosus as a single artery arising from the heart, from which arise the aorta, pulmonary artery and coronary arteries. There is always a coexisting ventricular septal defect, which the truncus overrides. Except for a right aortic arch, other congenital anomalies are uncommon and truncus arteriosus usually exists as an 'isolated' anomaly.

Several classifications have been advanced. Probably the most widely known is that of Collett & Edwards (1949), which describes four types of truncus. In Type 1 a common pulmonary trunk arises from the base of the truncus and gives rise to the right and left pulmonary arteries (Fig. 25.2). In Type 2 the right and left pulmonary arteries arise close together from the posterior wall of the truncus, and in Type 3 the right and left pulmonary arteries arise from the sides of the truncus. Type 4 refers to an anomaly in which there are no true proximal pulmonary arteries, pulmonary blood supply being via systemic-pulmonary collateral arteries. This latter entity has been termed a 'solitary aortic trunk' and is considered in Chapter 18 as a variety of tetralogy of Fallot with pulmonary atresia.

Clinical course

The clinical course of a patient with persistent truncus arteriosus is largely determined by the magnitude of pulmonary blood flow. Pulmonary

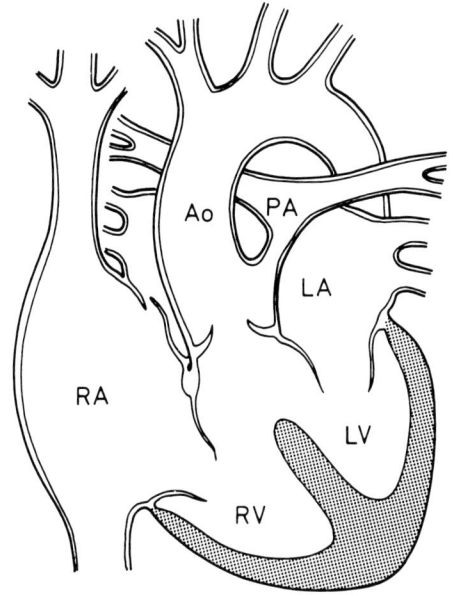

Fig. 25.2 Diagram of Type I truncus arteriosus.

flow depends, in turn, upon the size of the pulmonary arteries, the presence of pulmonary artery stenosis and the level of pulmonary vascular resistance. If pulmonary arteries are large and unobstructed, congestive heart failure occurs when pulmonary resistance falls during the first or second month of life. In such patients cyanosis is usually mild or even absent but tachypnea, poor feeding and slow growth are evident. Most of these infants die within the first year of life unless surgical intervention is successful (Marcelletti et al, 1976). Truncal valve stenosis occurs but is rare (Lee et al, 1973). On the other hand, truncal valve insufficiency is occasionally present and may be severe, adding to the already considerable hemodynamic burden of high pulmonary blood flow (Gelband et al, 1972). In the occasional infants with large pulmonary blood flow who survive infancy, pulmonary vascular resistance eventually rises, reducing pulmonary blood flow and increasing cyanosis. The total workload of the heart decreases, at least temporarily, and there may be a period of relative well-being until rising pulmonary vascular resistance further reduces pulmonary blood flow and produces marked arterial unsaturation and intense cyanosis. In an occasional case of truncus arteriosus one pulmonary artery is absent. If the remaining pulmonary artery is not stenotic, high pulmonary vascular resistance tends to develop unusually rapidly and irreversible pulmonary vascular disease is an inevitable consequence.

There is less pulmonary blood flow in individuals with relatively hypoplastic pulmonary arteries or with localized pulmonary artery stenosis. In such patients cyanosis is more intense, since there is, in general, an inverse relationship between pulmonary blood flow and the degree of arterial unsaturation. With an 'ideal' degree of pulmonary artery stenosis, pulmonary blood flow is high enough to prevent marked cyanosis, yet not so high as to lead to congestive heart failure. Relatively long survival is possible under these unusual circumstances.

Physical findings

General

The physical examination is also influenced by the magnitude of pulmonary blood flow. If flow is very large the infant will have the tachypnea and hepatomegaly of congestive heart failure and will be underweight if congestive heart failure is chronic. An infant with decreased pulmonary blood flow is not likely to be in heart failure but will be intensely cyanotic.

If total pulmonary vascular resistance is low, there will be a large diastolic run-off from the truncus, causing brisk or even bounding peripheral pulses and a corresponding increase in measured pulse pressure. The apical impulse is usually active since large pulmonary blood flow implies a volume overload of the left ventricle. There may or may not be a left parasternal lift. The jugular venous pulse is normal.

Auscultation

Heart sounds. The first heart sound is normal and the second heart sound is usually loud and single at the high left sternal border. The loudness of the second sound is explained by the proximity of the truncal valve to the anterior chest wall. The truncal valve closure sound may be prolonged and very rarely two components may be heard and demonstrated phonocardiographically, presumably because of asynchronous closure of different cusps of the truncal valve. A third heart sound is common in cases with increased pulmonary blood flow.

An early systolic ejection sound is one of the most consistent and useful auscultatory signs of persistent truncus arteriosus, and may emanate from the truncal valve or from the dilated truncus itself. It may be maximal at the apex or at the low left sternal border and does not vary with respiration.

Murmurs. A variety of murmurs may occur in patients with truncus arteriosus. Perhaps the most common is a mid and high left sternal border diamond-shaped systolic murmur caused by increased flow across the truncal valve (rarely to actual truncal valve stenosis). In some cases the systolic murmur is loud and maximal at the low left sternal border, closely simulating the murmur of a ventricular septal defect. A high pitched decrescendo diastolic murmur along the left sternal border signals the presence of truncal valve regurgitation. This murmur begins with the second heart sound and extends a variable distance into diastole. A rumbling apical diastolic murmur of relative mitral stenosis is often present in cases with increased pulmonary blood flow. If there is also a prominent low left sternal border systolic murmur, the auscultatory resemblance to a large ventricular septal defect is considerable. The early systolic ejection sound and bounding peripheral pulses which are characteristic of truncus arteriosus are useful differential features.

A continuous murmur is not common in truncus arteriosus, being especially rare in Type 1. Pulmonary artery stenosis occasionally generates a continuous murmur in Types 2 or 3.

Summary

In summary, truncus arteriosus is an anomaly in which a single arterial trunk gives rise to the pulmonary arteries, the aorta and the coronary arteries. The clinical course is determined by the level of pulmonary blood flow; very large flow inducing congestive heart failure in early infancy and restricted flow causing intense cyanosis. Important physical findings include an early systolic ejection sound, increased arterial pulses, and a variety of murmurs including a left sternal border systolic murmur, a decrescendo diastolic murmur of truncal regurgitation, an apical diastolic rumble of relative mitral stenosis and, rarely, a continuous murmur generated by pulmonary artery stenosis.

CARDIAC NEOPLASMS

Cardiac neoplasms are uncommon at any age but are especially rare in childhood. When they occur they may be intramural or intracavitary.

ATRIAL MYXOMA

Clinical course

The most common intracavitary tumor is the myxoma, a pedunculated growth which most commonly arises from the atrial septum near the fossa ovalis. It extends into the left atrium in 75 percent of cases and into the right atrium in the remainder. Myxomas may cause difficulty either by embolizing or by obstructing blood flow into or out of an atrium. The first sign of an atrial tumor may be sudden unexpected embolic occlusion of an artery supplying a limb or the brain or a diffuse shower of emboli to muscles or skin, rarely simulating polyarteritis nodosa. If the tumor is in the right atrium, the first sign may be the appearance of congestive heart failure, with hepatomegaly, jugular venous distention and peripheral edema. If it is in the left atrium, presentation may be with dyspnea and pulmonary edema. The onset of congestive failure may be gradual or abrupt and dramatic. An unreported 10-year-old patient from our institution was well until he developed severe dyspnea the day before admission. On admission, he had generalized pulmonary rales but no murmur could be heard. Chest roentgenograms showed an extensive patchy infiltrate that was interpreted as pneumonia. Death occurred ten hours after admission and at autopsy a myxoma was found to nearly fill the left atrial cavity. Another 10-year-old boy, reported by Neches et al (1974), developed signs and symptoms of an upper respiratory tract infection a week before admission. Exertional dyspnea and orthopnea appeared and became increasingly severe. On admission to hospital tachycardia, tachypnea and mild respiratory distress were present. The presence of an apical systolic murmur and cardiac enlargement and pulmonary venous congestion on chest roentgenogram led to a tentative diagnosis of acute rheumatic fever with mitral regurgitation. Complete clearing of the chest roentgenogram and abatement of dyspnea with a single dose of a diuretic was inconsistent with this diagnosis and led to cardiac catheterization. A large left atrial myxoma was demonstrated and was subsequently successfully removed surgically.

Physical findings

Growth and development are usually normal in a patient with an atrial myxoma, since the tumor produces few hemodynamic effects until embolization occurs or until it becomes large enough to obstruct an atrioventricular valve orifice. If embolization occurs before the tumor reaches a critical size, abnormal physical findings may be limited to those caused by sudden occlusion of a peripheral artery or an artery supplying the brain. Nonembolic consequences of an atrial myxoma depend upon the site of the tumor. With the more common left atrial variety the most important differential diagnosis is rheumatic heart disease with mitral valve involvement. There may be considerable resemblance to mitral stenosis, with an apical diastolic murmur, a loud pulmonic closure sound and a right ventricular lift suggestive of pulmonary hypertension. In other patients there is an apical pansystolic murmur of mitral regurgitation, with or without signs of pulmonary hypertension. If the myxoma is within the right atrium signs include peripheral edema, distended neck veins, hepatomegaly and a murmur of tricuspid regurgitation or of tricuspid stenosis. The differential diagnosis of right atrial myxoma includes chronic constrictive pericarditis, cardiomyopathy and tricuspid stenosis. (The absence of signs of mitral valve disease practically rules out rheumatic tricuspid stenosis.) In a patient with a left atrial myxoma there may be less dyspnea in one position than another, indicating variable severity of mitral orifice obstruction by the pedunculated tumor. The variability of the murmurs associated with atrial myxomas, especially with change in position, should be stressed.

A low pitched early diastolic sound may be present in a patient with either a right or left atrial myxoma (Nasser et al, 1972). The sound is usually loudest at the apex and has the same timing as a third heart sound. It has been referred to as a 'tumor plop' and is presumably generated as the tumor reaches the end of its tether and its motion is suddenly checked during early diastole (Pitt et al, 1967). A loud protodiastolic sound in a patient suspected of having tight mitral stenosis should suggest a myxoma, since an apical gallop is not an expected finding in a patient with significant mitral obstruction.

Summary

In summary, an atrial myxoma is a potentially disabling or even fatal intracardiac tumor which is curable if diagnosed. It should be considered in any patient with sudden unexplained arterial occlusion or with what seems to be atypical tricuspid or mitral valve disease. Fortunately, echocardiography has proven to be a very reliable means of screening for left atrial myxoma.

INTRAMURAL TUMORS

Fibroma and rhabdomyoma are the two most common intramural tumors. Rhabdomyomata are usually associated with tuberous sclerosis. Intramural tumors may be silent, producing no signs or symptoms, or may cause obstruction, most commonly subaortic or subpulmonic stenosis, but occasionally tricuspid or mitral stenosis. Congestive heart failure may result if there is extensive myocardial involvement. Arrhythmias may also occur.

UHL'S ANOMALY

Uhl's anomaly, or parchment right ventricle as it is sometimes called, is characterized anatomically by deficiency of right ventricular myocardium (Uhl, 1952). If the process is patchy it may be of no clinical or hemodynamic significance and be discovered only at post mortem examination (Gould et al, 1967). If the lack of right ventricular myocardium is generalized, the major hemodynamic consequence is lack of right ventricular mechanical systole, the right ventricle functioning as a capacious conduit. Congestive heart failure may be evident in early childhood but in some cases symptoms are surprisingly mild even into early adult life.

Cyanosis occurs if there is right to left shunting across a patent foramen ovale. The precordium is quiet and arterial pulses are normal unless there is frank congestive heart failure. Large 'A' waves may be present in the jugular venous pulse. The most striking auscultatory finding is the softness of the heart sounds. Since right atrial, right ventricular and pulmonary artery pressure tracings are nearly identical one would not expect audible tricuspid or pulmonic components of the first and second heart sounds, respectively. The mitral and aortic components are soft because of the large right ventricle interposed between the source of the sound and the chest wall (Zuberbuhler & Blank, 1970). Third and fourth heart sounds are not present and there is no murmur.

UNIVENTRICULAR HEART

The anomaly

The term 'univentricular heart' will be used to describe the spectrum of anomalies to be discussed here. (The alternative terms 'single ventricle', 'common ventricle' and 'double inlet left ventricle' are confusing because they are used differently by different authors.) Univentricular hearts have one feature in common: the atrioventricular valves have no dividing interventricular septum between them and connect to the same ventricular chamber. This definition leaves wide latitude for variation in ventricular chamber morphology, ventricular outflow arrangement and associated anomalies.

With outlet chamber

Two major types of univentricular hearts will be considered. In the most common variety both right and left atrioventricular valves (or a common atrioventricular valve) connect to a large ventricular chamber which anatomically approximates a left ventricle. This 'left' ventricle supports one great artery directly (usually the pulmonary artery), and communicates through the bulbo-ventricular foramen with an outflow chamber, which supports the other great artery (usually the aorta). This outlet chamber anatomically approximates the outlet portion of the right ventricle. Since the outlet chamber is most commonly located to the left of the main chamber, and since it usually supports the aorta, the great artery relationship is similar to that in 'corrected' transposition (Fig. 25.3).

Without outlet chamber

The other important but far less common variety of univentricular heart can be thought of as an exceptionally large ventricular septal defect. More or less complete right and left ventricular zones exist but are separated by only a rim of septum — or not at all (Fig. 25.4). Pulmonic stenosis is the most important anatomic variable in either variety of univentricular heart, since its presence or absence largely determines the clinical course.

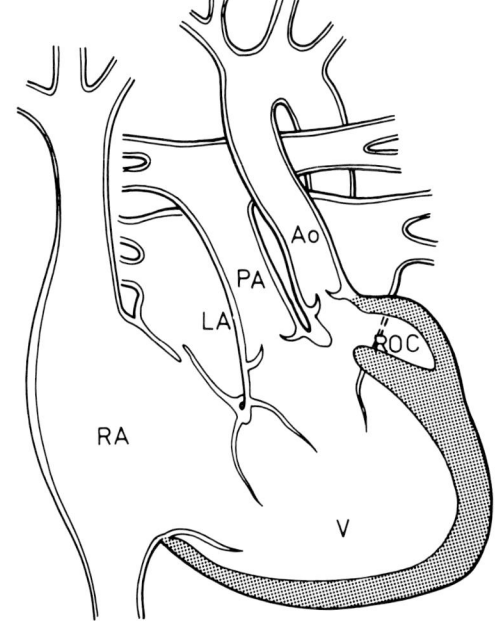

Fig. 25.3 Diagram of univentricular heart with outlet chamber (ROC) and ventriculo-arterial discordance.

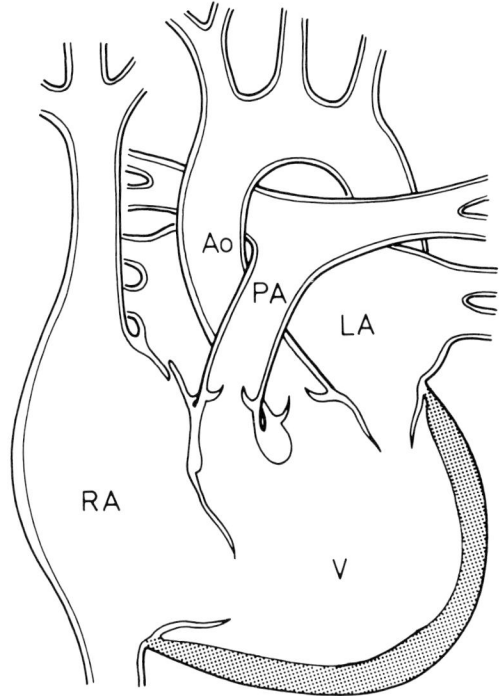

Fig. 25.4 Diagram of univentricular heart without outlet chamber.

Clinical course

Univentricular heart is one of the least clinically 'diagnosable' varieties of congenital heart disease. The clinical picture ranges from the desperately ill newborn who is either intensely cyanotic or in intractable congestive heart failure to the mildly cyanotic and nearly asymptomatic young adult (rare). The most important anatomic determinant of the clinical course is pulmonic stenosis. If there is no stenosis, congestive heart failure occurs in early infancy as pulmonary vascular resistance falls and permits very large pulmonary blood flow. If pulmonic stenosis is severe, pulmonary blood flow is quite limited and cyanosis is intense. If there is pulmonary atresia, pulmonary blood flow will be dependent upon patency of the ductus arteriosus, since sizable systemic-pulmonary collateral arteries are uncommon with univentricular heart. As in all ductus dependent anomalies, newborns with univentricular heart and pulmonary atresia are intensely cyanotic and unstable, succumbing quickly unless a systemic-pulmonary shunt can be surgically established. If there is an 'ideal' degree of pulmonic stenosis — enough to prevent excessive pulmonary blood flow and congestive heart failure but not enough to severely limit pulmonary flow and cause intense cyanosis — the clinical course may be relatively benign, with few symptoms and only mild cyanosis for several years. Although squatting or hypercyanotic spells may occur in patients with univentricular heart and pulmonic stenosis (Marin-Garcia et al, 1974), they are much less common than with tetralogy of Fallot. Atrioventricular valve insufficiency may eventually develop and the resulting atrial dilatation contributes to the development of atrial arrhythmias, especially atrial fibrillation. Ventricular arrhythmias may appear in late childhood or adolescence and may be the cause of death. Angina has been reported in patients with associated subaortic stenosis (Somerville et al, 1974) and infectious endocarditis and brain abscess are occasional complications. Even in patients with relatively favorable anatomy, survival is rarely beyond the second or third decade.

Physical findings

With the exception of cyanosis there are no physical findings directly attributable to 'univentricular heart', and even cyanosis is dependent upon the degree of associated pulmonic stenosis or pulmonary vascular disease. It may even be inapparent if pulmonary stenosis is mild or absent and pulmonary blood flow large. Congestive heart failure is also related to the degree of pulmonic stenosis (or, more precisely, to the lack of it). The jugular venous pulse is not remarkable unless there is severe tricuspid regurgitation and arterial pulses and blood pressure are normal unless there is an associated coarctation of the aorta. There is often a precordial bulge, especially if there is little or no pulmonic stenosis. Precordial motion is variable, the apical impulse tending to be normal if there is pulmonic stenosis and active if there is large pulmonary blood flow. The second heart sound may be single, especially if pulmonic stenosis is quite severe or if there is marked pulmonary hypertension. (Since the aortic valve usually underlies the high left sternal border a loud single second heart sound is not evidence of pulmonary hypertension, nor is a palpable systolic impulse in that area.) The second sound may be split if there is mild pulmonic stenosis. A third heart sound is common if there is increased pulmonary blood flow. Since pulmonic stenosis is usually subvalvar a pulmonic early systolic ejection sound is not common.

A variety of murmurs may be present in patients with univentricular heart. A systolic murmur of pulmonic stenosis is most common and is usually maximal along the mid or high left sternal border. It is crescendo-decrescendo and, as in patients with tetralogy of Fallot, the intensity and duration of the murmur tend to vary inversely with the severity of the obstruction, being loud and relatively long with moderate pulmonic stenosis and short and soft when pulmonary stenosis is very severe. A low left sternal border pansystolic murmur may signal the presence of tricuspid regurgitation and an apical systolic murmur suggests mitral regurgitation, although the murmur of pulmonic stenosis may be well heard anywhere along the left sternal border and even at the apex. The mid diastolic apical rumble of relative mitral stenosis is common if there is markedly increased pulmonary blood flow. Aortic regurgitation is rare with univentricular heart but hypertensive pulmonic regurgitation generates a similar high pitched decrescendo diastolic murmur along the left sternal border. The continuous murmur of a patent ductus arteriosus may be present in a newborn with univentricular heart and pulmonary atresia and is usually soft and high pitched.

REFERENCES

Ainger L E, Pate J W 1963 Rupture of a sinus of Valsalva aneurysm in an infant. American Journal of Cardiology 11 : 547

Brickman R D, Wilson L, Zuberbuhler J R, Bahnson H T 1970 Cor triatriatum: clinical presentation and operative treatment. Journal of Thoracic and Cardiovascular Survey 60 : 523

Bulkley B H, Hutchins G M, Ross R S 1975 Aortic sinus of Valsalva aneurysms simulating primary right-sided valvular heart disease. Circulation 52 : 696

Collett R W, Edwards J E 1949 Persistent truncus arteriosus: a classification according to anatomic types. Surgical Clinics of North America 29 : 1245

Edwards J E, Burchell H B 1956 Specimen exhibiting the essential lesion in aneurysm of the aortic sinus. Proceedings of the Staff Meetings of the Mayo Clinic 31 : 407

Gelband H, Van Meter S, Gersony W M 1972 Truncal valve abnormalities in infants with persistent truncus arteriosus. Circulation 45 : 397

Gould L, Guttman B, Carrasco J, Lyon A F 1967 Partial absence of right ventricular musculature. American Journal of Medicine 42 : 636

Jegier W, Gibbons J E, Wiglesworth F W 1963 Cor Triatriatum: clinical, hemodynamic and pathological studies: surgical correction in early life. Pediatrics 31 : 255

Lee M H, Bellon E M, Liebman J, Perrin E V 1973 Truncal valve stenosis. American Heart Journal 85 : 397

London S B, London R E 1961 Production of aortic regurgitation by unperforated aneurysm of the sinus of Valsalva. Circulation 24 : 1403

Marcelletti C, McGoon D C, Mair D D 1976 The natural history of truncus arteriosus. Circulation 54 : 108

Marin-Garcia J, Tandon R, Moller J H, Edwards J E 1974 Single ventricle with transposition. Circulation 49 : 994

Nasser W K, Davis R H, Dillon J C, Tavel M E, Helman C H, Feigenbaum H, Fisch C 1972 Atrial myxoma. American Heart Journal 83 : 810

Neches W H, Park S C, Lenox C C, Zuberbuhler J R, Siewers R D 1974 Left atrial myxoma: clinical presentation suggesting acute myocarditis. Journal of the American Medical Association 229 : 1906

Perloff J K 1978 The clinical recognition of congenital heart disease, 2nd edn. Saunders, Philadelphia, p 596

Pitt A, Pitt B, Schaefer J, Criley J M 1967 Myxoma of the left atrium — hemodynamic and phonocardiographic consequences of sudden tumor movement. Circulation 36 : 408

Sakakibara S, Konno S 1962 Congenital aneurysm of the sinus of Valsalva. Anatomy and classification. American Heart Journal 63 : 405

Somerville J, Becu L, Ross D 1974 Common ventricle with acquired subaortic obstruction. American Journal of Cardiology 34 : 206

Uhl H S 1952 Previously undescribed congenital malformation of the heart: Almost total absence of myocardium of right ventricle. Bulletin Johns Hopkins Hospital 91 : 197

Zuberbuhler J R, Blank E 1970 Hypoplasia of right ventricular myocardium. American Journal of Roentgenology, Radium Therapy and Nuclear Medicine 110 : 491

Differential diagnosis

This chapter deals with three diagnostic problems in the field of children's heart disease. They include the cyanotic newborn, the infant with congestive heart failure and the asymptomatic child with a murmur. Not all children with murmurs and not even all children who are cyanotic or who are in congestive heart failure have heart disease, but many do. Sorting out cardiac from non-cardiac disease, arriving at a reasonable clinical diagnosis, and arranging for invasive study with the appropriate degree of alacrity are challenging problems faced by physicians who care for infants and children.

THE CYANOTIC NEWBORN

In the neonate, cyanosis is not always due to congenital heart disease. It may also be caused by depressed central nervous system respiratory drive, by pulmonary disease or be related to marked polycythemia. The differentiation of cardiac from non-cardiac cyanosis is of obvious importance and can usually be accomplished by non-invasive means. If cyanosis is thought to be of cardiac origin, cardiac catheterization is mandatory, but even so, clinical diagnosis is of considerable importance since the urgency of invasive study varies. An infant with tetralogy of Fallot and pulmonary atresia whose pulmonary circulation is via sizable systemic-pulmonary collateral arteries, for instance, is likely to be quite stable. On the other hand, a newborn with pulmonary atresia and pulmonary blood flow via a patent ductus arteriosus tends to be quite unstable and requires emergency cardiac catheterization and early surgery. In addition, cardiac catheterization is likely to be safer and more definitive if an accurate clinical diagnosis permits the selection of optimum hemodynamic and angiographic techniques. In this chapter the physical, electrocardiographic and roentgenographic findings which are of most help in differentiating cardiac from non-cardiac cyanosis and which are most useful in attempting a specific cardiac diagnosis will be reviewed. It must be emphasized that clinical examination and invasive study are complimentary portions of the overall evaluation of the cyanotic infant with congenital heart disease.

DIFFERENTIAL DIAGNOSIS

Central nervous system

Depression of the respiratory center is probably the most common cause of cyanosis in the newborn, and is most frequently caused by maternal oversedation during labor. If air exchange is improved by stimulating the infant or by assisting ventilation, the cause of the arterial unsaturation is removed and cyanosis disappears. Cyanosis which resolves promptly and completely with improved ventilation with room air is almost always on a central nervous system basis.

Pulmonary

There are a number of pulmonary problems which can cause cyanosis. Tracheobronchial obstruction, pneumothorax, pulmonary hypoplasia or atelectasis, diaphragmatic hernia and parenchymal abnormalities such as pneumonia, aspiration or hyaline membrane disease are examples. An inability to completely oxygenate blood passing through the lungs is common to each. It is usually possible to clinically differentiate pulmonary from cardiac causes of cyanosis, using information obtained from the physical examination, the chest roentgenogram, the electrocardiogram and the echocardiogram. In an occasional newborn, the differentiation can be made only at cardiac catheterization.

Physical examination

The physical examination may or may not be helpful in differentiating pulmonary from cardiac causes of cyanosis. The presence of a murmur, abnormal pulses or abnormal precordial motion may point to cardiac disease. An occasional infant with cyanotic congenital heart disease, however, has little on physical examination to suggest a cardiac etiology of his cyanosis. In such an infant the differential diagnosis may be quite difficult. Both the infant with cardiac cyanosis and one with pulmonary disease may be tachypneic or be in severe respiratory distress. Intercostal retraction is more common with pulmonary disease but can occur in the cardiac infant. Pulmonary rales are very rarely present in the newborn with a congenital cardiac anomaly and their presence is strong evidence for pulmonary disease. It must be noted that important pulmonary disease, even a pneumothorax or extensive consolidation, may not be evident on physical examination.

Chest roentgenogram

The chest roentgenogram may be very useful in differential diagnosis. A pulmonary etiology of the cyanosis may be obvious, especially if a pneumothorax, extensive consolidation, cystic disease or the air bronchogram and ground glass appearance of hyaline membrane disease are present. Alternatively, there may be roentgenographic evidence of congenital heart disease. A right aortic arch points to tetralogy of Fallot or to persistent truncus arteriosus; marked cardiac enlargement is more consonant with cardiac than pulmonary disease. The contour of the heart may also point to a cardiac anomaly; the concave left upper border of tetralogy of Fallot or the 'egg on a string' contour sometimes seen with transposition of the great arteries are examples. Increased or decreased pulmonary vascular markings also favor a diagnosis of cardiac disease.

Electrocardiogram

An electrocardiogram which shows the right axis deviation and right ventricular hypertrophy expected in the newborn period does not help in differentiating pulmonary from cardiac causes of cyanosis. But left ventricular predominance or an axis of less than 90 degrees or more than 210 degrees argues for the presence of a cardiac anomaly.

Oxygen administration

The administration of oxygen may be helpful in differential diagnosis. While cardiac cyanosis may lessen in oxygen, a dramatic change is not usual. In contrast, the cyanosis of pulmonary disease may disappear entirely. If an infant is placed in an oxygen rich environment, an arterial oxygen tension of more than 100 mmHg makes cyanotic congenital heart disease unlikely; a tension of more than 200 mmHg practically rules it out.

Echocardiogram

The echocardiogram is normal in neonates with pulmonary disease and may be either normal or abnormal with cardiac disease. An abnormal echocardiogram may suggest a cardiac anomaly capable of causing cyanosis, but a normal one is less conclusive. It certainly does not rule out cyanotic congenital heart disease.

Polycythemia

In the neonate, the rubor of marked polycythemia can simulate cyanosis and there may occasionally be actual arterial unsaturation due to right to left shunting through the foramen ovale. A hemoglobin of more than 20 g percent is suggestive.

Cardiac

Quite a large number of cardiovascular anomalies and combinations of anomalies can produce cyanosis, but these fall into only a few broad groups. One group includes patients with a combination of right heart obstruction and right to left shunting through a septal defect proximal to the obstruction. Examples include tetralogy of Fallot, tetralogy of Fallot with pulmonary atresia, pulmonary atresia or critical pulmonary stenosis with intact ventricular septum, and tricuspid atresia. A second group of patients is cyanotic because of an abnormal vascular connection; ventriculo-arterial discordance (complete transposition of the great arteries) or total anomalous pulmonary venous return. A third group of cyanotic neonates have severe left heart obstruction, most commonly either aortic or mitral atresia or an interrupted aortic arch.

Once a clinical diagnosis of cyanotic congenital heart disease is made or strongly suspected in a neonate, cardiac catheterization is almost always indicated. Since the urgency of invasive study varies in different entities, an accurate clinical diagnosis is important. Fortunately, cyanotic infants can usually be placed in one of the above groups on the basis of the clinical examination. The physical findings which, if present, are most likely to be useful include a high left sternal border systolic murmur, a low left sternal border systolic murmur, a continuous murmur, and abnormal pulses. The intensity of the second heart sound at the high left sternal border and its splitting or singularity are also very important. On electrocardiogram, the frontal plane axis and ventricular predominance are most useful. Pulmonary vascularity is probably the most important roentgenographic finding, although the estimation of vascular markings on chest roentgenogram has many pitfalls. Faulty radiographic technique may either over- or under-emphasize markings, and even with ideal technique there is considerable inter- and intra-observer variation. Nonetheless, vascular markings are quite helpful in subclassifying cyanotic congenital heart disease. Cardiac size and contour and sidedness of the aortic arch are other useful roentgenographic features.

Normal or decreased pulmonary vascular markings

Differential diagnosis. The newborn normally has less pulmonary vascular markings than the older child or adult. Consequently, it is easier to be sure of increased than decreased markings in this age group. With normal or decreased markings, right heart obstruction is the most likely cardiac etiology of cyanosis. Specific diagnostic possibilities include tetralogy of Fallot with or without pulmonary atresia, pulmonary atresia or critical pulmonic stenosis with an intact ventricular septum, Ebstein's anomaly of the tricuspid valve and persistent fetal circulation. (The latter is a heterogenous group of newborns with increased pulmonary vascular resistance and right to left shunting through a patent foramen ovale and/or a patent ductus arteriosus.)

Physical findings. In a cyanotic full term newborn with normal or decreased pulmonary vascular markings a continuous murmur at the high left sternal border implies the presence of pulmonary atresia. The atresia may be isolated or associated with a ventricular septal defect, transposition of the great arteries, or a univentricular heart. The continuous murmur originates in a patent ductus arteriosus or, less commonly, in systemic-pulmonary collateral arteries. (Collateral arteries are well heard over the posterior thorax while the murmur of a patent ductus is well localized to the high left sternal border and subclavicular area.) A high left sternal border systolic murmur in a cyanotic newborn implies incomplete right ventricular outflow tract obstruction, most commonly tetralogy of Fallot or isolated valvar pulmonic stenosis. A systolic murmur which is loudest at the low left sternal border most commonly indicates tricuspid regurgitation, since a ventricular septal defect is usually silent in patients with cyanotic congenital heart disease. (Complete transposition of the great arteries is a major exception to this rule.) The murmur of tricuspid regurgitation is most common in neonates with pulmonary atresia and intact ventricular septum or with a primary abnormality of the tricuspid valve such as Ebstein's anomaly. The second heart sound is rarely split in this group, since the pulmonic closure sound is inaudible in cyanotic patients with tetralogy of Fallot, critical pulmonic stenosis, or pulmonary atresia. Audible splitting occasionally occurs with persistent fetal circulation and may be present with Ebstein's anomaly.

A midline liver suggests situs ambiguous, and in the presence of decreased pulmonary vascular markings, dextro-isomerism (asplenia) is more likely than levo-isomerism (polysplenia). Cardiac anomalies are complex and usually include severe pulmonic stenosis or pulmonic atresia.

Electrocardiogram. Right axis deviation and right ventricular hypertrophy are the expected electrocardiographic findings in the neonate and are not helpful in differential diagnosis. Left ventricular preponderance with left axis deviation suggests a univentricular heart with or without tricuspid atresia. Left ventricular predominance with an axis greater than zero degrees is most consistent with pulmonic atresia and intact ventricular septum, but also occurs in an occasional newborn with critical pulmonic stenosis.

Chest roentgenogram. Cardiomegaly rules out a diagnosis of tetralogy of Fallot, while a right aortic arch argues strongly for a tetralogy or persistent truncus arteriosus. A concave left upper cardiac border also suggests tetralogy of Fallot with or without pulmonary atresia. Dextrocardia with visceral situs solitus (isolated dextrocardia) suggests a complex cardiac malformation.

Echocardiogram. The echocardiogram may be very useful in differential diagnosis. Helpful findings in this group include the large overriding aorta of tetralogy of Fallot, the diminutive right ventricle of pulmonary atresia and intact ventricular septum, the large right ventricle and tricuspid valve of Ebstein's anomaly and a common anterior leaflet which crosses the septum in a complete endocardial cushion defect. Contrast echocardiography may also be very useful in localizing the right to left shunt to atrial or ventricular level. The echocardiogram is normal in neonates with persistent fetal circulation.

Increased pulmonary vascular markings

Differential diagnosis. Most cyanotic newborns with increased pulmonary vascular markings have either an abnormal vascular connection (transposition of the great arteries, total anomalous venous return) or severe left heart obstruction (mitral or aortic atresia, interrupted aortic arch).

Physical findings. Pulses are normal in patients with transposition, anomalous venous return and mitral atresia, but are decreased or absent with aortic atresia. (Strikingly diminished pulses combined with the mottling and poor capillary filling of very low cardiac output make a diagnosis of aortic atresia very likely. Myocardial disease may also be accompanied by diminished pulses, poor cutaneous blood flow and congestive heart failure but, in contrast to aortic atresia, the right ventricular impulse is not increased.) Leg pulses may be decreased with an interrupted aortic arch, but may be equal to or even stronger than arm pulses if the ductus is widely patent. A split second heart sound rules out aortic atresia but may be heard with other entities in this group, being more common with mitral atresia and with total anomalous pulmonary venous return than with complete transposition of the great arteries. The intensity of cyanosis varies somewhat among the anomalies in this group, typically being most intense with transposition of the great arteries. It may also be striking in patients with total anomalous pulmonary venous connection if there is marked obstruction to pulmonary venous return. In patients with transposition there is often no murmur, while in total anomalous pulmonary venous return a soft systolic murmur is almost always present at the base and over the back. In addition, a continuous hum may be heard over the anomalous channel. A similar hum may accompany mitral atresia, being generated at a restrictive inter-atrial communication and being heard along the lower sternum. Respiratory variation of the hum of anomalous venous return or mitral atresia is useful in differentiating it from the continuous murmur of a patent ductus arteriosus or of systemic-pulmonary collateral arteries.

Electrocardiogram. The electrocardiogram is not particularly useful in differential diagnosis within this group, almost always showing right axis deviation and right ventricular hypertrophy.

Chest roentgenogram. The chest roentgenogram may show the characteristic but not particularly common 'egg on a string' contour of transposition. The 'snowman' contour of total anomalous pulmonary venous return to the left innominate vein is not usually present in the neonate, developing only over the first few weeks or months of life.

Echocardiogram. The echocardiogram may or may not be helpful in a cyanotic neonate with increased pulmonary vascular markings. It is most likely to be diagnostic with aortic atresia, particularly if a very small aorta and diminutive mitral valve are visualized. It may or may not be helpful with other entities in this group, including transposition of the great arteries and total anomalous pulmonary venous return.

Summary

In summary, cyanosis in the neonatal period may be cardiac but may also arise from central nervous system or pulmonary abnormalities or may be related to polycythemia. When congenital heart disease is suspected in a cyanotic neonate, clinical diagnosis is an important preliminary to cardiac catheterization. If transposition of the great arteries or a ductus dependent lesion is suspected, cardiac catheterization should be done as an emergency procedure.

CONGESTIVE HEART FAILURE IN INFANCY

In infants, the clinical picture of congestive heart failure is quite different from that expected in adults. In any age group, however, the manifestations of failure can be thought of as being due to elevation of right or left atrial pressure or to diminished cardiac output. In older children and adults the signs of elevated right atrial pressure include jugular venous distension, an enlarged liver and dependent edema. Of these, only hepatomegaly is commonly present in the infant with congestive heart failure. (Edema is rare except with profound failure, and when present tends to be generalized rather than dependent. Neck veins are difficult to see in infants and are not usually visibly distended with failure.) In adults, the signs of elevated left atrial pressure include tachypnea, respiratory distress and rales. Tachypnea is almost always present in the infant in failure and respiratory distress may be evident as well. Rales are uncommon. In any age group, signs of decreased cardiac output may be present, and include weak peripheral pulses, cold clammy skin and poor capillary filling. In summary, then, the infant in congestive heart failure has a large liver, breathes abnormally, and if the failure is sufficiently severe has evidence of low cardiac output.

In the neonate, congestive heart failure is usually due to cardiovascular disease. An important exception is the infant of a diabetic mother, who may have many of the signs of congestive heart failure in the absence of structural cardiac abnormality. The heart and liver are commonly large and pulmonary vascular markings may be increased on the chest roentgenogram. There may also be tachypnea. Since glucose is the sole substrate for myocardial metabolism in the newborn, and since it is commonly diminished in the infant of a diabetic mother, there may be diminished myocardial function as well as organomegaly. Signs of congestive heart failure may also be present in an infant with sepsis, although the picture of shock is more common. An uncommon degree of lethargy or some predisposition to sepsis such as premature rupture of membranes or a maternal febrile illness may point to the correct diagnosis.

A rather large number of cardiac anomalies and combinations of anomalies can cause congestive heart failure in infancy. Congestive heart failure and cyanosis often coexist, although one or the other may predominate. Whatever the etiology, management of the infant with congestive heart failure may be quite difficult. Failure is first treated with a digitalis preparation (usually digoxin) with or without diuretics, and cardiac catheterization is then usually advisable. (Although some infants can be maintained on anti-congestive therapy, recurrent failure is common. Obviously, cardiac catheterization is less hazardous if done when failure is under control.) Although the clinical evaluation rarely obviates the necessity for cardiac catheterization, it is still of considerable importance. There is need to be both selective and expeditious in the performance of the invasive study, since infants in this general category may be quite ill at the time of cardiac catheterization. Too much contrast medium, for instance, may aggravate the failure, and angiograms that are most likely to be diagnostic should be done first. A left heart catheterization may be difficult in this age group but is mandatory if the clinical evaluation points to a left heart anomaly. Some cardiac anomalies are rare and may not be identified during a 'routine' cardiac catheterization unless the clinical examination suggests their presence. An example of the latter is a large intracranial arteriovenous fistula. If the diagnosis is suspected clinically it can easily be confirmed at invasive study, and such clues as high oxygen saturation in the superior vena cava or uncommonly large carotid or vertebral arteries are unlikely to go unnoticed.

In this section an exhaustive treatment of differential diagnosis by noninvasive means will not be attempted, but certain physical, roentgenographic and electrocardiographic findings which are often helpful in differential diagnosis will be discussed.

Physical findings

Pulses

The quality of the peripheral pulses is perhaps the single most helpful physical finding in differential diagnosis of the infant with congestive heart failure.

Decreased. Diminished peripheral pulses are expected in the presence of congestive failure. They are most consistently and profoundly depressed if there is aortic atresia. In this entity the entire systemic output is via the pulmonary artery and a patent ductus arteriosus; although pulses may be normal shortly after birth, they weaken and disappear as the ductus closes. Pulses are also generally diminished with critical aortic stenosis and with severe myocardial disease. Pulses tend to be normal in infants with transposition of the great arteries, total anomalous pulmonary venous return or ventricular septal defect until the infant is in extremis. The asymmetrical pulses of coarctation are diagnostic.

Increased. In the presence of congestive heart failure, an increase in the amplitude of peripheral pulses suggests a decrease in total systemic resistance. A patent ductus arteriosus is the most common cause of low systemic resistance, but a persistent truncus arteriosus must also be considered. It is suggested by an early systolic ejection sound or by a right aortic arch on chest roentgenogram. A large systemic arteriovenous fistula, another source of low systemic resistance, may also cause congestive heart failure in early infancy. The diagnosis should be considered if increased pulses and congestive heart failure coincide in an infant. The head is the most common site of such a fistula and a continuous bruit over the cranium should always be sought.

Regurgitation of blood from the aorta to the left ventricle may cause congestive heart failure in infancy and here, also, pulses are increased. Isolated severe aortic regurgitation is exceedingly rare in this age group. An aortico-left ventricular tunnel is an equally rare anomaly which may simulate aortic regurgitation. It is important because it is potentially correctable, even in early infancy. In the clinical setting of congestive failure and increased peripheral pulses, a to and fro murmur along the left sternal border suggests the diagnosis. Differentiation from persistent truncus arteriosus with truncal regurgitation is angiographic.

Blood pressure

Blood pressure determination in both arms and legs is mandatory in an infant with congestive heart failure. Asymmetry points to coarctation of the aorta. Systemic hypertension not due to coarctation of the aorta but severe enough to produce heart failure is rare, but may be caused by renal artery stenosis.

Murmurs

A systolic murmur, depending on its location, may suggest left or right ventricular outflow tract obstruction, a ventricular septal defect, or tricuspid or mitral regurgitation. With mitral regurgitation or a ventricular shunt large enough to cause congestive heart failure, an apical mid diastolic murmur of relative mitral stenosis is expected. A mid diastolic murmur at the low left sternal border, on the other hand, suggests relative tricuspid stenosis and occurs with total anomalous pulmonary venous return or with any very large left to right shunt at atrial level. A to and fro murmur along the left sternal border may emanate from tricuspid regurgitation and relative tricuspid stenosis, from an aortico-left ventricular tunnel, or from an absent pulmonic valve. In the latter entity pulses are normal; the diagnosis is suggested by hugely dilated proximal right and left pulmonary arteries on the chest roentgenogram.

A continuous murmur at the left base most commonly indicates a patent ductus arteriosus. Other continuous murmurs which may be heard in an infant in congestive failure include the hum occasionally heard over the anomalous channel in an infant with total anomalous pulmonary venous return, the murmur of a restrictive interatrial septal defect in an infant with mitral atresia, and the murmur arising in large systemic-pulmonary collateral arteries.

Chest roentgenogram

Cardiomegaly is expected on the chest roentgenogram of an infant with congestive heart failure. It is quite unusual, in fact, for congestive failure to be present without considerable cardiac enlargement. Exceptions to this general rule include infants with total anomalous pulmonary venous return with severe obstruction, infants with paroxysmal supraventricular tachycardia, or those with mitral stenosis. In each of these entities congestive heart failure may occur without cardiomegaly.

Pulmonary vascular markings are usually increased in infants with congestive failure and it is sometimes possible to differentiate pulmonary venous from pulmonary arterial plethora. Increased arterial markings are characteristic of left to right shunts in general, of transposition of the great arteries, and of total anomalous pulmonary venous return without obstruction. Increased pulmonary venous markings, on the other hand, are expected with total anomalous pulmonary venous return with obstruction and with left ventricular inlet obstruction such as cor triatriatum, mitral stenosis or atresia, or pulmonary vein stenosis. If pulmonary vascular markings are decreased, severe right ventricular outflow tract obstruction with intact ventricular septum (critical pulmonic stenosis, pulmonary atresia) or Ebstein's anomaly of the tricuspid valve should be considered.

In the setting of congestive heart failure, a right aortic arch is most commonly associated with a persistent truncus arteriosus.

Electrocardiogram

In the infant in congestive heart failure, the electrocardiogram may show either left or right ventricular hypertrophy. Isolated aortic stenosis and isolated coarctation of the aorta usually show electrocardiographic evidence of left ventricular hypertrophy, while aortic atresia, interruption of the aortic arch and coarctation with ventricular septal defect or patent ductus arteriosus usually show right ventricular hypertrophy. Left ventricular hypertrophy is also common with aortic runoff lesions such as patent ductus arteriosus, systemic arteriovenous fistula, aortic regurgitation or aortico-left ventricular tunnel. Most patients with myocardial abnormalities also have left ventricular hypertrophy on the electrocardiogram. The combination of a superior axis and left ventricular predominance in an infant in failure suggests a univentricular heart, with or without tricuspid atresia. Glycogen storage disease (Pompe) should be considered if there is a short PR interval. ST-T wave abnormalities often accompany the left ventricular hypertrophy of severe left ventricular outflow obstruction or of myocardial disease, but rarely that due to a left to right shunt. Right ventricular hypertrophy is expected with many anomalies that produce congestive heart failure and is not a helpful finding in differential diagnosis. (An accompanying superior axis suggests an atrioventricular canal but is not pathognomonic.)

Echocardiogram

Echocardiographic findings which may be diagnostically useful in the infant in congestive heart failure include the atrioventricular valve abnormalities seen in an endocardial cushion defect, the dilated left ventricle and poor left ventricular wall motion of myocarditis or 'congestive' cardiomyopathy, the septal thickening and systolic anterior motion of hypertrophic cardiomyopathy, and the late tricuspid valve closure of Ebstein's anomaly of the tricuspid valve.

Age

The age at which congestive heart failure appears is a helpful differential point. Failure in the first week of life is the rule with aortic atresia and is common with coarctation of the aorta, total anomalous pulmonary venous return with obstruction, and with a large systemic arteriovenous fistula. Failure is rare in the first month of life with a simple left to right shunt at any level. (An important exception is the premature infant with a patent ductus arteriosus.)

Summary

In summary, congestive heart failure in early infancy is most commonly related to a structural cardiovascular abnormality but may occasionally have a non-cardiac cause. Congestive failure should be treated before cardiac catheterization is attempted, but if treatment is unavailing invasive study should be carried out forthwith. The clinical examination is no substitute for cardiac catheterization in the infant with congestive heart failure, but the more accurate the clinical diagnosis before the performance of the invasive study, the more likely it is that the study will provide a precise anatomic and physiologic diagnosis without harm to the infant.

THE ASYMPTOMATIC CHILD WITH A MURMUR

The asymptomatic child with an incidentally discovered cardiac murmur is a very common clinical problem. Many normal children fall into this group, as do most children with minor cardiac defects and many with major anomalies of considerable hemodynamic importance. Not every apparently healthy child with a murmur can be referred to a pediatric cardiac center, and careful appraisal of the clinical findings is still the best basis for appropriate referral. For example, an asymptomatic child suspected of having a significant obstructive lesion such as aortic or pulmonic stenosis or coarctation of the aorta should be promptly referred, as should one with a septal defect resulting in a large left to right shunt, even though symptoms may be absent. On the other hand, there is no need for referral of a child with a very small ventricular septal defect, and no urgency about referral of a child with mild aortic or pulmonic stenosis. The identification of these anomalies is important, however, so that prophylaxis against infectious endocarditis may be instituted. A mild rheumatic valvar lesion may not require referral, but should be recognized so that prophylaxis against future streptococcal infections can be begun.

Some system of classifying murmurs is required, and since most murmurs are first heard by a non-cardiologist the classification should be simple and should not deal with auscultatory minutiae. The following system is a very simple one indeed, being based only on the timing, loudness and location of murmurs. Even the non-cardiologist should be able to decide whether a murmur is loud or soft, where it falls in the cardiac cycle, and where it is of maximal intensity. In the following discussion, systolic murmurs are first considered and these are discussed by location and by loudness. A similar process is then followed with diastolic and continuous murmurs. (Chapter 3 includes a discussion of how murmurs can be accurately timed and their point of maximal intensity localized on the chest wall.)

Systolic murmurs

Basal

Loud. The only common sources of loud basal systolic murmurs are right or left ventricular outflow tract obstruction. The murmur of aortic stenosis is usually loudest at the high right sternal border and that of pulmonic stenosis at the high left sternal border. Certain associated features further help in the differential diagnosis. The murmur of aortic stenosis characteristically radiates well to the neck while that of pulmonic stenosis radiates less well to the neck and better to the left posterior thorax. Both aortic and pulmonic valvar stenosis very commonly generate early systolic ejection sounds and these, too, are of differential value. The high pitched ejection sound of pulmonic stenosis is maximal at the high left sternal border and varies with the phase of respiration. (If the first heart sound itself is absent or soft at the base, the ejection sound of pulmonic stenosis may seem to be the first heart sound. Its high pitch and clicking quality and its respiratory variation should serve to identify it.) The ejection sound of aortic stenosis does not vary during the respiratory cycle, is of the same pitch as the first heart sound and is maximal near the apex.

If a thrill accompanies a basal systolic murmur, the outflow tract obstruction may or may not be severe, but the presence of a basal thrill mandates a chest roentgenogram and electrocardiogram. A normal heart size is the usual finding, even with rather severe aortic or pulmonic stenosis, but dilatation of the aorta or of the main and left pulmonary arteries are useful diagnostic clues. A normal electrocardiogram is reassuring in children with pulmonic stenosis, since the high right ventricular pressure of severe pulmonic stenosis is usually reflected as right ventricular hypertrophy. A normal electrocardiogram is common, however, in the child with significant aortic stenosis. Here, the presence of a thrill serves as an indicator for cardiac catheterization. In summary, a child with a loud basal systolic murmur almost always has organic heart disease and should be referred to a cardiac center for evaluation. The referral should be urgent if an infant has such a murmur.

Soft. A soft basal systolic murmur is a very common clinical finding. The murmur usually originates at the aortic or pulmonic valve and can be generated by mild obstruction or by rapid flow, either related to a cardiovascular anomaly or to fever, exercise, or some other cause of increased cardiac output. A soft basal systolic murmur may also be heard in normal children at rest. In the clinical setting of an apparently healthy child, the most likely specific diagnostic possibilities include mild aortic or pulmonic stenosis, an interatrial septal defect, coarctation of the aorta or an innocent murmur. The systolic murmur itself is similar in each of these entities and is not helpful in the differential diagnosis, serving only to call attention to the possibility of cardiac disease. Certain associated findings, however, are very useful in differentiating the various entities which can produce a soft basal systolic murmur. Coarctation of the aorta is recognized by finding weaker pulses and lower blood pressure in the legs than in the arms. Mild valvar aortic or pulmonic stenosis is almost always accompanied by an early systolic ejection sound and, in addition, the systolic murmur becomes strikingly louder with exercise. An interatrial septal defect is the congenital cardiovascular anomaly which is most commonly diagnosed in adult life, simply because it is the one most frequently missed during childhood. The high left sternal border systolic murmur of an interatrial defect is soft and is indistinguishable from the murmur of mild valvar pulmonic stenosis or from an innocent pulmonic murmur. The associated findings are characteristic, if somewhat subtle, and should be sought in any child with such a systolic murmur. The second heart sound is abnormally split in almost all children with an interatrial septal defect with significant left to right shunting. In most, the second sound is fixedly split throughout the respiratory cycle. In some, the width of splitting varies slightly with respiration but there is audible end expiratory splitting. In patients with an interatrial defect a soft medium pitched mid-diastolic murmur is often present at the low left sternal border and results from increased diastolic flow across the tricuspid valve. This murmur is subtle and never heard unless carefully sought. If the triad of a soft high left sternal border systolic murmur, a fixedly split second heart sound and a low left sternal border diastolic murmur are present, there is little doubt of the diagnosis. The diagnosis of an innocent basal systolic murmur is one of exclusion, being made when pulses are normal, an ejection sound absent, the second heart sound physiologically split and diastole clear.

Low left sternal border

Loud. In an apparently healthy child a loud lower left sternal border systolic murmur usually emanates from a ventricular septal defect. There may or may not be an associated thrill and the shunt may range from trivial to large. If the left to right shunt is large, pulmonary blood flow will be increased and there will be a large diastolic flow across the mitral valve, resulting in the low pitched mid diastolic apical rumble of relative mitral stenosis. (The presence of such a distolic murmur suggests pulmonary blood flow at least twice systemic blood flow.) A chest roentgenogram and an electrocardiogram should be obtained in every child with a loud low left sternal border systolic murmur. If these are normal and if there is no apical diastolic murmur, there is no urgency about referral, since a ventricular septal defect often closes spontaneously. (Spontaneous closure is signaled first by a softening of the systolic murmur and then by its shortening and eventual disappearance.) A low left sternal border functional murmur may occasionally be loud, and must then be differentiated from the murmur of a ventricular septal defect (see below). Rarely, a loud low left sternal border systolic murmur may be due to subvalvar aortic stenosis or to tricuspid regurgitation (Chs. 12 & 16).

Soft. A soft mid or low left sternal border systolic murmur may be innocent or may originate at a ventricular septal defect. A very small ventricular defect with trivial flow or a very large one with equal right and left ventricular peak systolic pressure may each produce a soft systolic murmur. When the defect is tiny the murmur may be pansystolic or confined to early systolic, but is always high pitched. The soft murmur of a very large ventricular septal defect is less high pitched, ends well before the second heart sound and is accompanied by the physical findings of pulmonary hypertension.

The differential between a tiny ventricular septal defect and an innocent murmur depends upon the characteristic quality of the latter, often described as 'vibratory' or 'twanging string'. The loudness of the innocent murmur often varies from time to time, becoming especially prominent with febrile illnesses. Rarely, an innocent murmur may be very loud and even be accompanied by a thrill, but the quality remains characteristic. Tricuspid regurgitation produces a soft low left sternal border systolic murmur, but it is very rare in children, particularly asymptomatic ones.

Apical

A systolic murmur which is maximal at the apex is almost always due to mitral regurgitation. The murmur is most often holosystolic but may be late systolic, especially if the regurgitation is related to mitral leaflet prolapse. The systolic murmur itself tells little about the severity of the regurgitation, but the apical impulse is over-active when mitral regurgitation is severe. Also, with severe regurgitation a low pitched mid-diastolic rumble is heard at the apex and represents the increased diastolic mitral flow which is an inevitable consequence of major systolic reflux to the left atrium. A chest roentgenogram and electrocardiogram should be obtained in any child with an apical systolic murmur. If mitral regurgitation is severe, the chest roentgenogram will show cardiomegaly and often increased pulmonary vascular markings as well. The electrocardiogram may show left atrial enlargement (especially if regurgitation is rheumatic) as well as left ventricular hypertrophy. A superior axis should suggest the possibility of an endocardial cushion defect, the most common non-rheumatic cause of mitral regurgitation in childhood. In a partial endocardial cushion defect the murmur of mitral regurgitation may be more obvious than the pulmonary flow murmur of the atrial septal defect itself.

Back

A systolic murmur may be as loud or louder over the posterior thorax than over the precordium. A prominent posterior murmur may arise in pulmonary arteries, either because of rapid flow (e.g. interatrial septal defect) or because of pulmonary artery stenosis. With either increased flow or stenosis the systolic murmur is heard at the base anteriorly, in the axillae and across the back. If the second heart sound is physiologically split and if there is no low left sternal border diastolic murmur, an interatrial septal defect of sufficient size to produce a murmur over the back is unlikely. In this situation, pulmonary artery stenosis is a more likely diagnosis. Posterior murmurs may also arise in systemic-pulmonary collateral arteries or in the systemic collateral arteries accompanying a coarctation, but in such patients other evidence of organic heart disease is always present.

Diastolic murmurs

Diastolic murmurs usually indicate semilunar valve regurgitation or atrioventricular valve stenosis. The latter may be relative or organic. The diastolic murmurs of relative tricuspid and mitral stenosis which accompany atrial or ventricular shunts or severe tricuspid or mitral regurgitation always have accompanying systolic murmurs which have been dealt with above. The apical diastolic murmur of organic mitral stenosis is rare in childhood. The diastolic murmur of isolated pulmonic regurgitation is also quite rare, leaving only the murmur of aortic regurgitation for consideration. The murmur of aortic regurgitation is high pitched, decrescendo, maximal at the mid left sternal border and begins with the aortic component of the second heart sound. It may be quite soft and is easily missed. The murmur is usually louder with the patient sitting and leaning forward with the breath held in expiration and is accentuated even more with sudden squatting. If aortic regurgitation is severe, peripheral signs of a widened pulse pressure will be present. Aortic regurgitation is usually rheumatic and is then often accompanied by mitral regurgitation. Aortic regurgitation may also be associated with a bicuspid aortic valve or with a ventricular septal defect. Patients with aortic regurgitation should be referred to a center for evaluation.

Continuous murmurs

In an apparently healthy child, a continuous murmur most often arises in a patent ductus arteriosus or is a jugular venous hum. In each situation the murmur is well heard at the base and may be loud or soft. Although intensity of a venous hum can be varied with head turning or unilateral pressure over jugular veins, these maneuvers may be resisted by the child or may be equivocal. It is easier to simply have the child lie down. A venous hum disappears; the murmur of a patent ductus arteriosus is unchanged. If a patent ductus is present and is small, pulses are normal and are of no help in differential diagnosis.

A continuous murmur at the mid or low left sternal border is not likely to be due to a patent ductus arteriosus. It may represent instead a coronary-cardiac fistula or ventricular septal defect with coexistent aortic regurgitation. (In the latter complex the murmur is made up of similarly pitched systolic and early diastolic murmurs but may sound 'continuous' at the mid left sternal border. The separate systolic and diastolic components may be identifiable higher or lower along the left sternal border or along the right sternal border.)

Other rarer causes of continuous murmurs include systemic or pulmonary arteriovenous fistulae, a sequestered pulmonary lobe with arterial stenosis, systemic-pulmonary collateral arteries or localized pulmonary artery stenosis. Unless a continuous murmur can be clearly shown to be a jugular venous hum, referral is mandatory.

Index

A

A waves, 7
  atrioventricular block, in, 8, 9
  etiology of, 8
  PR interval, effect of, 9
  pulmonary hypertension, in, 145, 146
  pulmonary stenosis, in, 64, 66
  tricuspid atresia, in, 107
  tricuspid stenosis, in, 102
  Uhl's anomaly, in, 162
Amyl nitrite
  murmur of aortic regurgitation, and, 84, 92
  murmur of mitral stenosis, and, 84, 92
Aneurysm
  membranous septum, 41
  right ventricular outflow tract, 14
  sinus of Valsalva, 157, 158
    patent ductus arteriosus, versus, 50
    rupture of, 50
Angina
  anomalous origin of left coronary artery, in, 139
  aortic stenosis, in, 79
  coronary-cardiac fistula, in, 137
  pulmonary hypertension, and, 145
  tricuspid atresia and transposition of the great arteries, in, 108
  univentricular heart, in, 163
Anomalous muscle bundle, 68
Anomalous origin of coronary artery, *see* Coronary artery, anomalous
Anomalous pulmonary venous connection
  anatomy, 56
  clinical course, 56, 57
  continuous hum, 50, 58
  cyanosis, 56, 57
  differential diagnosis, 50, 58
  heart sounds, 57, 58
  murmurs, 58, 168
  partial, 58
  precordial motion, 57
  pulmonary venous obstruction, 56, 57

Aortic atresia
  anatomy, 113
  clinical course, 113, 114
  critical aortic stenosis, versus, 78
  cyanosis, 114
  differential diagnosis, 115
  heart sounds, 115
  jugular venous pulse, 114
  murmurs, 115
  precordial motion, 114, 115, 168
  pulses, 114, 115, 168
Aortic regurgitation
  acute, 85, 86
  aortic stenosis, associated with, 78
  associated anomalies, 83, 86, 88
  clinical course, 83
  ejection sound, 84
  heart sounds, 83, 84, 86
  murmurs, 83, 84, 86, 88
  precordial motion, 83
  pulses, 83, 86
  sinus of Valsalva aneurysm and, 157
  suprasternal notch pulse in, 14
  tetralogy of Fallot with, 119
Aortic stenosis, subvalvar
  anatomy, 78
  classification, 78
  hypertrophic, 79, 80
  intramural tumor, due to, 161
  murmurs, 79
  pulses, 78
  tricuspid atresia and, 108
  univentricular heart and, 78
Aortic stenosis, supravalvar, 80, 82
Aortic stenosis, valvar
  anatomy, 75
  aortic regurgitation, associated with, 78
  critical, 78
  ejection sound, 76, 78
  heart sounds, 75, 76
  murmurs, 76–78
  precordial motion, 75, 78
  pulses, 75
  thrill, 77
Aortico-left ventricular tunnel, 88
Aortico-pulmonary window, 49
Arrhythmia
  Ebstein's anomaly of the tricuspid valve and, 103

  in utero, 136
  intramural tumor and, 161
  univentricular heart and, 163
  Wolff-Parkinson-White syndrome and, 154
Arterial pulse, *see* Pulse, arterial
Arteriovenous fistula, *see* Fistula, systemic arteriovenous
Ascites in constrictive pericarditis, 143
Asplenia, *see* Situs ambiguous
Atrial myxoma, 160, 161
Atrial septal defect
  anomalous venous return, and, 34
  associated anomalies, effect of, 38
  classification, 34
  clinical course, 34, 35
  heart sounds, 36
  mitral regurgitation, and, 34
  murmurs, 35, 36
  ostium primum type, 34
  ostium secundum type, 34
  precordial motion, 35
  pulmonary hypertension, 37, 38
  sinus venosus type, 34
Atrioventricular block
  classification, 152
  clinical course, 152
  complete, 153
  corrected transposition of the great arteries and, 130, 132, 133
  etiology, 152
  heart sounds, 153
  incomplete, 153
  jugular venous pulse, 153
  murmurs, 153
Atrioventricular canal, *see* Endocardial cushion defect
Atrioventricular septal defect, 45
Auscultation, *see also* individual anomalies, 15
Austin Flint murmur, 84
  versus murmur of mitral stenosis, 84, 92

B

Bacterial endocarditis, *see* Infectious endocarditis
Barlow's syndrome, *see* Mitral valve prolapse

Bicuspid aortic valve and coarctation of the aorta, 59
Blood pressure
  asymmetry of, 11
  coarctation of the aorta, in, 59, 60
  determination of, 11
  differential diagnosis of congestive heart failure in infancy, and, 170
  flush, 11
  respiration, effect of, 11
  supravalvar aortic stenosis, in, 80, 82
Brain abscess
  pulmonary arteriovenous fistula, in, 137
  pulmonary hypertension, in, 145
Branham's sign, 134
Bronchial obstruction and absent pulmonic valve, 71
Bundle branch block, heart sounds, in, 153, 154

C

C waves, 7
Cannon waves, 8, 9, 153
Carvallo's sign, 101, 147
Cervical loop aorta, 14
Cleft mitral valve, see Mitral valve cleft
Clicks (see also Sounds, ejection)
  mid-systolic, 28
  patent ductus arteriosus, and, 48
  prolapsing mitral valve, and, 94, 96
Coanda effect, 80, 82
Coarctation of the aorta
  anatomy, 59
  associated anomalies, 59, 62
  blood pressure, 59, 60
  clinical course, 59, 62
  collateral arteries, 60, 62
  differential cyanosis, 62
  heart sounds, 60
  mitral atresia and, 112
  mitral valve abnormality, and, 59, 62, 89
  murmurs, 62
  precordial motion, 60
  pulses, 59, 60, 62
  retroesophageal subclavian artery, and, 60
  suprasternal notch pulsation, 14
  tricuspid atresia and, 108
Collateral arteries
  coarctation of the aorta, in, 60, 62
  intercoronary, with anomalous left coronary artery, 139
  systemic-pulmonary
    patent ductus arteriosus, versus, 50, 167
    tetralogy of Fallot, in, 117, 120
Common atrium, 55
Congestive heart failure (see also individual anomalies)
  age of onset of, 171
  contrast media and, 169
  feeding, effect on, 4

growth, effect on, 4
in utero, differential diagnosis of, 136
infancy, in, 169–172
infant of diabetic mother and, 169
respiratory pattern of, 5
therapy of, 169
Constrictive pericarditis, 143
Cor triatriatum, 156
Coronary artery, anomalous origin of, 138–140
Coronary-cardiac fistula, see Fistula, coronary-cardiac
Corrected transposition of the great arteries
  anatomy, 129, 130
  associated anomalies, 130–132
  clinical course, 130
  heart sounds, 131–133
  murmurs, 132, 133
  nomenclature, 130
  precordial motion, 131
Corrigan's pulse, 83
Cyanosis
  absent pulmonic valve, in, 71
  anemia, effect of, 5
  anomalous pulmonary venous connection, in, 56, 57
  aortic atresia, in, 114
  aortic stenosis, critical, in, 78
  central nervous system disease, and, 165
  common atrium, in, 55
  differential
    coarctation of the aorta, in, 62
    patent ductus arteriosus, in, 48
    transposition of the great arteries, in, 126
  differential diagnosis of, in newborn, 165
  Ebstein's anomaly, in, 102, 103
  endocardial cushion defect, in, 54
  fistula, arteriovenous, in
    pulmonary, 136, 137
    pulmonary artery—left atrial, 137
    systemic, 134
  general, 5
  mitral atresia, in, 111–113
  mitral stenosis, in, 89
  polycythemia, with, 165
  pulmonary atresia and intact ventricular septum, in, 110
  pulmonary disease, in, 165, 166
  pulmonary hypertension, in, 145
  pulmonary stenosis, in, 64, 67
  tetralogy of Fallot, in, 116, 117, 119–121
  tetralogy of Fallot with pulmonary atresia, in, 121, 122
  transposition of the great arteries, in, 123–126, 128
  tricuspid atresia, in, 108
  tricuspid regurgitation, in, 99
  tricuspid stenosis, in, 102
  truncus arteriosus, in, 159
  Uhl's anomaly, in, 162

univentricular heart, in, 163
Cyanotic spells, see Hypercyanotic spells

D

Dextrocardia, 168
Differential cyanosis, see Cyanosis, differential
Double chamber right ventricle, 68
Down's syndrome, 51
Duroziez's sign, 84, 85, 158
Dysplastic pulmonary valve, 64, 65

E

Ebstein's anomaly
  anatomy, 102
  arrhythmias, 103
  clinical course, 102, 103
  corrected transposition of the great arteries and, 130
  cyanosis, 102, 103
  heart sounds, 103, 105
  jugular venous pulse, 103
  murmurs, 105
  neonate, in the, 106, 167
  precordial motion, 103
  tricuspid regurgitation, with, 99
  tricuspid stenosis, with, 101
Echocardiogram, in differential diagnosis of
  congestive heart failure in infancy, 171
  cyanosis in the newborn, 166, 168, 169
Electrocardiogram, in differential diagnosis of
  congestive heart failure, 171
  cyanosis in the newborn, 166–168
Ellis Van Creveld syndrome, 55
Emboli, from atrial myxoma, 160, 161
Endocardial cushion defect
  anatomy, 51
  associated anomalies, 54
  classification, 52
  common atrium, 55
  complete, 53, 54
  Down's syndrome and, 51
  mitral regurgitation, with, 51–53
  partial, 52, 53
  situs ambiguous and, 51
  transitional form of, 52
Endocardial fibroelastosis, 139

F

Fibroma, intramural, 161
First heart sound, see Sounds, heart, first
Fistula, coronary—cardiac, 137, 138
  patent ductus arteriosus, versus, 50
  sinus of Valsalva aneurysm, versus, 158
Fistula, pulmonary arteriovenous, 136, 137
Fistula, pulmonary—left atrium, 137

Fistula, systemic arteriovenous, 134–136
  patent ductus arteriosus, versus, 50
  venous hum, versus, 150
Floppy mitral valve, see Mitral valve prolapse
Foramen ovale, 34
Friedreich's sign, 143

G

Gallop (see also Sounds, heart, third and fourth)
  atrial, 26
  respiration, effect of, 25
  summation, 26
  ventricular, 25, 26
Glycogen storage disease, 171
Graham Steell murmur, 147
Growth, effect of heart disease on, 4

H

Hepatic pulse, 9
  hepatic arteriovenous fistula, in, 134
  pulmonary stenosis, in, 64
  transmitted impulse, versus, 9
  tricuspid atresia, in, 107
  tricuspid regurgitation, in, 99
Hepatojugular reflux, 10
Hereditary hemorrhagic telangiectasia, 136
Hypercyanotic spells, 117, 119
Hypertension
  coarctation of aorta, in, 60
  etiology of, 11
Hypertrophic subaortic stenosis, see Aortic stenosis, subvalvar
Hypoplastic right ventricle
  pulmonary atresia, in, 109
  tricuspid atresia, in, 107

I

Incidence of congenital heart disease, 1
Infectious endocarditis
  aortic regurgitation, 83
  mitral regurgitation, 93
  pulmonary regurgitation, 71
  tricuspid regurgitation, 99
Infundibular pulmonary stenosis, see Pulmonary stenosis, subvalvar
Interatrial septal defect, see Atrial septal defect
Interrupted aortic arch, 168
Interventricular septal defect, see Ventricular septal defect
Intramural cardiac tumor, 161

J

Jugular venous hum, see Venous hum, jugular
Jugular venous pulse
  A wave, 7
  arterial pulse, versus, 7
  arteriovenous fistula, in, 10
  atrial myxoma, in, 161
  atrioventricular block, in, 153
  C wave, 7
  constrictive pericarditis, in, 9, 10, 143
  corrected transposition of the great arteries, in, 133
  Ebstein's anomaly, in, 103
  endocardial cusion defect, in, 52
  infants, in, 7
  intracranial arteriovenous fistula, in, 134, 135
  Kussmaul sign, 9
  mitral atresia, in, 112
  position, effect of, 7
  pulmonary atresia, in, 110
  pulmonary hypertension, in, 145, 146
  pulmonary stenosis, in, 64
  tetralogy of Fallot, in, 118
  transposition of the great arteries, in, 124, 127, 128
  tricuspid atresia, in, 107, 108
  tricuspid regurgitation, in, 99
  tricuspid stenosis, in, 102
  Uhl's anomaly, in, 162
  V wave, 7

K

Knock, pericardial, 26, 143
Korotkoff sounds, 11
Kussmaul sign, 9, 10, 143

L

Lutembacher's syndrome, 89

M

Mammary souffle, 136, 150, 151
  patent ductus arteriosus, versus, 49
  systemic arteriovenous fistula, versus, 136
Marfan's syndrome, 83
Mid systolic click, see Click, mid systolic
Mitral arcade, 89
Mitral atresia
  anatomy, 110, 111
  associated anomalies, 111, 112
  clinical course, 111
  cyanosis, 111–113
  heart sounds, 112
  jugular venous pulse, 112
  murmurs, 112, 168
  precordial motion, 112
  pulses, 112
Mitral regurgitation
  acute, 95
  anomalous origin of left coronary artery, in, 139
  associated anomalies, 93, 96, 98
  clinical course, 93
  critical aortic stenosis, in, 78
  differential diagnosis, 95, 96
  endocardial cushion defect, in, 51–53
  etiology, 93
  heart sounds, 94, 95
  left atrial myxoma, in, 161
  mitral valve prolapse, due to, 93, 94
  murmurs, 93, 94
  precordial motion, 94
  pulmonary hypertension, 95
  pulses, 95
  systolic click, 94, 96
Mitral stenosis
  anatomy, 89
  associated anomalies, 89, 91
  clinical course, 89
  cyanosis, 89
  differential diagnosis, 91, 92, 161
  heart sounds, 90, 91
  intracardiac tumor, and, 161
  murmurs, 91
    Austin Flint murmur, versus, 84
    relative mitral stenosis, versus, 84, 91, 92
  precordial motion, 89
  relative
    atrioventricular septal defect, in, 45
    complete endocardial cushion defect, in, 54
    mitral regurgitation, in, 96
    patent ductus arteriosus, in, 48
    ventricular septal defect, in, 43
Mitral valve cleft, 51
Mitral valve prolapse, see also Mitral regurgitation, 93, 94, 96
Moderator band, 68
Mongolism, see Down's syndrome
Mortality rate in congenital heart disease, 1
Murmur
  anomalous origin of left coronary artery, in, 139
  anomalous pulmonary venous connection, in, 58
  aortic atresia, in, 115
  aortic regurgitation, in, 83, 84, 86, 88
  aortic stenosis, in, 76–80
  apical systolic, differential diagnosis of, 174
  atrial myxoma, in, 160, 161
  atrial septal defect, in, 35, 36
  basal systolic, differential diagnosis of, 172, 173
  carotid, in normals, 150
  classification of, 172
  coarctation of the aorta, in, 62
  common atrium, in, 55
  congestive heart failure, in differential diagnosis of, 170, 171
  continuous
    anomalous origin of left coronary artery, in, 139
    anomalous pulmonary venous connection, in, 58
    coarctation of the aorta, in, 62
    congestive heart failure, in differential diagnosis of, 170, 171

Murmur (contd.)
  continuous (contd.)
    cor triatriatum, in, 156
    coronary-cardiac fistula, in, 50, 137, 138
    cyanosis, in differential diagnosis of, 167, 168
    differential diagnosis of, 175
    fistula, arteriovenous, in
      intracranial, 134, 135
      pulmonary, 137
      systemic, 134–136
    fistula, coronary-cardiac, in, 137
    mitral atresia, in, 112, 113
    mitral stenosis, in, 91
    patent ductus arteriosus, in, 47–49
    pulmonary artery stenosis, in, 69
    pulmonary atresia, in, 110
    pulmonary vein stenosis, in, 157
    sinus of Valsalva aneurysm, in, 50, 158
    tetralogy of Fallot, in, 119, 120
    tetralogy of Fallot with pulmonary atresia, in, 122
    transposition of the great arteries, in, 125, 127, 128
    truncus arteriosus, in, 160
    univentricular heart, in, 164
    ventricular septal defect plus aortic regurgitation, in, 44, 88
  cor triatriatum, in, 156
  corrected transposition of the great arteries, in, 132
  cranial, 150
  cyanosis, in differential diagnosis of, 167, 168
  diastolic
    anomalous origin of left coronary artery, in, 139
    anomalous pulmonary venous connection, in, 58
    aortic regurgitation, in, 83, 84, 86, 88
    atrial myxoma, in, 161
    atrial septal defect, in, 35, 36
    coarctation of the aorta, in, 62
    cor triatriatum, in, 156
    coronary—left ventricular fistula, in, 138
    corrected transposition of the great arteries, in, 132
    differential diagnosis of, 174, 175
    Ebstein's anomaly, in, 105
    endocardial cushion defect, in, 53, 54
    hypertrophic subaortic stenosis, in, 79
    mitral atresia, in, 112
    mitral regurgitation, in, 94
    mitral stenosis, in, 91
    patent ductus arteriosus, in, 48
    pulmonary atresia, in, 110
    pulmonary hypertension, with, 147
    pulmonary regurgitation, in, 73, 91
    pulmonary versus aortic regurgitation, 73, 88
    tetralogy of Fallot, in, 119, 121
    transposition of the great arteries, in, 125
    tricuspid regurgitation, in, 101
    tricuspid stenosis, in, 102
    truncus arteriosus, in, 160
    univentricular heart, in, 164
    ventricular septal defect, in, 43
  Ebstein's anomaly, in, 105, 106
  endocardial cushion defect, in, 53, 54
  fistula, arteriovenous, in
    intracranial, 134, 135
    pulmonary, 137
    systemic, 134–136
  fistula, coronary-cardiac, 137, 138
  functional, 149, 150
  genesis of, 29
  grading of, 30, 31
  hypertrophic subaortic stenosis, in, 79, 80
  innocent, 149, 150
  localization of, 31
  loudness of, 16, 29, 30
  low left sternal border systolic, differential diagnosis of, 173, 174
  mitral atresia, in, 112
  mitral regurgitation, in, 93–96
  mitral stenosis, in, 91, 92
  patent ductus arteriosus, in, 47–49
  pericardial rub, versus, 141
  pharmacologic manipulation of
    aortic regurgitation versus mitral stenosis, 84, 92
    hypertrophic subaortic stenosis, in, 80
    mitral regurgitation, in, 96
  physical manipulation of
    aortic regurgitation, in, 84
    hypertrophic subaortic stenosis, in, 80
    mitral regurgitation, in, 96
    mitral stenosis, in, 91
    ventricular septal defect, in, 42
  pitch of, 31
  posterior thoracic systolic, differential diagnosis of, 174
  pulmonary artery stenosis, in, 69, 150
  pulmonary atresia, in, 110
  pulmonary hypertension, in, 147
  pulmonary regurgitation, in, 73
  pulmonary stenosis, in, 64, 66–69
  pulmonary vein stenosis, in, 157
  quality of, 33
  radiation of, 16
  shape of, 32, 33
  sinus of Valsalva aneurysm, in, 158
  Still's, 150
  subvalvar aortic stenosis, in, 79
  subvalvar pulmonary stenosis, in, 68
  tetralogy of Fallot, in, 118–121
  tetralogy of Fallot with pulmonary atresia, in, 122
  timing of, 31, 32
  to and fro
    aortico-left ventricular tunnel, in, 88, 170
    differential diagnosis of, 170
    pulmonary regurgitation, in, 73
  transposition of the great arteries, in, 125–128
  tricuspid atresia, in, 108
  tricuspid regurgitation, in, 100, 101
  tricuspid stenosis, in, 102
  truncus arteriosus, in, 160
  univentricular heart, in, 164
  valvar aortic stenosis, in, 76–78
  valvar pulmonary stenosis, in, 66, 67
  ventricular septal defect, in, 39–45
Mustard's operation for transposition of the great arteries, 126, 127
Myocardial infarction, anomalous origin of left coronary artery, in, 139

N
Noonan's syndrome, 64

O
Opening snap
  characteristics, 28
  differentiation from split second sound, 29
  mitral, 28, 29, 90, 91
  tricuspid, 29, 102
Oxygen test in differential diagnosis of cyanosis, 166

P
Papillary muscle dysfunction
  anomalous origin of left coronary artery, and, 139
  mitral valve prolapse and, 94
Parachute mitral valve, 89
Parchment right ventricle, see Uhl's anomaly
Partial anomalous pulmonary venous connection, see Anomalous pulmonary venous connection, partial
Partial atrioventricular canal, see Endocardial cushion defect, partial
Partial endocardial cushion defect, see Endocardial cushion defect, partial
Patent ductus arteriosus
  aortic atresia and, 113, 114
  associated anomalies, 48, 49
  cervical arteriovenous fistula, versus, 135
  clinical course, 46
  coronary-cardiac fistula, versus, 138
  differential diagnosis, 49, 50
  heart sounds, 47
  jugular venous hum, versus, 150

Patent ductus arteriosus (*contd.*)
  maternal rubella and, 46
  murmurs, 47–49
  precordial motion, 46, 48
  prematurity and, 46
  pulmonary atresia and, 109, 110
  pulmonary hypertension, 48
  pulses, 46
  reversed flow, 48
  sinus of Valsalva aneurysm, versus, 158
  transposition of the great arteries and, 125
Pericardial effusion, 141
Pericardial knock, 26, 143
Pericardial rub, 141
Pericardial tamponade, 141, 142
Pericarditis, acute, 141
Pericarditis, constrictive, 143
Persistent fetal circulation, 167
Physical examination, general approach, 6
Physiologic pulmonary artery stenosis, *see* Pulmonary artery stenosis
Pistol shot pulse, *see* Pulse, arterial
Polycythemia, 166
Polysplenia, *see* Situs ambiguous
Pompe's disease, 171
Post ductal coarctation, *see* Coarctation, anatomy
Post pericardiotomy syndrome, 141, 143
Precordial motion
  anomalous origin of left coronary artery, in, 139
  anomalous pulmonary venous connection, in, 57
  aortic atresia, in, 114, 115
  aortic regurgitation, in, 83
  aortic stenosis, in, 75, 78, 79
  apical impulse, 13
  atrial septal defect, in, 35
  coarctation of the aorta, in, 14, 60
  constrictive pericarditis, in, 143
  cor triatriatum, in, 156
  corrected transposition of the great arteries, in, 131
  Ebstein's anomaly of the tricuspid valve, in, 103
  endocardial cushion defect, in, 52, 54
  fistula, systemic arteriovenous, in, 134
  general, 11, 12
  hypertrophic subaortic stenosis, in, 79
  mitral atresia, in, 112
  mitral regurgitation, in, 94
  mitral stenosis, in, 89
  parasternal impulse, 13
  patent ductus arteriosus, in, 46, 48
  presystolic impulse
    aortic stenosis, valvar, in, 75
    hypertrophic subaortic stenosis, in, 79
  pulmonary artery pulsation, 14, 37, 54, 146
  pulmonary atresia, in, 110
  pulmonary hypertension, with, 146
  pulmonary regurgitation, in, 72
  pulmonary stenosis, in, 64
  sinus of Valsalva aneurysm, in, 158
  suprasternal notch pulsation, 14, 60
  tetralogy of Fallot, in, 118, 121
  tricuspid atresia, in, 108
  tricuspid regurgitation, in, 14, 99, 100
  tricuspid stenosis, in, 102
  transposition of the great arteries, in, 124, 126
  truncus arteriosus, in, 159
  univentricular heart, in, 163
  ventricular aneurysm, in, 14
  ventricular septal defect, in, 39
Preductal coarctation, *see* Coarctation, anatomy
Preexcitation syndrome, *see* Wolff-Parkinson-White syndrome
Prematurity and patent ductus arteriosus, 46
Primary pulmonary hypertension, *see* Pulmonary hypertension, primary
Pseudo truncus arteriosus, *see* Tetralogy of Fallot, pulmonary atresia
Pulmonary artery banding, 69
Pulmonary artery pulsation, 14, 37, 54, 146
Pulmonary artery stenosis, 69
  patent ductus arteriosus, versus, 50
  physiologic, 69, 150
  surgical band, 69
Pulmonary arteriovenous fistula, *see* Fistula, pulmonary arteriovenous
Pulmonary atresia with intact ventricular septum
  anatomy, 109
  clinical course, 109, 110
  cyanosis, 110
  heart sounds, 110
  jugular venous pulse, 110
  murmurs, 110
  precordial motion, 110
  tricuspid regurgitation, and, 99
  tricuspid stenosis, and, 101
Pulmonary emboli, as cause of pulmonary hypertension, 144
Pulmonary hypertension
  atrial septal defect, in, 37, 38, 144
  clinical course, 145
  cor triatriatum, in, 156
  corrected transposition of the great arteries, in, 131, 132
  cyanosis, 145
  ejection sound, 147
  endocardial cushion defect, in, 54
  etiology of, 144
  heart sounds, 146, 147
  jugular venous pulse, 145, 146
  mitral regurgitation, acute, in, 95
  mitral stenosis, in, 89
  murmurs, 147
  precordial motion, 146
  primary, 144
  pulmonary vein stenosis, in, 157
  secondary, 144, 145
  transposition of the great arteries, in, 126
  tricuspid regurgitation, and, 99
  ventricular septal defect, in, 39–41
Pulmonary—left atrial fistula, 137
Pulmonary regurgitation
  associated anomalies, 71
  clinical course, 71
  corrected transposition of the great arteries, in, 132
  cyanosis, 71
  endocardial cushion defect, in, 54
  heart sounds, 72, 73
  infectious endocarditis and, 71
  mitral stenosis, in, 91
  murmurs, 73
  precordial motion, 72
  tetralogy of Fallot, in, 119
Pulmonary stenosis (*see also* Pulmonary stenosis—valvar, subvalvar and supravalvar, and Pulmonary artery stenosis)
  associated anomalies, 64, 65
  clinical course, 64
  corrected transposition of the great arteries and, 130, 132
  cyanosis, 64, 67
  heart sounds, 64
  hepatic pulse, 64
  jugular venous pulse, 64
  mitral atresia and, 111
  murmurs, 64
  neonate, in the, 67
  Noonan's syndrome and, 64
  precordial motion, 64
  transposition of the great arteries and, 123, 124, 126
  tricuspid atresia and, 107, 108
Pulmonary stenosis, subvalvar
  anatomy, 67, 68
  heart sounds, 68
  intramural tumor, due to, 161
  murmur, 68
  sinus of Valsalva aneurysm, and, 157
Pulmonary stenosis, supravalvar
  see also Pulmonary artery stenosis, 69
Pulmonary stenosis, valvar
  anatomy, 65
  dysplastic valve, 64, 65
  ejection sound, 66
  heart sounds, 65, 66
  murmur, 66, 67
Pulmonary vascular resistance
  atrial septal defect, in, 144
  newborn with ventricular septal defect, in, 39, 144, 145
  normal newborn, in, 39

INDEX

Pulmonary vascular resistance (*contd.*)
  patent ductus arteriosus, in, 46, 48
  truncus arteriosus, in, 159
Pulmonary vein stenosis, 156, 157
Pulmonary venous obstruction
  anomalous pulmonary venous
    connection, in, 56, 57
  transposition of the great arteries, in,
    126, 128
Pulse, arterial
  amplitude, 10
  aortic atresia, in, 114, 115, 168
  aortic regurgitation, in, 83, 86
  aortic stenosis, in, 75, 78, 79
  bifid
    aortic regurgitation, in, 83
    hypertrophic subaortic stenosis,
      in, 79, 80
  carotid
    cervical arteriovenous fistula, in,
      134
    intracranial arteriovenous fistula,
      in, 134, 135
  coarctation of the aorta, in, 60, 62
  congestive heart failure, in
    differential diagnosis of, in
      infancy, 169, 170
  cyanosis, in differential diagnosis of,
    168
  femoral, delay, 10
  fistula, coronary-cardiac, in, 137
  fistula, systemic arteriovenous, in,
    134
  hypertrophic subaortic stenosis, in,
    79, 80
  interrupted aortic arch, in, 168
  mitral atresia, in, 112
  mitral regurgitation, in, 95
  paradoxic, 11, 142, 143
  patent ductus arteriosus, in, 46
  pericardial tamponade, in, 142
  pistol shot, 83, 158
  sinus of Valsalva aneurysm, in, 158
  subvalvar aortic stenosis, in, 78
  symmetry of, 10
  transposition of the great arteries
    with patent ductus arteriosus,
    in, 125
  tricuspid atresia, in, 108
  truncus arteriosus, in, 159
  valvar aortic stenosis, in, 75, 78
  ventricular septal defect, in, 39
Pulse, venous, *see* Jugular venous
    pulse; Hepatic pulse
Pulsus bisfiriens, *see* Pulse, arterial,
    bifid
Pulsus paradoxus, *see* Pulse, arterial,
    paradoxic

Q
Quincke's pulse, 83

R
Rendu-Osler-Weber syndrome, 136
Rhabdomyoma, 161

Roentgenogram, chest
  congestive heart failure, in
    differential diagnosis of, 171
  cyanosis, in differential diagnosis of,
    166–168
Rubella syndrome
  patent ductus arteriosus in, 46
  pulmonary artery stenosis in, 64, 65

S
Sail sound, 105
Schone's syndrome, 89
Secondary pulmonary hypertension, *see*
    Pulmonary hypertension,
    secondary
Sepsis, 169
Single atrium, 55
Sinus of Valsalva aneurysm, *see*
    aneurysm, sinus of Valsalva
Situs ambiguous, 51, 167, 168
'Snow man' configuration on chest
    roentgenogram, 168
Sounds, heart
  anomalous pulmonary venous
    connection, in, 57, 58
  aortic atresia, in, 115
  aortic regurgitation, in, 84, 86
  aortic stenosis, in, 75, 76, 79
  atrial myxoma, in, 161
  atrial septal defect, in, 36, 37
  atrioventricular block, in, 153
  bundle branch block, in, 153, 154
  common atrium, in, 55
  corrected transposition of the great
    arteries, in, 131–133
  cyanosis, in differential diagnosis of,
    167, 168
  Ebstein's anomaly of the tricuspid
    valve, in, 103, 105, 106
  ejection,
    aortic
      aortic stenosis, valvar, in, 76, 78
      characteristics of, 27, 28
      genesis of, 28
      split first sound, differentiation
        from, 28
      tetralogy of Fallot, in, 118
      tetralogy of Fallot with
        pulmonary atresia, in, 122
    pulmonary
      atrial contraction, effect on, 27,
        66
      characteristics of, 27
      genesis of, 26, 27
      pulmonary hypertension, with,
        147
      pulmonary stenosis, in, 66
      respiration, effect of, 27, 66
      tetralogy of Fallot, in, 118
      truncus arteriosus, in, 160
  endocardial cushion defect, in, 53, 54
  first
    genesis of, 17
    loudness of, 18–20
      acute aortic regurgitation, in, 86

  aortic atresia, in, 115
  atrial septal defect, in, 37
  atrioventricular block, in, 153
  corrected transposition of the
    great arteries, in, 132, 133
  endocardial cushion defect, in,
    53
  mitral atresia, in, 112
  mitral regurgitation, in, 95
  mitral stenosis, in, 90, 92
  Uhl's anomaly, in, 162
  splitting of, 17, 18
  fistula, systemic arteriovenous, in,
    134
  fourth
    aortic stenosis, in, 75, 76
    differentiation from first sound—
      ejection sound sequence, 26
    Ebstein's anomaly, in, 105
    genesis of, 26
    hypertrophic subaortic stenosis,
      in, 79, 80
    left ventricular, 26
    mitral regurgitation, in, 95, 98
    pulmonary hypertension, with,
      147
    pulmonary stenosis, in, 65
    right ventricular, 26
  genesis of, 17
  mitral atresia, in, 112, 113
  mitral regurgitation, in, 94, 95
  mitral stenosis, in, 90, 92
  patent ductus arteriosus, in, 47
  pericardial tamponade, in, 142
  pulmonary artery stenosis, in, 69
  pulmonary atresia, in, 110
  pulmonary hypertension, with, 146,
    147
  pulmonary regurgitation, in, 72, 73
  pulmonary stenosis, in, 64–66, 68, 69
  second
    genesis of, 20
    loudness of, 25
      atrial septal defect, in, 36, 37
      mitral stenosis, in, 90
      pulmonary artery stenosis, in, 69
      pulmonary regurgitation, in, 72
      pulmonary stenosis, in, 65, 68,
        69
    single, 23, 24
    splitting of, 20, 22
      fixed, 22, 23, 36, 37
      impedance, role of, 24, 25
      paradoxic, 23, 24, 47, 75, 128,
        154, 155
      pulmonary hypertension and,
        146, 147
      right ventricular function, role
        of, 25
  tetralogy of Fallot, in, 118, 120, 121
  tetralogy of Fallot with pulmonary
    atresia, in, 122
  third
    atrial myxoma, in, 161
    atrioventricular block, in, 153

Sounds, heart (*contd.*)
  third (*contd.*)
    anomalous origin of left coronary artery, in, 139
    Ebstein's anomaly, in, 105
    fistula, systemic arteriovenous, in, 134
    genesis of, 25
    mitral regurgitation, in, 94, 95
    mitral stenosis, in, 90
    normal, versus gallop, 25
    pulmonary hypertension, with, 147
    tricuspid atresia, in, 108
    tricuspid regurgitation, in, 100
    truncus arteriosus, in, 160
    transposition of the great arteries, in, 124–126, 128
    tricuspid atresia, in, 108
    tricuspid regurgitation, in, 100
    truncus arteriosus, in, 159, 160
    Uhl's anomaly, in, 162
    univentricular heart, in, 163, 164
    ventricular septal defect, in, 40
    Wolff-Parkinson-White syndrome, in, 154, 155
Stethoscope, 14
Still's murmur, 150
Stokes-Adams attacks, 152
Subacute bacterial endocarditis, *see* Infectious endocarditis
Subvalvar aortic stenosis, *see* Aortic stenosis, subvalvar
Subvalvar pulmonary stenosis, *see* Pulmonary stenosis, subvalvar
Supracristal ventricular septal defect, *see also* Ventricular septal defect
  aortic regurgitation, and, 44, 86, 88
Supravalvar aortic stenosis, *see* Aortic stenosis, supravalvar
Supravalvar pulmonary stenosis, *see* Pulmonary stenosis, supravalvar
Systemic venous obstruction following Mustard operation, 126, 127
Systolic clicks, *see* Clicks

T

Tamponade, *see* Pericardial tamponade
Tetralogy of Fallot
  anatomy, 116
  clinical spectrum, 116, 117
  cyanosis, 116, 117, 119–121
  ejection sound, 118, 120
  heart sounds, 118, 120, 121
  jugular venous pulse, 118
  murmurs, 118–121
  precordial motion, 118, 121
  pulmonary atresia, and, 121, 122, 138
  pulses, 118
  spells, in, 117, 119
Thrill
  aortic stenosis, valvar, in. Indication for cardiac catheterization, 77
  carotid, in normals, 150
  detection of, 30
  jugular venous, in normals, 150
  suprasternal notch, in coarctation of the aorta, 60
Transposition of the great arteries
  anatomy, 123
  clinical course, 123
  cyanosis, 123–126, 128
  corrected, *see* Corrected transposition of the great arteries
  heart sounds, 124–126, 128
  jugular venous pulse, 124, 127, 128
  murmurs, 125–128
  patent ductus arteriosus, and, 125
  postoperative findings, 126, 127
  precordial motion, 124, 126
  pulmonary hypertension, 126
  pulmonary stenosis, and, 123, 124, 126
  pulses, 125
  tricuspid atresia, and, 108
  tricuspid regurgitation, and, 128
  ventricular septal defect, and, 125
Traube's sign, 83
Tricuspid atresia
  anatomy, 107
  clinical course, 107, 108
  coarctation of the aorta, with, 108
  cyanosis, 108
  heart sounds, 108
  hepatic pulse, 107
  jugular venous pulse, 107, 108
  murmurs, 108
  precordial motion, 108
  pulmonary stenosis, with, 107, 108
  transposition of the great arteries, and, 108
Tricuspid regurgitation
  anatomy, 99
  associated anomalies, 99
  atrial myxoma, due to, 161
  clinical course, 99
  cyanosis, 99
  functional, 99
  heart sounds, 100
  hepatic pulse, 99
  iatrogenic, 99
  jugular venous pulse, 99
  mitral atresia, in, 112
  mitral stenosis, in, 91
  murmurs, 100, 101
  neonate, in the, 167
  precordial motion, 14, 99, 100
  pulmonary atresia, in, 109, 110
  pulmonary stenosis, in, 67
  sinus of Valsalva aneurysm and, 157
  transient, 99
  transposition of the great arteries, in, 126, 128
  univentricular heart, in, 164
Tricuspid stenosis
  anatomy, 101
  associated anomalies, 101, 102
  atrial myxoma and, 161
  cyanosis, 102
  intramural tumor, due to, 161
  jugular venous pulse, 102
  murmur, 102
  precordial motion, 102
  pulmonary atresia, in, 109, 110
  relative,
    atrial septal defect, in, 35, 36
    atrioventricular septal defect, in, 45
    tricuspid regurgitation, in, 101, 110
Truncus arteriosus
  classification, 158
  clinical course, 158, 159
  cyanosis, 159, 160
  ejection sound, 160
  heart sounds, 159, 160
  murmur, 160
  patent ductus arteriosus, versus, 49
  precordial motion, 159
  pulses, 159
Tumor, cardiac, 160, 161
Tumor 'plop,' 161
Tunnel subaortic stenosis, *see* Aortic stenosis, subvalvar
Turner's syndrome, 59

U

Uhl's anomaly, 161, 162
Univentricular heart
  anatomy, 162
  clinical course, 163
  heart sounds, 163, 164
  murmur, 164
  precordial motion, 163
  subaortic stenosis, and, 78
  tricuspid atresia, and, 107

V

V waves, 7
  etiology of, 9
  pulmonary hypertension, in, 146
  tricuspid regurgitation, in, 99
Valsalva maneuver, effect on murmur of:
  hypertrophic subaortic stenosis, 80
  mitral atresia, 112
  mitral stenosis, 91
  prolapsing mitral valve, 96
  pulmonary arteriovenous fistula, 137
  ventricular septal defect, 42, 43
Venous hum
  anomalous pulmonary venous connection, in, 50, 58
  jugular, 150
    arteriovenous fistula, versus, 150
    patent ductus arteriosus, versus, 49, 150
Ventricular septal defect
  aortic regurgitation and, 44, 86, 88
  associated anomalies, effect of, 43
  classification of, 41
  clinical course, 39

Ventricular septal defect (*contd.*)
  corrected transposition of the great arteries and, 130–132
  differential diagnosis, 43, 44
  heart sounds, 40
  murmurs, 39–45
  precordial motion, 39
  pulmonary vascular resistance, 39
  pulses, 39
  transposition of the great arteries and, 125
Ventriculo-arterial discordance, *see* Transposition of the great arteries

W

Water-hammer pulse, 83
William's syndrome, 80
Wolff-Parkinson-White syndrome, 154, 155
  Ebstein's anomaly, and, 103